Pain Management

Editor

DAVID SANCHEZ-MIGALLON GUZMAN

VETERINARY CLINICS OF NORTH AMERICA: EXOTIC ANIMAL PRACTICE

www.vetexotic.theclinics.com

Consulting Editor
JÖRG MAYER

January 2023 • Volume 26 • Number 1

ELSEVIER

1600 John F. Kennedy Boulevard • Suite 1800 • Philadelphia, Pennsylvania, 19103-2899
http://www.vetexotic.theclinics.com

**VETERINARY CLINICS OF NORTH AMERICA: EXOTIC ANIMAL PRACTICE Volume 26, Number 1
January 2023 ISSN 1094-9194, ISBN-13: 978-0-323-98657-1**

Editor: Stacy Eastman
Developmental Editor: Axell Ivan Jade M. Purificacion

Veterinary Clinics of North America: Exotic Animal Practice (ISSN 1094-9194) is published in January, May, and September by Elsevier, Inc., 360 Park Avenue South, New York, NY 10010-1710. Subscription prices are $305.00 per year for US individuals, $614.00 per year for US institutions, $100.00 per year for US students and residents, $355.00 per year for Canadian individuals, $739.00 per year for Canadian institutions, $370.00 per year for international individuals, $739.00 per year for international institutions, $100.00 per year Canadian students/residents, and $165.00 per year for international students/residents. To receive student/resident rate, orders must be accompanied by name of affiliated institution, date of term, and the *signature* of program/residency coordinator on institution letterhead. Orders will be billed at individual rate until proof of status is received. Foreign air speed delivery is included in all *Clinics* subscription prices. All prices are subject to change without notice. **POSTMASTER:** Send address changes to *Veterinary Clinics of North America: Exotic Animal Practice*, Elsevier Health Sciences Division, Subscription Customer Service, 3251 Riverport Lane, Maryland Heights, MO 63043. **Customer Service: Telephone: 1-800-654-2452** (U.S. and Canada); **1-314-447-8871** (outside U.S. and Canada). **Fax: 1-314-447-8029. E-mail: journalscustomerservice-usa@ elsevier.com (for print support); journalsonlinesupport-usa@elsevier.com (for online support).**

Reprints. For copies of 100 or more of articles in this publication, please contact the Commercial Reprints Department, Elsevier Inc., 360 Park Avenue South, New York, New York 10010-1710. Tel.: 212-633-3874; Fax: 212-633-3820; E-mail: reprints@elsevier.com.

Veterinary Clinics of North America: Exotic Animal Practice is covered in *MEDLINE/PubMed (Index Medicus).*

Contributors

CONSULTING EDITOR

JÖRG MAYER, Dr med vet, Msc
Diplomate, American Board of Veterinary Practitioners (Exotic Companion Mammals); Diplomate, European College of Zoological Medicine (Small Mammals); Diplomate, American College of Zoological Medicine; Associate Professor of Zoological Medicine, Department of Small Animal Medicine and Surgery, University of Georgia College of Veterinary Medicine, Athens, Georgia, USA

EDITOR

DAVID SANCHEZ-MIGALLON GUZMAN, LV, MS
Diplomate, European College of Zoological Medicine (Avian, Small Mammal); Diplomate, American College of Zoological Medicine; Diplomate, American Board of Veterinary Practice (Avian); Exotic Animal Medicine and Surgery, Professor of Clinical Zoological Companion Animal Medicine and Surgery, Department of Medicine and Epidemiology, School of Veterinary Medicine, University of California, Davis, Davis, California, USA

AUTHORS

ALESSIA CENANI, DVM, MS
Diplomate, American College of Veterinary Anesthesia and Analgesia; Assistant Professor of Clinical Anesthesiology, Department of Surgical and Radiographical Sciences, School of Veterinary Medicine, University of California, Davis, Davis, California, USA

RICARDO DE MATOS, LMV, MSC
Diplomate, American Board of Veterinary Practitioners, Avian Focus; Diplomate, European College of Zoological Medicine (Avian, Small Mammal); Associate Clinical Professor, Section of Zoological Medicine, Department of Clinical Sciences, Cornell University College of Veterinary Medicine, Ithaca, New York, USA

LINDSEY FRY, DVM, cVMA, CVPP, CCRP
Red Sage Integrative Veterinary Partners, Fort Collins, Colorado, USA

TARA M. HARRISON, DVM, MPVM, CVA
Diplomate, American College of Zoological Medicine; Diplomate, American College of Veterinary Preventive Medicine; Diplomate, European College of Zoological Medicine (Zoo Health Management); Exotic Animal Medicine Service, North Carolina State University, College of Veterinary Medicine, Raleigh, North California, USA

MICHELLE G. HAWKINS, VMD
Diplomate, American Board of Veterinary Practitioners (Avian Practice); Department of Medicine and Epidemiology, School of Veterinary Medicine, University of California, Davis, Davis, California, USA

RONALD B. KOH, DVM, MS, CVA, CCRP, CVMMP, CVCH, CVFT
Diplomate, American College of Veterinary Sports Medicine and Rehabilitation;
Integrative Medicine Service, UC Davis Veterinary Medical Teaching Hospital, School of
Veterinary Medicine, University of California, Davis, Davis, California, USA

LA'TOYA V. LATNEY, DVM, CertAqV
Diplomate, European College of Zoological Medicine; Diplomate, American Board of
Veterinary Practitioners (Reptile/Amphibian); Avian and Exotic Medicine and Surgery, The
Animal Medical Center, New York, New York, USA

MATTHEW C. LEACH, BSc (Hons), MSc, PhD
School of Natural and Environmental Sciences, Newcastle University, Agriculture
Building, Newcastle Upon Tyne, United Kingdom

CHRISTOPH MANS, Dr med Vet
Diplomate, American College of Zoological Medicine; Department of Surgical Sciences,
School of Veterinary Medicine, University of Wisconsin-Madison, Madison, Wisconsin,
USA

NICOLE A. MIKONI, DVM
William R. Pritchard Veterinary Medical Teaching Hospital, School of Veterinary Medicine,
University of California, Davis, Davis, California, USA

AMY L. MILLER, BSc (Hons), PhD
School of Health and Life Sciences, Teesside University, Middlesbrough Tower,
Middlesbrough, United Kingdom

RHONDA OATES, DVM, MPVM
Diplomate, American College of Laboratory Animal Medicine; Associate Director,
Research and Teaching Animal Care Program, Campus Veterinary Services, University of
California, Davis, Davis, California, USA

VANESSA L. OLIVER, DVM, MSc
Diplomate, American College of Laboratory Animal Medicine; Associate University
Veterinarian, Adjunct Assistant Professor, Department of Comparative Biology and
Experimental Medicine, Faculty of Veterinary Medicine, University of Calgary, Alberta,
Canada

SARAH OZAWA, DVM
Diplomate, American College of Zoological Medicine; Clinical Assistant Professor,
Department of Clinical Sciences, College of Veterinary Medicine, North Carolina State
University, Raleigh, North Carolina, USA

DANIEL S.J. PANG, BVSC, PhD
Diplomate, European College of Veterinary Anaesthesia and Analgesia; Diplomate,
American College of Veterinary Anesthesia and Analgesia; MRCVS, Associate Professor,
Department of Veterinary Clinical and Diagnostic Sciences, Faculty of Veterinary
Medicine, University of Calgary, Calgary, Alberta, Canada; Department of Clinical
Sciences, Faculty of Veterinary Medicine, Université de Montréal, Québec, Canada

JOANNE PAUL-MURPHY, DVM
Diplomate, American College of Zoological Medicine; Diplomate, American College of
Animal Welfare; Department of Medicine and Epidemiology, School of Veterinary
Medicine, University of California, Davis, Davis, California, USA

OLIVIA A. PETRITZ, DVM
Diplomate, American College of Zoological Medicine; Assistant Professor of Avian and Exotic Animal Medicine, Department of Clinical Sciences, North Carolina State University, College of Veterinary Medicine, Raleigh, North Carolina, USA

JONATHAN A.C. ROQUES, BSC, MSC, PhD
Researcher, Department of Biological and Environmental Sciences, University of Gothenburg, Gothenburg, Sweden

JESSICA RYCHEL, DVM, cVMA, CCRP
Diplomate, American College of Veterinary Sports Medicine and Rehabilitation; Red Sage Integrative Veterinary Partners, Fort Collins, Colorado, USA

MIRANDA J. SADAR, DVM
Diplomate, American College of Zoological Medicine; Assistant Professor, Avian, Exotic, and Zoological Medicine, Service Head, Department of Clinical Sciences, College of Veterinary Medicine and Biomedical Sciences, Colorado State University, Fort Collins, Colorado, USA

DAVID SANCHEZ-MIGALLON GUZMAN, LV, MS
Diplomate, European College of Zoological Medicine (Avian, Small Mammal); Diplomate, American College of Zoological Medicine; Diplomate, American Board of Veterinary Practice (Avian); Exotic Animal Medicine and Surgery, Professor of Clinical Zoological Companion Animal Medicine and Surgery, Department of Medicine and Epidemiology, School of Veterinary Medicine, University of California, Davis, Davis, California, USA

NICO SCHOEMAKER, DVM, PhD
Diplomate, European College of Zoological Medicine (Avian, Small Mammal); Division of Zoological Medicine, Department of Clinical Sciences, Faculty of Veterinary Medicine, Utrecht University, Utrecht, the Netherlands

KURT K. SLADKY, MS, DVM
Diplomate, American College of Zoological Medicine; Diplomate, European College of Zoological Medicine (Zoo Health Management and Herpetology); University of Wisconsin-Madison, School of Veterinary Medicine, Madison, Wisconsin, USA

LYNNE U. SNEDDON, BSC (HONS), PhD
Department of Biological and Environmental Sciences, University of Gothenburg, Gothenburg, Sweden

DANIELLE K. TARBERT, DVM
Staff Veterinarian, Companion Exotic Animal Medicine and Surgery Service, Veterinary Medical Teaching Hospital, School of Veterinary Medicine, University of California, Davis, Davis, California, USA

YVONNE VAN ZEELAND, DVM, MVR, PhD, CPBC
Diplomate, European College of Zoological Medicine (Avian, Small Mammal); Division of Zoological Medicine, Department of Clinical Sciences, Faculty of Veterinary Medicine, Utrecht University, Utrecht, the Netherlands

Contents

Preface: Exotic Animal Pain Management   xiii

David Sanchez-Migallon Guzman

Pain Recognition in Fish   1

Lynne U. Sneddon and Jonathan A.C. Roques

Empirical evidence has demonstrated that fish experience pain, and so to ensure their good welfare, it is vital that we can recognize and assess pain. A range of general, behavioral, and physiologic indicators can be used when assessing pain in fish. Many of these can be used at the tank side and are termed operational welfare indicators, whereas some require further computer or laboratory analysis. Behavioral indicators are valid and have been shown to profoundly differ between nonpainful and painful treatments in fish. However, these are not universal, and species-specific differences exist in behavioral responses to pain.

Treatment of Pain in Fish   11

Kurt K. Sladky

This chapter provides an overview of our current understanding of clinical analgesic use in fish. Recently, the efficacy and pharmacokinetics of several analgesic drugs for use in fish have been investigated, and the most important data indicates that μ-opioid agonist drugs (e.g, morphine) are consistently effective as analgesics across fish species. In addition, bath application of some analgesic drugs may be useful, which affords multiple methods for delivering analgesics to fish. Although few published studies of non-steroidal anti-inflammatory drugs administered to fish show promise, we have much to learn about the analgesic efficacy of most drugs in this class.

Pain Recognition in Reptiles   27

La'Toya V. Latney

Advances in reptile cognitive research would help to (1) better qualify behavioral responses to pain experiences, (2) monitor welfare impacts, and (3) model analgesic studies with ecologically relevant insight to better qualify interventional responses. The focus of future analgesic studies in reptiles require the continued elucidation of the opiate systems and the given variations across taxa in efficacy in nociceptive tests.

Treatment of Pain in Reptiles   43

Kurt K. Sladky

This chapter provides an overview of our current understanding of clinical analgesic use in reptiles. Currently, μ-opioid agonist drugs are the standard of care for analgesia in reptiles. Reptile pain is no longer considered a necessary part of recovery to keep the reptile from becoming active too early. Rather, treating pain allows for the reptile to begin normalizing their behavior. This recognition of pain and analgesia certainly benefits our reptile patients and greatly improves reptile welfare, but it also benefits our students and house officers, who will carry the torch and continue to demand excellence in reptile medicine.

Pain Recognition and Assessment in Birds   65

Nicole A. Mikoni, David Sanchez-Migallon Guzman, and Joanne Paul-Murphy

The recognition and assessment of pain in avian species are crucial tools in providing adequate supportive care in clinical, laboratory, zoologic, rehabilitation, and companion animal settings. With birds being a highly diverse class of species, there is still much to be determined regarding how to create specific criteria to recognize and assess pain in these animals. This article provides a clinical review on the physiology of pain in birds, observed behavioral and physiologic alterations with pain, how different sources and degrees of pain can alter behaviors observed, and how this information can be applied in a clinical setting.

Treatment of Pain in Birds   83

David Sanchez- Migallon Guzman and Michelle G. Hawkins

This article provides an overview of the current understanding of evidence-based clinical analgesic use in birds. The field of avian analgesia has dramatically expanded during the last 20 years, affording more options for alleviating both acute and chronic pain. These options include opioids, nonsteroidal anti-inflammatory drugs, local anesthetics, and/or other drugs like gabapentin, amantadine, and cannabinoids, acting at different points in the nociceptive system thereby helping to provide greater pain relief while reducing the risk of adverse effects when combined.

Pain Recognition in Rodents   121

Vanessa L. Oliver and Daniel S.J. Pang

Available methods for recognizing and assessing pain in rodents have increased over the last 10 years, including the development of validated pain assessment scales. Much of this work has been driven by the needs of biomedical research, and there are specific challenges to applying these scales in the clinical environment. This article provides an introduction to pain assessment scale validation, reviews current methods of pain assessment, highlighting their strengths and weaknesses, and makes recommendations for assessing pain in a clinical environment.

Treatment of Pain in Rats, Mice, and Prairie Dogs   151

Rhonda Oates and Danielle K. Tarbert

Recent myomorph and sciuromorph rodent analgesia studies are reviewed and evaluated for potential clinical application. Differences between laboratory animal studies and clinical use in diseased animals are discussed. Analgesia classes reviewed include local anesthetics, nonsteroidal anti-inflammatories, acetaminophen, opioids, and adjuvants such as anticonvulsants. Routes of administration including sustained-release mechanisms are discussed, as are reversal agents. Drug interactions are reviewed in the context of beneficial multimodal analgesia as well as potential adverse effects. Dosage recommendations for clinical patients are explored.

Hystricomorph Rodent Analgesia   175

Miranda J. Sadar and Christoph Mans

Limited information on the analgesic efficacy and safety of even clinically commonly used analgesic drugs in guinea pigs and chinchillas is available. Buprenorphine and meloxicam are currently the most common analgesics routinely used to treat painful conditions in guinea pigs and chinchillas. Hydromorphone has also shown to be an effective analgesic drug in these species, with limited adverse effects. Tramadol in chinchillas does not provide analgesia even at high doses, and no information is available on the efficacy of this drug in guinea pigs. Multimodal analgesic protocols should be considered whenever possible.

Pain Recognition in Rabbits   187

Amy L. Miller and Matthew C. Leach

Rabbits typically undergo at least one painful procedure during their lifetime and appropriate methods of assessment are essential to reduce or alleviate pain. Various methods of assessing pain in rabbits have been investigated, with the validity of spontaneous behavior and grimace scale scoring being the most studied to date. Assessment of pain is challenging, compounded by rabbits being a prey species that display freezing behavior in the presence of unfamiliar caregivers. Here we discuss some key changes in rabbits that can be used in the assessment of pain and provide some practical suggestions to ensure that the assessment can be carried out effectively.

Treatment of Pain in Rabbits   201

Sarah Ozawa, Alessia Cenani, and David Sanchez-Migallon Guzman LV

Rabbits occupy facets of veterinary medicine spanning from companion mammals, wildlife medicine, zoologic species, and research models. Therefore, analgesia is required for a variety of conditions in rabbits and is a critical component of patient care. Considerations when selecting an analgesic protocol in rabbits include timing of administration, route of administration, degree or anticipated pain, ability to access or use controlled drugs, systemic health, and any potential side effects. This review focuses on pharmacologic and locoregional management of pain in rabbits and emphasizes the need for further studies on pain management in this species.

Pain Recognition in Ferrets   229

Yvonne van Zeeland and Nico Schoemaker

Recognition and accurate assessment of the severity of pain can be challenging in ferrets as they are unable to verbally communicate, and often hide their pain. Pain assessment relies on the assessment of behavioral, physiologic, and other clinical parameters that serve as indirect indicators of pain. Assessment of physiologic and clinical parameters requires handling, which results in changes in these parameters. Behavioral parameters can be assessed less invasively by observing the patient. Due to their nonspecificity, correct interpretation may be challenging. Just as in other species, a grimace scale seems to be the most helpful tool in recognizing pain in ferrets.

Treatment of Pain in Ferrets   245

Olivia A. Petritz and Ricardo de Matos

Ferrets often require pain management as part of comprehensive veterinary care. Recognition and objective quantification of pain, such as the ferret grimace scale, are the first steps of an analgesic plan. As in other species, a multimodal approach to pain management is preferred, which includes combining analgesic drugs of multiple classes and/or techniques to affect different areas of the pain pathway. This article reviews the current published literature on analgesic medications in domestic ferrets, including specific drugs, doses, dosing intervals, and routes of administration.

Acupuncture in Zoological Companion Animals   257

Ronald B. Koh and Tara M. Harrison

Over the past years, the concept of pain management in veterinary medicine has evolved and led to the establishment of a new concept of multimodal approach to pain management, as the current standard of care. The use of multimodal analgesia combining pharmacologic and nonpharmacologic techniques not only helps optimize the quality and efficacy of analgesia but also may prevent the development of chronic or persistent pain. During the past decade, acupuncture has become more popular and evolved into one of the most used forms of integrative medicine interventions and nonpharmacologic therapeutic options for pain management in humans and animals in North America and Europe. There is ample evidence from basic and clinical research for acupuncture is effective in the treatment of acute and chronic pain by influencing neural networks of the nervous system. While in the modern days' veterinary acupuncture has been predominantly used in horses and dogs, its popularity in zoologic companion animals (ZCA) has increased in recent years as an adjunct therapy for treating musculoskeletal, neurologic, and gastrointestinal disorders due to its minimal invasiveness and low risk of adverse events. The integrative use of acupuncture has become even more important with the increasingly limited use of opiates in veterinary medicine due to the opiate crisis. The purpose of this article aims to provide guidance for using acupuncture for pain management in ZCA in clinical practice, based on available information and recommendations from experienced veterinary acupuncturists.

Physical Rehabilitation in Zoological Companion Animals   281

Ronald B. Koh, Jessica Rychel, and Lindsey Fry

Animal physical rehabilitation is one of the fast-growing fields in veterinary medicine in recent years. It has become increasingly common in small animal practice and will continue to emerge as an essential aspect of veterinary medicine that plays a vital role in the care of animals with physical impairments or disabilities from surgery, injuries, or diseases.1 This is true now more than ever because of the increasing advances in lifesaving treatments, the increased lifespan of companion animals, and the growth of chronic conditions, of which many are associated with movement disorders. The American Association of Rehabilitation Veterinarians (AARV) defines APR as "the diagnosis and management of patients with painful or functionally limiting conditions, particularly those with injury or illness related to the neurologic and musculoskeletal systems." Rehabilitation not only focuses on recovery after surgical procedures but also on improving the function and quality of life in animals suffering from debilitating diseases such as arthritis or neurologic disorders. The overall goal of APR is to decrease pain, reduce edema, promote tissue healing, restore gait and mobility to its prior activity level, regain strength, prevent further injury, and promote optimal quality of life. Typically, a multimodal approach with pharmaceutical and nonpharmaceutical interventions is used by APR therapists to manage patients during their recovery. The purpose of this article aims to provide knowledge and guidance on physical rehabilitation to help veterinarians in the proper return of their patients with ZCA safely after injury and/or surgery.

VETERINARY CLINICS OF NORTH AMERICA: EXOTIC ANIMAL PRACTICE

FORTHCOMING ISSUES

May 2023
Dermatology
Dario d'Ovidio and Domenico Santoro, *Editors*

September 2023
Critical Care
Lily Parkinson, *Editor*

RECENT ISSUES

May 2022
Cardiology
Michael Pees, *Editor*

January 2022
Sedation and Anesthesia of Zoological Companion Animals
Miranda J. Sadar and João Brandão, *Editors*

SERIES OF RELATED INTEREST

Veterinary Clinics of North America: Small Animal Practice
Available at: https://www.vetsmall.theclinics.com/

THE CLINICS ARE NOW AVAILABLE ONLINE!
Access your subscription at:
www.theclinics.com

Preface

Exotic Animal Pain Management

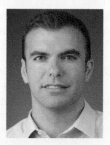

David Sanchez-Migallon Guzman, LV,
MS, Dipl ECZM (Avian, Small
Mammal), Dipl ACZM
Editor

With an increase in the life expectancy of our exotic patients and the increased demand in the quality of patient care, the recognition and treatment of pain in our patients
have gained more importance in our daily practice. We are faced now with clients that
are emotionally connected and more educated in the diagnosis and treatment of pain,
with higher expectations regarding pain management. While much progress has been
made and we feel like we can treat pain in these species, exotic animal pain management is still in an early stage of development when compared with what is known in
canine, feline, and, of course, human patients.

   This issue of the *Veterinary Clinics of North America: Exotic Animal Practice*, with 14
articles and 26 authors, who are experts in their field, covers pain recognition and treatment in fish; reptiles; birds; rabbits; guinea pigs and chinchillas; rats, mice, gerbils,
hamsters, and prairie dogs; ferrets as well as acupuncture and physical therapy in
these species. The information presented here evidences the significant advances
that our field has experienced in this area since the last issue of the *Veterinary
Clinics of North America: Exotic Animal Practice* was published in 2011, with a very
large number of behavioral, pharmacokinetics, pharmacodynamics, safety, and toxicologic studies as well as evaluation of locoregional techniques and case reports.
The dosages presented in the tables of these articles represent in many instances
the ones evaluated in the studies referenced and not necessarily recommended dosages or drugs in a given case. When indicated, these drugs and dosages should be
applied under close observation for analgesic effectiveness and safety.

   I would like to encourage clinicians to consult with board-certified colleagues in
anesthesia and pain management when evaluating and treating exotic patients with
pain as well as document these cases and promote research in this area. We also
can learn a lot from other groups like the International Veterinary Academy of Pain

Vet Clin Exot Anim 26 (2023) xiii–xiv
https://doi.org/10.1016/j.cvex.2022.10.001
vetexotic.theclinics.com
1094-9194/23/© 2022 Elsevier Inc. All rights reserved.

Management, where the foundational aspects of pain management can be learned and ultimately improve the care of our patients.

I would like to thank all the authors for their effort and contribution to this issue, and we hope that the reader will find the information presented here educational and clinically applicable. It was our goal to help clinicians keep up with the increasing new information in this area and present it in a friendly manner. Last, I would like to thank Elsevier for the opportunity given to serve as a guest editor of this issue and for their support and guidance. It has been a great pleasure, and I look forward to contributing to the *Veterinary Clinics of North America: Exotic Animal Practice* in the future.

David Sanchez-Migallon Guzman, LV, MS, Dipl ECZM (Avian, Small Mammal),
Dipl ACZM
Department of Medicine and Epidemiology
School of Veterinary Medicine
University of California Davis
Davis, CA 95616, USA

E-mail address:
guzman@ucdavis.edu

Pain Recognition in Fish

Lynne U. Sneddon, BSc (Hons), PhD[a],*,
Jonathan A.C. Roques, BSc, MSc, PhD[a,b]

KEYWORDS

• Fishes • Nociception • Pain • Stress • Welfare • Zebrafish • Rainbow trout

KEY POINTS

• Invasive procedures that cause tissue damage give rise to pain in fish.
• Behavioral and physiological indicators can be used for pain assessment in fish.
• Pain indicators are species-specific in fish.

INTRODUCTION

The first characterization of nociceptors in a teleost (bony) fish, the rainbow trout (*Oncorhynchus mykiss*) was published in 2002.[1] Since then numerous empirical studies have demonstrated the capacity for pain in teleost fish using neuroanatomical, electrophysiological, molecular, physiological, imaging, and behavioral techniques.[2–4] Besides rainbow trout, several other species of fish have been investigated, including Atlantic salmon (*Salmo salar*),[5,6] goldfish (*Carassius auratus*)[6–8], common carp (*Cyprinus carpio*),[7] Nile and Mozambique tilapia (*Oreochromis niloticus, O mossambicus*),[9,10] piauçu (*Leporinus macrocephalus*),[11] and zebrafish (*Danio rerio*).[7,12–14] Given that there are well over 30,000 species of fish and studies so far have shown profound differences in response to pain between species, more research is needed to explore species-specific differences. Painful stimuli, such as mechanical cutting, high temperature, and algogenic chemicals result in profound changes in behavior in fish and in some cases physiological parameters are altered.[2–4,15] Common to all fish species tested so far is significant changes in behavior that in some cases can be prevented by the use of analgesia (pain relief).[16] The acceptance of pain in fish naturally has implications for their treatment.[16,17] In the context of scientific experimentation, fish are protected by legislation in many countries, including the European Union (EU), and researchers using fish models are legally required to avoid, minimize, and alleviate pain when pain is not the study's goal.[18,19] However, there is still a lack of data on analgesic use in fish and there is a need for the development of pain

a Department of Biology and Environmental Sciences, University of Gothenburg, Medicineragatan 18A, Gothenburg 413 90, Sweden; b SWEMARC, the Swedish Mariculture Research Center, University of Gothenburg, 18A, Gothenburg 413 90, Sweden
* Corresponding author.
E-mail address: Lynne.sneddon@bioenv.gu.se

Vet Clin Exot Anim 26 (2023) 1–10
https://doi.org/10.1016/j.cvex.2022.07.002
1094-9194/23/© 2022 Elsevier Inc. All rights reserved.

assessment strategies. Fishes are now used in large numbers across the globe in laboratory experiments and are the second most commonly used animal in the EU.[17,20] In particular, zebrafish have become a popular model species adopted in a range of experimental contexts and, in some countries and regions, account for approximately 50% of all fish used in experiments. Therefore, there is a real need to identify indicators of pain to assess pain in fish in the laboratory and veterinary contexts.

Fish are subject to a range of invasive procedures in the laboratory, including injections, Passive Integrated Transponder (PIT) tagging (where a tag is inserted through the abdomen into the intraperitoneal cavity), fin clipping (where part of a fin is removed for genomic screening, individual recognition or the study of fin amputation), surgery (eg, implant of biologgers, heart damage, optic nerve crush, spinal lesions), infection studies where diseases can be necrotic, genetic modifications leading to potentially painful phenotypes (eg, osteoarthritis), and gamete collection.[14,17] Any tissue damage caused by these procedures may give rise to pain and poor welfare. To assess pain during and after these events, a number of indicators as described later can be used either at the tank side and so are operational welfare indicators (OWIs) or require further analyses and, as such, are laboratory welfare indicators (LabWIs).[20,21]

RECOGNIZING PAIN IN FISH

Pain assessment cannot be generalized because it is expressed differently between individual animals. This means there is no gold standard indicator to measure pain in animals or indeed fish.[22] Responses to "painful treatment" will differ between species and between individuals, as well as be specific to each type of pain.[7,23,24] Therefore, pain can only be evaluated by measuring a range of indirect parameters, including general changes in appearance and alterations in behavior and physiology (**Table 1**).

General changes in appearance or demeanor can be reflected in the physical appearance of the animal or can be assessed by measuring the animal's biological functioning and gauging any changes as a result of pain. These indirect measurements are a consequence of prolonged responses in physiological or behavioral parameters due to the painful event. General indicators, such as the overall physical condition of the fish, the presence of lesions, demeanor, and body or fin posture, make a contribution to the assessment of pain, but they alone do not determine whether the animal is in pain. Pain is inherently stressful and, as such, physiologic indicators of stress can assist in understanding the extent to which pain affects welfare and homeostasis. More importantly, changes in biological function traits can be used more effectively to determine if an animal is pain-free; if the animals exhibit normal behavior and demeanor, no significant stress responses, are healthy and disease-free, reproduce normally, and grow normally, then there is likely no pain.

Physiological indicators can be indirect, such as ventilation rate (the rate of the beating of the operculum that covers the gills) or be direct measures of stress responsiveness at a specific time (such as cortisol or metabolites like glucose). Biochemical or other clinical parameters can be measured in the individual animal, and changes can be recorded when the animal experiences pain. As stated earlier, pain elicits a stress response which involves the release of cortisol because of the activity of the hypothalamic–pituitary–interrenal axis and elicits the release of adrenalin and noradrenalin via the sympathetic nervous system.[24,25] Damaged tissue also activates immune responses and the release of inflammatory mediators.[3] However, caution does need to be applied to physiologic indicators when assessing pain in fish, because it may not be easy to distinguish between pain itself from the inherent stress response

Table 1
A list of indicators that can be used to assess pain in fishes

Types	Indicators	Species	References
General	Presence of lesions or wounds may be painful	*D. rerio*	Martins et al,[35] 2016
	Change in coloration and/or position of fins	*D. rerio*	Martins et al,[35] 2016
	Increased mucus production	*D. rerio*	Dash et al,[36] 2018, Martins et al,[35] 2016
	Reduced or no food consumption	*O. mykiss*	Sneddon,[15] 2003
	Reduced weight	*C. carpio*	Harms et al,[37] 2005
Behavioral	No response to food	*D. rerio*	Martins et al,[35] 2016
	Loss of equilibrium or struggle to maintain balance	*D. rerio* *C. carpio* *O. mykiss*	Martins et al,[35] 2016 Reilly et al,[7] 2008
	Altered use of tank space compared with normal use (eg, time spent in the bottom, reduced exploration, wall hugging, or thigmotaxis)	*D. rerio* *O. niloticus*	Costa et al,[38] 2019 Deakin et al,[14] 2019 Schroeder and Sneddon,[39] 2017 Roques et al,[9] 2010
	Altered levels of activity (measured as eg, total distance traveled, time spent in activity, or swimming)	*D. rerio* *O. mykiss*	Deakin et al,[14] 2019 Correia et al,[41] 2011 Ashley et al,[28] 2009
	Altered swimming speed	*D. rerio* *O. mykiss*	Deakin et al,[14] 2019 Ashley et al,[28] 2009
	Erratic or sudden movements (eg, rapid unexpected changes in direction during swimming)	*D. rerio* *O. mossambicus*	White et al,[26] 2017, Maximino,[40] 2011 Roques et al,[10] 2012
	Lethargic or no response to external stimuli	*D. rerio*	Martins et al,[35] 2016
	Swim individually or away from group/shoal	*D. rerio*	Thomson et al,[31] 2019 Martins et al,[35] 2016
	No response to conspecifics	*D. rerio*	Martins et al,[35] 2016
	Rocking on pectoral fins	*C. carpio* *O. mykiss*	Reilly et al,[7] 2008, Sneddon,[15] 2003
	Rubbing hurt area against the substrate or tank walls	*C. carpio* *O. mykiss*	Reilly et al,[7] 2008, Sneddon,[15] 2003
	Administering analgesic returns behavior to normal	*O. mykiss*	Sneddon,[15] 2003 Deakin et al,[29][14,] 2019
	Body curve index (hunched position)	*D. rerio*	Costa et al,[38] 2019
	Tail "wafting" or tail beats performed whilst stationary	*D. rerio*	Schroeder and Sneddon,[39] 2017, Maximino,[40] 2011
	Freezing for prolonged periods (>30 s)	*D. rerio*	Costa et al,[38] 2019
	Increased aggression	*D. rerio*	Martins et al,[35] 2016
	Reduced complexity or fractal dimension of swimming trajectory	*D. rerio*	Deakin et al,[29] 2019
Physiological	Increased stress measured via cortisol levels	*D. rerio* *O. mykiss*	White et al,[26] 2017 Ashley et al,[28] 2009
	Ventilation rate or frequency of opercular (gill cover) beats altered	*D. rerio* *O. mykiss*	Ashley et al,[28] 2009, Reilly et al,[7] 2008
	Altered blood biochemistry	*C. carpio*	Harms et al,[37] 2005

Species where the indicator has been used is noted. OWIs have no highlight but behaviors or welfare indicators measures that require further computer or laboratory analysis are highlighted in gray or the text is gray.

caused by handling and the procedure itself, unless the physiological changes are more elevated than a typical stress response. For example, the ventilation rate in rainbow trout and zebrafish after painful treatment is elevated more than rates seen after stress.[7] Physiological parameters can change rapidly over very short periods, so they provide a snapshot of what is happening within the animal and may be influenced by the sampling method itself. That is, removing fish from water to obtain a blood sample causes stress. To circumvent this, White and colleagues sampled cortisol from the surrounding tank water containing zebrafish rather than disturbing the fish to obtain a sample.[26] This study found that painful treatment significantly elevated cortisol excretion.

Behavioral indicators are very valuable in pain assessment because many animals show detrimental changes in behavior during pain.[22] Any changes from the normal behavioral patterns of animals are easy to observe if they are profoundly different. This does rely on the carer or researcher having in-depth knowledge of what is considered normal for the species of fish under their care. Behavioral indicators, such as changes in activity, tank space use, and lack of feeding, can be used to evaluate the presence of pain in animals, and several have been proposed.[24] However, these indicators could be subject to different interpretations by each observer if the observers are not properly trained.[4,7,28] Even within species, there may be differences in the behavioral expression of pain due to intraspecific variation in behavior linked to bold, risk-taking individuals versus shy, risk-averse animals or due to social status within the group.[27,28,29] Many recent studies have shown that zebrafish exposed to pain are much less active with lengthy periods of immobility, use the bottom of the tank mostly, and swim much less (**Fig. 1**).[14,27,29,31] These are easily recognized behavioral changes by direct observation because healthy zebrafish are normally very

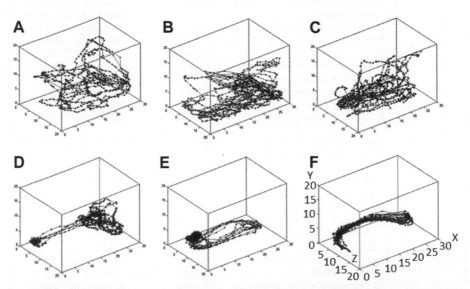

Fig. 1. Zebrafish 3D swimming trajectory plots (0–5 minutes sample taken from a 25 minutes recording at the 2 hours time point after treatment) of three control zebrafish (*A–C*) and three treatment zebrafish (*D*, 10% acid lip; *E*, fin clip; *F*, PIT tag). These plots demonstrate the reduction in space use and movement seen after painful treatment (*D, E,* and *F*; reproduced under a Creative Commons Attribution (CC BY) license from Deakin and colleagues 2019).[29]

active, using all of the tank space and swimming almost continuously. Additionally, performance of anomalous behaviors specific to pain has been observed in fish, including zebrafish.[2,4,30,32] For example, zebrafish engage in tail "wafting" after fin clipping, where part of the tail fin is removed, yet they are not swimming and are stationary when performing this behavior. Normal swimming is restored by the use of analgesia.[14,29,40]

SPECIES-SPECIFIC RESPONSES TO PAIN

Similarly to mammals, there are commonalities and differences in the behavioral responses to pain among fish species. Thus, it is vitally important to have a real insight into the normal behavior of a chosen species when deciding if there are changes during or after pain. For example, rainbow trout and zebrafish reduce activity, spend more time in the bottom of their tanks, increase their ventilation rate far above a stress response, and perform anomalous behaviors specific to painful treatment. In contrast, common carp exhibit no change in swimming or ventilation rate but do engage in anomalous behavior.[7] Whereas Nile tilapia subjected to fin clip actually increase their frequency of swimming,[9] and formalin injection in piauçu results in higher locomotor activity.[11] More research is needed to define OWIs and behavioral indicators for each species of fish.

AUTOMATED RECOGNITION OF PAIN

Recent studies have explored the use of artificial intelligence in the development of automated monitoring of zebrafish welfare during invasive laboratory procedures. Two new tools have been published that can detect the behavioral changes associated with pain, and they use video analysis to determine how much zebrafish behavior is altered.

The first tool is the fish behavior index (FBI), which uses real-time behavioral information to classify individual zebrafish as "healthy," "okay," "unhealthy" or "abnormal."[14] The FBI combines two factors: distance traveled and activity, and was developed by exploring the behaviors of healthy controls; fish subjected to a variety of laboratory procedures performed under anesthesia with behavior assessed before the treatment and afterward; fin clip; PIT tagging; subcutaneous injection of acetic acid at 1%, 5%, and 10% (a standard pain test in animals)[15,33]; and fin clip coupled with administration of analgesic drugs. All these procedures were conducted under anesthesia and the fish were allowed 30 minutes to recover before video analysis commenced. The study demonstrated that zebrafish still exhibited signs of pain after 6 hours when they were either fin clipped, PIT tagged, or injected with 5% and 10% acetic acid (**Fig. 2**). After 6 hours, only 1% acetic acid-injected fish had recovered. Some of the analgesics tested provided effective pain relief and prevented the decline in activity and distance traveled observed in fin-clipped fish. Exploration of the data demonstrated that at least a 10-minute real-time assessment was required to accurately measure pain responses. The FBI tool, therefore, would have utility in assessing pain in zebrafish who are held individually during genomic screening or those subject to invasive surgery that are held alone to promote healing. The software is freely available via links in the published study.[14]

The second tool, the Chromatic Fish Analyzer, assesses behavior in groups of zebrafish (each treatment had eight replicates of six fish per tank). In this case, measurements are made directly from videos where light saturation (proxy for activity), hue horizontally and vertically (position of fish in the tank) and clustering (closeness of fish within the group) are assessed.[31] In zebrafish, there is a reduction in activity and

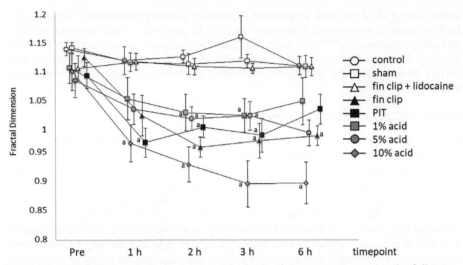

Fig. 2. Mean (±S.E.) fractal dimension (y-axis) of zebrafish trajectories under the following treatments: control, anesthetized and handled, fin clip and lidocaine, fin clip, PIT tag, 1%, 5%, and 10% acetic acid injected into the lip ($n = 7$ each group) over time. [a]Significant difference ($P < .05$) when comparing treatment groups with controls. Data points have been altered via jitter to reduce overlap (reproduced under a Creative Commons Attribution (CC BY) license from Deakin and colleagues 2019).[29]

enhanced use of the bottom of the tank after pain, and this was also observed in groups. Thus, these measures are applicable to the pain response. Indeed, groups of zebrafish where 1, 3, or 6 fish within each group received a fin clip dramatically reduced their activity and moved to the bottom of the tank compared with pretreatment behavior. Administration of analgesia was effective in preventing these changes in groups where 1 or 3 fish had been clipped but was less successful when all 6 fish were clipped. This may be because of the dose of the pain-relieving drug being insufficient. However, future studies should explore this as an explanation. Currently, this tool is under development and is not available for download. However, both of these monitoring software tools have the potential to increase the welfare of fish through accurate and rapid pain assessment.

ASSESSMENT OF PAIN

When determining the severity of pain, there are many guides or OWIs that can be used for mammals. For example, grimace scales in rodents where the extent of changes in facial expression is linked to how severe the pain may be.[34] This then assists the carer or veterinarian in making the decision with regard to pain relief. In fish, this is relatively understudied. To date, only one pain severity scale has been developed, and again, this is relevant to zebrafish (**Fig. 3**).[29] To develop the zebrafish pain scale, the fractal dimension of complex swimming trajectories of pain-free controls, anesthetized only fish, fin clipped, PIT tagged, 1%, 5%, and 10% acetic acid injected, and fin clip administered with pain relief, was calculated. In other animal groups, a decline in fractal dimension or complexity of movement has been linked to reduced welfare. On the zebrafish scale, the range of fractal dimensions of pain-free animals was comparable to those who were fin clipped and administered with pain relief. Those animals anesthetized and handled only reflect a stress response,

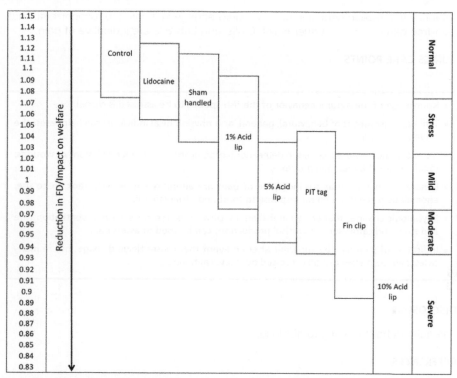

Fig. 3. Hypothetical fractal dimension (FD) welfare scale indicating the range of FD values associated with each treatment group [control, sham handled (anesthetized and handled only), fin clip and lidocaine, fin clip, PIT tag, 1%, 5%, and 10% acetic acid injected into the lip]. A decrease in FD value indicates a reduction in welfare and an arbitrary scale of intensity represents zebrafish welfare as normal, stressed, and in pain from mild to severe (reproduced under a Creative Commons Attribution (CC BY) license from Deakin and colleagues 2019).[29]

and this is followed by mild, moderate, and severe pain (see **Fig. 3**). Subcutaneous injection into the frontal lips with 10% acetic acid appeared to be the most painful treatment, but this scale does require information from other invasive procedures (eg, surgery) to produce a fully detailed and informative pain scale.

SUMMARY

Fishes exhibit pain responses to a variety of noxious and damaging stimuli, including mechanical damage, high temperature, and algogenic chemicals. Pain results in significant changes to general demeanor, physiology, and behavior and a range of behavioral and physiological indicators can easily be measured by the side of the tank by direct observation that represent OWIs or that can be measured by further video tracking analysis of behavior or measured in the laboratory (eg, stress hormones). Automated software tools may be especially useful in experimental facilities with large numbers of zebrafish, and future studies should investigate extrapolating the tools available to other laboratory species. The assessment of pain is particularly important when determining the use of analgesia to reduce pain. Therefore, veterinarians, researchers, and carers should engage in training to recognize normal, pain-free behaviors and further which OWIs and Lab WIs are indicative of pain.

CLINICS CARE POINTS

- Knowledge of the natural behavior of the fish species to be assessed is crucial.
- Tank-side assessment of behavioral, general, and physiological indicators can help assess the presence of pain.
- General indicators are changes in demeanor (color, posture); presence of lesions or wounds; rapid weight changes, and anorexia.
- Behavioral changes that are indicative of pain are alterations in activity, tank space use, anomalous behaviors, and no response to food and other stimuli.
- Physiologic changes that are greater than a typical stress response, such as ventilation rate and stress indicators such as cortisol production, can be used to assess pain.
- Indicators of pain may be apparent after an event that causes tissue damage, but in many cases, pain responses can be expressed over several hours.

DISCLOSURE

The authors have nothing to disclose.

REFERENCES

1. Sneddon LU. Anatomical and electrophysiological analysis of the trigeminal nerve in a teleost fish, *Oncorhynchus mykiss*. Neurosci Lett 2002;319(3):167–71.
2. Sneddon LU. Pain in aquatic animals. J Exp Biol 2015;218(7):967–76.
3. Sneddon LU. Comparative physiology of nociception and pain. Physiology 2018; 33:63–73.
4. Sneddon LU. Evolution of nociception and pain: evidence from fish models. Phil Trans R Soc B 2019;374(1785):20190290.
5. Nordgreen J, Garner JP, Janczak AM, et al. Thermonociception in fish: effects of two different doses of morphine on thermal threshold and post-test behaviour in goldfish (*Carassius auratus*). Appl Anim Behav Sci 2009;119(1–2):101–7.
6. Bjørge MH, Nordgreen J, Janczak AM, et al. Behavioural changes following intraperitoneal vaccination in Atlantic salmon (*Salmo salar*). Appl Anim Behav Sci 2011;133(1–2):127–35.
7. Reilly SC, Quinn JP, Cossins AR, et al. Behavioural analysis of a nociceptive event in fish: comparisons between three species demonstrate specific responses. Appl Anim Behav Sci 2008;114(1–2):248–59.
8. Dunlop R, Laming P. Mechanoreceptive and nociceptive responses in the central nervous system of goldfish (*Carassius auratus*) and trout (*Oncorhynchus mykiss*). J Pain 2005;6(9):561–8.
9. Roques JAC, Abbink W, Geurds F, et al. Tailfin clipping, a painful procedure: studies on Nile tilapia and common carp. Physiol Behav 2010;101(4):533–40.
10. Roques JAC, Abbink W, Chereau G, et al. Physiological and behavioral responses to an electrical stimulus in Mozambique tilapia (*Oreochromis mossambicus*). Fish Physiol Biochem 2012;38(4):1019–28.
11. Wolkers CPB, Junior AB, Menescal-de-Oliveira L, et al. GABAA-benzodiazepine receptors in the dorsomedial (Dm) telencephalon modulate restraint-induced

antinociception in the fish Leporinus macrocephalus. Physiol Behav 2015;147: 175–82.

12. Thomson JS, Deakin AG, Cossins AR, et al. Acute and chronic stress prevents responses to pain in zebrafish: evidence for stress-induced analgesia. J Exp Biol 2020;223(14):jeb224527.

13. de Abreu MS, Giacomini AC, Genario R, et al. Understanding early-life pain and its effects on adult human and animal emotionality: Translational lessons from rodent and zebrafish models. Neurosci Lett 2022;768:136382.

14. Deakin AG, Buckley J, AlZu'bi HS, et al. Automated monitoring of behaviour in zebrafish after invasive procedures. Sci Rep 2019;9(1):1–13.

15. Sneddon LU. The evidence for pain in fish: the use of morphine as an analgesic. Appl Anim Behav Sci 2003;83(2):153–62.

16. Sloman KA, Bouyoucos IA, Brooks EJ, et al. Ethical considerations in fish research. J Fish Biol 2019;94(4):556–77.

17. Sneddon LU. Pain in laboratory animals: A possible confounding factor? Altern Lab Anim 2017;45(3):161–4.

18. Sneddon LU, Halsey LG, Bury NR. Considering aspects of the 3Rs principles within experimental animal biology. J Exp Biol 2017;220(17):3007–16.

19. European Commission. Statistical report, SWD 204: executive summary parts A and B and Part C. Data of 2018 from 28 member states and Norway. European Union; 2018. Accessed February 24, 2022.

20. Noble C, Gismervik K, Iversen MH, et al. Welfare Indicators for farmed Atlantic salmon: tools for assessing fish welfare. In: Nofima. 2018. Available at: https://nofimaas.sharepoint.com/sites/public/Cristin/Welfare%20indicators%20for%20farmed%20Atlantic%20salmon%20-FishWell-%20November%202018%20-%20Web%20version.pdf. Accessed February 24, 2022.

21. Sneddon LU, Elwood RW, Adamo SA, et al. Defining and assessing animal pain. Anim Behav 2014;97:201–12.

22. Le Neindre P., Guémené D., Guichet J., et al. Animal pain: identifying, understanding and minimising pain in farm animals. Multidisciplinary scientific assessment, Summary of the expert report INRA: Paris. p. 98, 2009. Available at: https://www.inrae.fr/sites/default/files/pdf/05e1f915d62a32c84cf9865b9d6cba39.pdf. Accessed August 15, 2022.

23. Prunier A, Mounier L, Le Neindre P, et al. Identifying and monitoring pain in farm animals: a review. Animal 2013;7(6):998–1010.

24. Sneddon LU, Wolfenden DC, Thomson JS. Stress management and welfare. In: Schreck CB, Tort L, Farrell AP, et al, editors. Biology of stress in fish: fish physiology. London: Academic Press; 2016. p. 463–539.

25. Wendelaar Bonga SE. The stress response in fish. Physiol Rev 1997;77(3): 591–625.

26. White LJ, Thomson JS, Pounder KC, et al. The impact of social context on behaviour and the recovery from welfare challenges in zebrafish, Danio rerio. Anim Behav 2017;132:189–99.

27. Sneddon LU. Pain Perception in Fish: Evidence and Implications for the Use of Fish. J Conscious Stud 2011;18(9–10):209–29.

28. Ashley PJ, Ringrose S, Edwards KL, et al. Effect of noxious stimulation upon antipredator responses and dominance status in rainbow trout. Anim Behav 2009; 77(2):403–10.

29. Deakin AG, Spencer JW, Cossins AR, et al. Welfare challenges influence the complexity of movement: fractal analysis of behaviour in zebrafish. Fishes 2019;4(1):8.

30. Simonetti RB, Santos Marques L, Streit DP Jr, et al. Zebrafish (*Danio rerio*): ethics in animal experimentation. IOSR J Agric Vet Sci Ver 2016;9(7):2319–72.
31. Thomson JS, Al-Temeemy AA, Isted H, et al. Assessment of behaviour in groups of zebrafish (*Danio rerio*) using an intelligent software monitoring tool, the chromatic fish analyser. J Neurosci Methods 2019;328:108433.
32. Sneddon LU. Clinical anesthesia and analgesia in fish. J Exot Pet Med 2012; 21(1):32–43.
33. Martinez V, Coutinho S, Thakur S, et al. Differential effects of chemical and mechanical colonic irritation on behavioral pain response to intraperitoneal acetic acid in mice. Pain 1999;81(1–2):179–86.
34. NC3Rs. NC3Rs Grimace Scales 2022. In NC3Rs. 2022. Available at: https://nc3rs.org.uk/3rs-resources/grimace-scales. Accessed February 24, 2022.
35. Martins T, Valentim AM, Pereira N, et al. Anaesthesia and analgesia in laboratory adult zebrafish: a question of refinement. Lab Anim 2016;50(6):476–88.
36. Dash S, Das S, Samal J, et al. Epidermal mucus, a major determinant in fish health: a review. Iran J Vet Res 2018;19(2):72.
37. Harms CA, Lewbart GA, Swanson CR, et al. Behavioral and clinical pathology changes in koi carp (*Cyprinus carpio*) subjected to anesthesia and surgery with and without intra-operative analgesics. Comp Med 2005;55(3):221–6.
38. Costa FV, Rosa LV, Quadros VA, et al. Understanding nociception-related phenotypes in adult zebrafish: Behavioral and pharmacological characterization using a new acetic acid model. Behav Brain Res 2019;359:570–8.
39. Schroeder PG, Sneddon LU. Exploring the efficacy of immersion analgesics in zebrafish using an integrative approach. Appl Anim Behav Sci 2017;187:93–102.
40. Maximino C. Modulation of nociceptive-like behavior in zebrafish (*Danio rerio*) by environmental stressors. Psychol Neurosci 2011;4:149–55.
41. Correia AD, Cunha SR, Scholze M, Stevens ED. A Novel Behavioral Fish Model of Nociception for Testing Analgesics. Pharmaceuticals 2011;4(4):665–80.

Treatment of Pain in Fish

Kurt K. Sladky, MS, DVM, Dipl ACZM, Dipl ECZM (Zoo Health Management & Herpetology)

KEYWORDS

- Fish • Analgesia • Opioids • NSAIDs • Local anesthetics

KEY POINTS

- Analgesic drug administration in fish should be considered standard of care under clinical and research conditions, which are considered painful in other species.
- Based on current evidence, mu-opioid agonists are considered the most effective choice for analgesia in fish.
- Although limited data are available with respect to pharmacokinetics and/or pharmacodynamics of few non-steroidal anti-inflammatory drugs (NSAIDs) in a limited number of fish species, we know almost nothing about NSAID efficacy. Nevertheless, we tend to use NSAIDs in fish for painful or inflammatory conditions with the hope that it helps the fish to which it is administered.
- Preemptive administration of analgesics, for example, before a surgical procedure, should be considered an expectation of practice in fish clinical medicine and research.

INTRODUCTION

In the late 1990s, as a zoological medicine resident, I became interested in clinical fish analgesia while conducting a research project in which I was comparing the anesthetic efficacy of tricaine methanesulfonate (MS-222) with clove oil (active ingredient of which is eugenol) in red pacu (*Piaractus brachypomus*).[1] During that study, I used a hypodermic needle insertion as my method for inducing a painful reaction, as most fish species generally react to this noxious stimulus during routine blood sampling from the coccygeal vein. During my study, I found that few pacu reacted to the needle insertion if they were anesthetized with MS-222, but most reacted when anesthetized with eugenol even when the fish were characterized at a deep stage of anesthesia. At the time, this reactive behavior to a needle stick was concerning to me, as some veterinarians, aquaculturists and aquarists were using clove oil for quick and inexpensive sedation of fish, while also subjecting fish to relatively invasive procedures, including surgery. With these data in mind, I was motivated to start digging deeper in an attempt to understand efficacious analgesic drugs in fish. I endeavored to better understand

University of Wisconsin-Madison, School of Veterinary Medicine, 2015 Linden Drive, Madison, WI 53705 USA
E-mail address: kurt.sladky@wisc.edu

Vet Clin Exot Anim 26 (2023) 11–26
https://doi.org/10.1016/j.cvex.2022.07.003
1094-9194/23/© 2022 Elsevier Inc. All rights reserved.

how best to choose, and apply, analgesic drugs in fish medicine and surgery, as there were no evidence-based published data on analgesic use in fish before 2000.

By the early 2000s, fish pain perception became a hot, albeit controversial, topic in the literature,[2–4] and this interest in fish pain stimulated a subsequent interest in ameliorating pain-related behavior in fish through the application of analgesics. Despite the ongoing debate about whether fish are capable of feeling pain, many teleost (bony) and elasmobranch (cartilaginous) fish have the necessary neuro-anatomy, neurophysiology, and behavioral changes to meet the criteria for pain perception.[2,5–11] In response to stressors (eg, handling, noxious stimuli), fish develop avoidance behaviors, and undergo pain-related physiologic responses (eg, changes in opercular rate, heart rate, cardiac output, food consumption, activity, endogenous cortisol level, blood glucose, electrolytes, and blood gases).[1–3,5,9,12–17]

Although our understanding of pain and analgesia in fish has advanced since the early 2000s, there is still much to learn. For example, we know very little about individual analgesic drug safety and efficacy or appropriate doses to administer across the significant diversity of fish species; or how water temperature impacts analgesic drug metabolism. In addition, we know little about the duration of analgesic drug efficacy in different species, nor do we know the most appropriate routes of analgesic drug administration. However, our limited understanding of pain and analgesia in fish should not obscure our clinical decisions, and we should err on the side of fish well-being by assuming that conditions considered painful in humans and other mammals should be assumed to be potentially painful across all fish species. However, whenever possible, the choice and dosage of analgesics must be based on sound research. Unfortunately, sometimes the best we can do is extrapolate information from related, or even divergent, species. Therefore, pursuit of clinically relevant pain and analgesia research is critical for expanding our understanding of these issues in fish, and for improving the welfare of fish under our care. The objective of this article was to present evidence-based and clinically relevant analgesic data for use in captive fish.

GENERAL CONSIDERATIONS
Diversity of Fishes

It is estimated that there are currently greater than 36,000 species of fish worldwide, which is more species than all other vertebrate species, combined.[18] In addition, fish inhabit nearly every ecosystem on earth. With this in mind, how do we begin to understand efficacy of analgesic drugs across all fishes and aquatic environments? Obviously, the answer is that it is impossible, but we need to start somewhere, and as with many drugs used in zoologic medicine, anecdotal evidence, and extrapolation across species, and even Taxa, becomes the information on which we rely. Clearly, trying to describe and discuss analgesia across the multitude of fish species along with the variety of ecosystems within which fish inhabit, with varying water temperatures and water chemical characteristics, is beyond the scope of this article, but I mention these concerns as they should always remain in the back of our minds when thinking about the efficacy, pharmacokinetics, and pharmacodynamics of analgesic drugs in fish.

Methods of Administration

The administration of analgesics to fish can be accomplished via several routes.[11,19] Bath administration involves exposing the gills of the fish patient to a measured concentration of the drug that is solubilized in the water in which the fish resides or in which the fish is placed for treatment. Some of these drugs will cross the blood–brain barrier and affect the central nervous system of the fish. Bath administration is the most common method for anesthetizing fish as well, for example, by using drugs such as MS-222, which also happens to be the only US FDA-approved anesthetic drug for use in fish. An alternative to a bath is parenteral administration via a hypodermic needle injection, which is also a common method for administrating analgesics in fish. Needle injection can include intramuscular (IM), intravenous (IV), or intracoelomic (ICe) administration, as the subcutaneous (SC) space is less practical for use in fish drug administration due to lack of tissue elasticity. IM administration is typically accomplished by insertion of the needle into the epaxial muscles just ventral to the dorsal fin. Anecdotally, it is best to administer drugs in the front half of the body, much like reptiles, in order to avoid any potential hepatic first pass effect of drug elimination. ICe, commonly referred to as intraperitoneal (IP) in the literature, administration allows for larger volumes, but drug absorption may be diminished compared with IM. In addition, the ICe route makes it difficult to administer drugs in the front half of the body, and the process can be fraught with complications associated with needle insertion and administration into unintended organ systems within the coelom. IV administration of analgesics is less practical and not commonly used. Oral administration (PO) is an alternative to parenteral routes but typically requires oral gavage via feeding tubes, needles, or syringes. The absorption of drugs across the gastrointestinal tract of fish species is largely unknown and may be significantly different between herbivorous, carnivorous, and omnivorous teleosts and elasmobranchs.

CLINICAL ANALGESIA
Local Anesthetics

Local anesthetics are used frequently in veterinary medicine for a variety of diagnostic and therapeutic purposes, primarily as a local block to reduce potential pain from the procedure. However, in fish species local anesthetics are also used for sedation, anesthesia, and analgesia. Tricaine methansulfonate (ethyl-*m*-amino-benzoate methanesulfonate; MS-222) is an ester-type synthetic, benzocaine derivative that induces anesthesia in fish by blocking sodium channels in the neuronal membranes, thus reducing action potentials, and inducing muscle relaxation.[20] In fish species, MS-222 also functions more holistically, such that it crosses the blood-brain barrier blocking the action potential generation in sensory and motor systems as well as in central nervous circuits.[20] MS-222, sold as a powder, is administered to fish as a bath after being dissolved in dechlorinated water and buffered with sodium bicarbonate. Although the efficacy of MS-222 as an analgesic is not well substantiated from an evidence-based perspective, in red pacu anesthetized with MS-222 (200 mg/L), 14/15 pacu showed no behavioral response to a hypodermic needle insertion.[1] Similarly, when adult zebrafish were exposed to MS-222 (100 mg/L), there was no response to a tail pinch.[21] On the contrary, in the red pacu study, MS-222 was compared with bath eugenol as an analgesic, and 14/15 red pacu anesthetized with eugenol (100 or 200 mg/L) reacted dramatically to a hypodermic needle insertion.[1] Eugenol (4-allyl-2-methoxyphenol), a phenolic compound and the active ingredient in clove oil, is derived from the leaves and buds of the plant, *Eugenia caryophyllata*.[1] Because it is an oil, it must be mixed with ethanol to be used in water as a fish anesthetic. Although eugenol has many uses, it is thought to exert anesthetic properties by blocking sodium channels, much like MS-222, and there are many published data supporting its use as an anesthetic in fish. However, it is not known to cross the blood–brain barrier. In all, these data suggest that MS-222 likely has some analgesic efficacy at certain concentrations, whereas eugenol is likely not an analgesic. In support of this hypothesis, low concentrations (1–5 mg/L) of eugenol had no effect on pain-associated behavior in adult zebrafish (*Danio rerio*), which had acetic acid injected into their lips.[22] There are no other evidence-based, published studies supporting the use of eugenol or isoeugenol as an analgesic in fish. This is particularly concerning with the worldwide use of isoeugenol for fish anesthesia, including during invasive surgical procedures.

Other local anesthetics, such as lidocaine and benzocaine, have been used as both bath and parenteral anesthetics but few evidence-based, published data exist. In a study of rainbow trout (*Oncorhynchus mykiss*) subjected to noxious lip injections with acetic acid to induce pain-related behavior, local administration of lidocaine (1–2 mg/fish) was significantly more effective at blunting the nocifensive behavior when compared with carprofen or buprenorphine.[23] Using a caudal fin forceps pinch to induce a painful stimulus in adult zebrafish, a combination of lidocaine (100 μg/mL) and propofol (1.25 μg/mL) administered as a bath solution was as effective as MS-222 in reducing an avoidance response to the fin pinch.[21] Female zebrafish exposed to three different noxious stimuli (fin clip, PIT tag insertion IM, and acetic-acid lip injection) showed changes in behavior, such as decreased swimming, spending more time at the bottom of the tank, and decreased tank exploration; referred to as the Fish Behavioral Index by the authors.; lidocaine (5 mg/L bath) was the most effective drug at eliminating the abnormal behaviors associated with fin clipping.[24] In the same study, bupivacaine (0.25, 0.5, and 1 mg/L) was not effective as an analgesic drug, and the authors speculated that a higher dose may be necessary as lidocaine and bupivacaine have similar properties in other species with a differing duration of effects.[24] In larval zebrafish, lidocaine (5 mg/L) administered as a bath decreased behavioral changes induced by acetic acid added to the water of the fish.[25] Similarly, lidocaine (40 μM bath) dampened nocifensive behavioral changes in larval zebrafish after exposure to formalin in the water.[26] In total, of the local anesthetics available, the most consistently effective drugs for providing analgesia in fish appear to be lidocaine, in bath and parenteral form, and bath MS-222.

Opioids and Opioid-like Drugs

Parenteral morphine, a μ-receptor agonist, has been shown to be effective in ameliorating the adverse physiologic or behavioral reactions to noxious stimuli in goldfish (*Carassius auratus*), winter flounder (*Pseudopleuronectes americanus*) and trout, and to post-gonadectomy pain in koi (*Cyprinus carpio*) (**Table 1**).[10,17,27,28] After rainbow trout were injected with acetic acid in their lips, morphine (30 mg/fish IM) administration attenuated some of the behavioral responses that were observed in fish that did not receive morphine.[10] In a similar study, morphine (5 mg/kg IM) attenuated the avoidance behavior after lip injections of both acetic acid and formalin in silver catfish, and naloxone reversed this behavior.[29] In winter flounder, morphine (40 mg/kg ICe and IM) induced rapid bradycardia and decreased tachycardia associated with acetic-acid administration in the cheek of the fish.[17] Winter flounder also showed a transient bradycardia after morphine administration in the same study supporting the idea that a biological response indicates that μ-opioid receptors are present in fish.[17] In a comprehensive study of the effects of morphine on goldfish, the pharmacokinetics of plasma morphine were determined after bath morphine (0.12–48 mg/L water) and parenteral morphine (40 mg/kg IM and ICe), and the efficacy of morphine as an analgesic was compared as a bath (0.12–48 mg/L water) versus parenteral ICe administration at three doses (2, 20, and 40 mg/kg).[27] Results included the following: (1) there was a slow morphine uptake from water, as

Table 1
Evidence-based analgesics used in fish

Drug	Dosage or Concentration/Route	Comments	Refs
Local Anesthetics			
Bupivacaine	0.25, 0.5, 1.0 mg/L bath	Female zebrafish; blunted nocifensive response to fin clip, acetic acid injected into lips, and pit tag insertion IM	24
Eugenol	100–200 mg/L bath	Pacu; no evidence of analgesia	1
	1, 2, 5 mg/L bath	Zebrafish; no evidence of analgesia	22
Lidocaine	0.5, 1.0, 2.0 mg/fish administered into lips	Rainbow trout (females) administered acid in lips; analgesia at higher doses	23
	5 mg/L bath	Larval zebrafish; attenuated nocifensive response after exposure acetic and citric acid	25
	40 μM bath	Larval zebrafish; attenuated avoidance behavior after exposure to formalin	26
	5 mg/L bath	Larval zebrafish; attenuated nocifensive behavior after acetic and citric acid exposure	25
	5 mg/L bath	Female zebrafish; blunted nocifensive response to fin clip, acetic acid injected into lips, and pit tag insertion IM	24
Tricaine methanesulfonate (MS-222; Tricaine-S, Syndel USA)	100–200 mg/L bath	Pacu; antinociceptive reaction to needle stick	1
	100 mg/L bath	Adult zebrafish; antinociceptive when tail pinch was used to induce pain	21

(continued on next page)

Table 1
(continued)

Drug	Dosage or Concentration/Route	Comments	Refs
Opioids			
Butorphanol	0.4 mg/kg IM once	Koi/postoperative analgesia	33
	10 mg/kg IM once	Koi/postoperative analgesia/respiratory depression at this dose; temporary buoyancy issues in some individuals	28
	0.25–5 mg/kg IM once	Chain Dogfish; no effect on MAC of MS-222	34
	0.1, 0.2, 0.4 mg/kg IM once	Goldfish; reduced MAC of MS-222 at lowest dose, but no effect at 2 higher doses	32
Buprenorphine	0.01, 0.05, 0.1 mg/kg IM once	Rainbow trout (females) administered acid in lips; no analgesic effect at any dose	23
	5μM bath	Larval zebrafish; blocked nocifensive response to acute hot- and cold-water noxious stimuli	36
	0.1 μg/mL bath	Larval zebrafish; blocked nocifensive response to high voltage electrical noxious stimulus	35
	0.05 mg/kg IM	Rainbow trout; post-surgical bradycardia and bradypnea but no analgesia	37
Fentanyl	6μM bath	Larval zebrafish; attenuated avoidance behavior after exposure to formalin	26

Morphine	5 mg/kg IM once	Koi/analgesia	28
	5 mg/kg IM once	Silver catfish; attenuated nocifensive behavior after acetic acid and formalin injections into lips	29
	48 mg/L bath	Larval zebrafish; attenuated nocifensive behavior after acetic and citric acid exposure	25
	6.7 mg/kg ICe once	Rainbow trout/PD; attenuated the avoidance to facial electric shock; naloxone reversed this behavior	31
	40 mg/kg ICe or 17 mg/kg IV once	Winter flounder/analgesia after acetic acid administered in cheek; both doses caused significant bradycardia and prolonged (>48 h) increase in cardiac output; not recommended	17
	0.12–48 mg/L bath	Goldfish; PK and analgesic efficacy; detectable in plasma at highest concentrations; antinociceptive at highest concentrations	27
	40 mg/kg IM and ICe once	Goldfish; PK and analgesic efficacy; detectable in plasma with 37h half-life IM; not clearly antinociceptive	27
	2, 20, and 40 mg/kg ICe once	Goldfish; detectable in plasma, but not as significant as IM; not clearly antinociceptive	27
	10, 20, and 40 mg/kg IM once	Goldfish; reduced MAC of MS-222	32
	3 and 6 mg/kg IM	Zebrafish; attenuated avoidance behavior to acetic acid lip injections; behavior reversed with naloxone (6 mg/kg IM)	12
	48 mg/L bath	Larval zebrafish; attenuated nocifensive behavior to hot water and acetic acid injections, but not cold water	25
	3 and 48 mg/L bath	Female zebrafish; blunted nocifensive response to fin clip and acid injected into lips	24

(continued on next page)

Table 1
(continued)

Drug	Dosage or Concentration/Route	Comments	Refs
NSAIDS			
Aspirin (acetyl salicylic acid)	2.5 mg/L bath	Larval zebrafish; attenuated nocifensive behavior after acetic and citric acid exposure	25
Carprofen	1.0, 2.5, 5.0 mg/kg IM once	Rainbow trout (females) administered acid in lips; analgesia at higher doses	23
	2.5 mg/kg IM, PO, IV once	Rainbow trout/PK	41
Flunixin meglumine	2.2 mg/kg IM once	Nile tilapia/PK; plasma concentrations consistent with analgesia in mammals	43
	10 µg/fish bath	Larval zebrafish; no effect	25
	2, 4, 8 mg/L bath	Female zebrafish; blunted nocifensive response to fin clip, acetic acid injected into lips, and pit tag insertion IM	24
Ketoprofen	2 mg/kg IM once	Koi/postoperative analgesia	33
	3 mg/kg IM, IV once	Rainbow trout/PK; equivalent plasma concentrations for analgesia in mammals for at least 24h	40
	8 mg/kg IM once	Nile tilapia/PK; equivalent plasma concentrations for analgesia in mammals for at least 24h	40
	0.5, 1.0, and 2.0 mg/kg IM once	Goldfish; no effect on MAC of MS-222	32
	1.0, 2.0, and 4.0 mg/kg IM once	Chain dogfish; no effect on MAC of MS-222	34
Meloxicam	1 mg/kg IM, IV once	Nile tilapia/PK; rapid elimination; multiple daily treatments would be necessary	42
	1 mg/kg IM once	Nile tilapia/PK; rapid elimination from plasma, but metabolite detectable for up to 6 d	43

Robenacoxib (Onsior, Elanco)	2 mg/kg IM once	Rainbow trout/PK, PD; presumptive antinociceptive plasma concentration duration 3 d; analgesia after acetic acid administration to lips	44
Other Drugs			
Amitriptyline hydrochloride (tricyclic antidepressant)	0.5 μM bath	Larval zebrafish; no effects on acute hot and cold aversion	36
Clonidine hydrochloride (alpha-2-agonist)	5 μM bath	Larval zebrafish; blocked acute hot and cold aversion	36
Gabapentin	100 μM bath	Larval zebrafish; no effects on acute hot and cold aversion	36
Medetomidine	0.025 mg/kg IM once	Goldfish; decreased MAC of MS-222	32
Tramadol	50–100 nmol/g (approx. 13–25 mg/kg)	Common carp; analgesia after electrical noxious stimulus	38
	25–50 μg/fish	Larval zebrafish; no analgesia but hyperactivity and tachypnea at lower dose and 100% mortality at higher dose	39

Abbreviations: μM, micro-Molar; h, hours; IM, intramuscular; IV, intravenous; PO, oral; SC, subcutaneous.

measured in goldfish plasma, which increased with external concentration and with time available for uptake; (2) morphine was detectable in goldfish plasma after both ICe and IM administration and the half-life was 37 h; (3) bath morphine was analgesic at the highest concentration when acetic acid was injected into the cheek of fish, but the results were not as clear for the ICe and IM administered morphine making interpretation of morphine efficacy as an analgesic in this species more difficult.

Morphine efficacy may differ with experimental design, and plasma elimination appears to be temperature and species-dependent, with slower elimination in cold-water species[30] and more rapid elimination in rainbow trout compared with winter flounder.[17] Morphine (48 mg/L) administered as a bath, decreased behavioral changes after exposure to acetic-acid and hot-water baths in larval zebrafish, but had no effect on the fish when exposed to a cold-water bath.[25] This suggests that type of experimental model plays a role in how and when fish species will respond to specific noxious stimuli. In a study evaluating multiple analgesics as bath applications, nocifensive behaviors of female zebrafish subjected to a fin clip were attenuated after exposure to bath morphine (48 mg/L).[24] In adult zebrafish, morphine (3 and 6 mg/kg IM) administered 30 min before acetic-acid injections into the lips, attenuated the decreased activity observed in control fish receiving saline; naloxone (6 mg/kg IM) eliminated this response.[12] Similarly, zebrafish subjected to electrical shock to the face showed less avoidance behavior after morphine administration (6.7 mg/kg IM), and this lessened avoidance response was reversed after naloxone (30 mg/kg IM) administration.[31] Conversely, morphine was found to be ineffective at studied doses (40 and 50 mg/kg IM) in goldfish exposed to a thermal noxious stimulus, again, supporting the idea that the type of noxious stimulus may be important in determining the efficacy of an analgesic in fish.[30] Using the minimum inhibitory concentration (MAC) model for assessing analgesic efficacy, morphine (10, 20, and 40 mg/kg IM) reduced MAC of MS-222 in goldfish which was deemed necessary to attenuate response to an IM needle insertion in goldfish, therefore suggesting morphine may have analgesic properties.[32]

Fewer published data are available for butorphanol, a κ-opioid receptor agonist, and μ-antagonist, as an analgesic in fish. In koi, butorphanol (0.4 mg/kg IM), was effective at reducing postsurgical pain-related behavioral changes.[33] At higher doses butorphanol (10 mg/kg) provided more rapid return to normal behavior in koi undergoing gonadectomy but was associated with respiratory depression and abnormal buoyancy.[28] In this same study, morphine appeared to be a better choice as an analgesic with a more rapid return to activity and feeding, along with fewer untoward side effects.[28] In chain dogfish (Scyliorhinus retifer), an elasmobranch species, butorphanol (0.25–5 mg/kg IM) was not effective in reducing the MAC of MS-222.[34] Similarly, in a study using goldfish as subjects, a low dose of butorphanol (0.1 mg/kg IM) decreased the MAC of MS-222, but at slightly higher doses (0.2 and 0.4 mg/kg IM) increased the MAC of MS-222, making interpretation of analgesic properties ambiguous.[32] To date, the published data on morphine efficacy as an analgesic across several species of fish are compelling and provide the strongest evidence in support of its clinical application.

Other opioid or opioid-like drugs, buprenorphine (partial μ-opioid agonist) and tramadol (μ-opioid agonist with serotonin/norepinephrine reuptake-inhibition properties), have been studied in fish. Thus far, buprenorphine has shown equivocal results depending on laboratory model and route of administration used. IM buprenorphine (0.01, 0.05, and 0.1 mg/kg) did not provide evidence of analgesia in rainbow trout subjected to SC acetic-acid injections.[23] However, in zebrafish larvae, bath administered buprenorphine prevented stimulus-induced responses to noxious stimuli (eg, electrical, thermal, and SC acetic-acid administration), and these responses were eliminated when bath naloxone was administered before the buprenorphine.[35,36] In a study of larval zebrafish exposed to a hot- and cold-water noxious stimuli, buprenorphine (5 μM) as a bath diminished the behavioral response to the noxious thermal stimuli.[36] Similarly, larval zebrafish exposed to bath buprenorphine (0.1 μg/mL) showed diminished behavioral avoidance behaviors when an electrical noxious stimulus was applied to the fish.[35] However, at lower electrical voltages, this diminished avoidance was not observed. In a physiologic study, buprenorphine (0.05 mg/kg) administered IM to rainbow trout caused significant and prolonged bradycardia and bradypnea that lasted 4 to 5 days post-administration, suggesting that buprenorphine receptors are present and induce a biological response, but there was no evidence of analgesia.[37]

Results of tramadol as an analgesic in fish are also equivocal. Tramadol (50 μM/kg; or approximately 13 mg/kg) administered IM in common carp (*C carpio*) induced a prolonged (greater than 2 h), dose-dependent analgesic response to a noxious electrical stimulus, whereas still maintaining normal swimming and other behaviors.[38] However, in a study using zebrafish, tramadol (25 μg/fish, IM) caused hyperactivity and tachypnea, and at 50 μg/fish IM caused 100% mortality.[39] These conflicting data may be due to species or dose–response differences, but also highlight that caution must be exercised when making analgesic decisions in some species.

Fentanyl, a synthetic μ-opioid agonist that is considered to be 80 to 100 times the potency of morphine, has been used experimentally in one fish model. Fentanyl (6 μM bath) attenuated nocifensive behavioral reactions to formalin added to water in larval zebrafish.[26] Fentanyl also caused respiratory depression in the same zebrafish subjects, and naloxone reversed this effect, again supporting the presence of μ-opioid receptors in zebrafish through the establishment of biological activity. These data corroborate with the morphine data that μ-opioid receptor agonists are a logical choice when considering opioid analgesic drugs in fish.

Non-steroidal Anti-inflammatory Drugs

There are very few data in the literature with respect to nonsteroidal analgesic efficacy or anti-inflammatory activity in fish species, primarily because efficacy is difficult to measure (**Table 1**). However, in those studies in which untoward consequences associated with nonsteroidal anti-inflammatory drug (NSAID) administration were documented, there are no evidence-based data to suggest that individual drugs or doses are unsafe. Acetylsalicylic acid (aspirin) administered as a bath (2.5 mg/L) prevented the predrug administration hypoactivity associated with water exposure to 0.1% or higher acetic acid in zebrafish.[25] In koi, ketoprofen (2 mg/kg IM) was not effective at reducing postsurgical pain-related behavioral changes but did reduce postsurgical muscle damage.[33] Similarly, in chain dogfish, ketoprofen (1–4 mg/kg IM) was not effective in reducing the MAC of MS-222, suggesting a possible lack of analgesic properties using this methology.[34] However, in a pharmacokinetic study of ketoprofen in Nile tilapia (*Oreochromis niloticus*) (8 mg/kg IM) and rainbow trout (3 mg/kg IM and IV), plasma concentrations were above those considered analgesic in mammals for at least 24 h.[40] Carprofen (2.5 and 5 mg/kg) administered IM to rainbow trout appeared to normalize behavior (increase activity and decrease respiratory rate) after acetic acid was administered SC in lips, but decreased activity was observed at the higher dose, making any conclusions equivocal.[23] In goldfish, ketoprofen (0.5, 1, and 2 mg/kg IM) significantly reduced the MAC of MS-222, suggesting a possible analgesic response.[32]

With NSAIDs, pharmacokinetics and pharmacodynamics are easier to measure in fish than efficacy but interpretation of plasma concentrations as efficacious is more complex when compared to mammalian plasma concentrations. The pharmacokinetics of carprofen (2.5 mg/kg) administered IV, IM, and PO were evaluated in rainbow trout broodstock.[41] The half-life of the IV, IM, and PO routes was 30.66 h, 46.11 h, and 41.08 h, respectively, which was similar to those mammalian species studied. A newer NSAID, meloxicam, used extensively in mammals and birds, has not been systematically studied for efficacy as an analgesic in fish species. However, in a pharmacokinetic study, the data showed that plasma meloxicam was eliminated more rapidly in Nile tilapia compared with mammals when administered both IM and IV at 1 mg/kg.[42] In that study, meloxicam (1 mg/kg) administered IM achieved plasma concentrations equivalent to analgesic concentrations in mammals for approximately 5 h, which would imply requiring multiple doses within every 24-h period.[42] These data were replicated in a separate study using Nile tilapia administered meloxicam (1 mg/kg, IM and PO); meloxicam and its primary metabolite never reached clinically relevant plasma or tissue concentrations and were eliminated rapidly from plasma.[43] Of interest was that the primary metabolite of meloxicam, 5'Hydroxy-desmethyl-meloxicam, was detectable in plasma up to 6 days postdrug administration for both IM and oral routes, which may indicate a possible longer-acting drug depot effect.[43] Similar to the Nile tilapia studies, after rainbow trout broodstock were administered meloxicam (1 mg/kg IV, IM, and PO), the IM route provided good bioavailability, but a relatively short mean half-life of 4.55 h.[44] Those same trout receiving IV and PO meloxicam had low plasma concentration bioavailability and a shorter half-life than the IM route. However, unlike the teleost studies, three recent studies of meloxicam pharmacokinetics in elasmobranch species show longer half-lives and greater bioavailability. In yellow stingrays (*Urobatis jamaicensis*), meloxicam pharmacokinetics were compared between IM (1 mg/kg) and PO (2 mg/kg) routes.[45] The half-life of the IM route was slightly longer (5.75 h) compared with the aforementioned teleost studies, but the PO route half-life was 15.46 h and reached clinically relevant plasma concentrations (compared with mammalian effective concentrations) suggesting that oral meloxicam (2 mg/kg q 24 h) may be beneficial in this species. Similarly, undulate skates (*Raja undulata*) administered meloxicam (1.5 mg/kg IM) had clinically relevant plasma concentrations for approximately 8 to 12 h.[46] Comparable results were achieved in nursehound sharks (*S stellaris*) administered meloxicam (1.5 mg/kg IM), in which plasma concentrations reached clinically relevant levels for approximately 8 to 12 h.[47] In all of the meloxicam studies, there were no observed adverse effects directly associated with meloxicam administration. With the availability of meloxicam in most veterinary hospitals it seems prudent to continue evaluating its efficacy in multiple fish species at different water temperatures.

Flunixin meglumine, another NSAID commonly used in mammals, has also been evaluated pharmacokinetically in two teleost species. The pharmacokinetics of flunixin meglumine (2.2 mg/kg IM) were evaluated in Nile tilapia and plasma concentrations were relatively high by 12 h postdrug administration and remained detectable for 96 h, although concentrations were below clinically relevant plasma concentrations (compared with mammals) by 24 h post-administration.[43] In an efficacy study evaluating multiple analgesics as bath applications, the nocifensive behavior of female zebrafish subjected to a fin clip were unchanged after exposure to bath flunixin meglumine (2, 4, and 8 mg/L).[24] More recently, robenacoxib (2 mg/kg IM) has been shown to be antinociceptive in rainbow trout after acetic-acid lip injections, and the clinically relevant plasma concentrations (compared with mammals) lasted up to 3 days after a single IM dose.[48] More NSAID efficacy and pharmacokinetic studies are needed across a variety of fish species, as NSAID use is a staple of clinical veterinary medicine.

Other Drugs

A few other classes of drugs have been evaluated as analgesics in fish. Alpha-2 agonists, such as medetomidine, generally induce sedation in those fish species studied but analgesic activity has not been clearly shown **(Table 1)**.[11] In goldfish, medetomidine (0.025 mg/kg IM), had a minimal effect on decreasing MAC of MS-222, suggesting a possible, yet negligible, analgesic effect.[32] Using a thermal nociceptive model in zebrafish and measuring behavior after the fish were exposed to either cold or hot water as noxious stimuli, with and without the immersion-based drugs, both clonidine (0.5 μM bath; an alpha-2 adrenergic agonist) and amitriptyline (5 μM bath; a tricyclic antidepressant and used for neuropathic pain) diminished the behavioral response to thermal noxious stimuli, but gabapentin (100 μM bath) did not.[36] No significant differences were observed when the zebrafish were exposed to cold water. These results suggest that more experimentation is necessary to determine whether other anesthetic and anti-inflammatory drugs may be analgesic candidates for use in fish.

Summary

The field of clinical fish analgesia has progressed in the past 20 years and many clinicians have developed an acute awareness of the necessity for providing analgesics to fish under conditions deemed painful in other species. Based on current data, typical bath anesthetics used in fish may provide some level of analgesia (eg, MS-222 and lidocaine), but might best be supplemented with additional analgesics before invasive procedures. For acutely painful conditions, choosing a μ-opioid agonist, such as morphine, in addition to an NSAID, such as carprofen, ketoprofen or meloxicam (even though we have little evidence of efficacy) may benefit the welfare of the fish patient by having it return to normal behavior more rapidly, thereby reducing morbidity and mortality. For more chronic and debilitating disease conditions in fish, data are essentially absent, and our understanding of the efficacy and safety of long-term use of NSAIDs and other analgesic drugs is completely inadequate. Although the field of fish analgesia has progressed, we still have much to learn, and anecdotal evidence and extrapolation of drugs and dosages remain salient for the near future.

DISCLOSURE

Nothing to disclose.

REFERENCES

1. Sladky KK, Swanson CR, Stoskopf MK, et al. Comparative efficacy of tricaine methanesulfonate and clove oil for use as anesthetics in red pacu (*Piaractus brachypomus*). Am J Vet Res 2001;62:337–42.

2. LU Sneddon. Pain perception in fish: indicators and endpoints. ILAR J 2009;50: 338–42.

3. Braithwaite VA, Boulcott P. Pain perception, aversion and fear in fish. Dis Aquat Organ 2007;75:131–8.

4. Rose JD. The neurobehavioral nature of fishes and the question of awareness and pain. Rev Fish Sci 2002;10:1–38.

5. Weber ES. Fish analgesia: pain, stress, fear aversion, or nociception? Vet Clin North Am Exot Anim Pract 2011;14:21–32.

6. Chandroo KP, Duncan IJH, Moccia RD. Can fish suffer?: perspectives on sentience, pain, fear and stress. Appl Anim Behav Sci 2004;86:225–50.

7. Volpato GL, Goncalves-de-Freitas E, Fernandes-de-Castilho M. Insights into the concept of fish welfare. Dis Aquat Organ 2007;75:165–71.
8. Chandroo KP, Yue S, Moccia RD. An evaluation of current perspectives on consciousness and pain in fishes. Fish Fish 2004;5:281–95.
9. Dunlop R, Millsopp S, Laming P. Avoidance learning in goldfish (*Carassius auratus*) and trout (*Oncorhynchus mykiss*) and implications for pain perception. Appl Anim Behav Sci 2006;97:255–71.
10. LU Sneddon, Braithwaite VA, Gentle MJ. Novel object test: Examining nociception and fear in the rainbow trout. J Pain 2003;4:431–40.
11. Neiffer DL, Stamper MA. Fish sedation, analgesia, anesthesia, and euthanasia: considerations, methods, and types of drugs. ILAR J 2009;50:343–60.
12. Correia AD, Cunha SR, Scholze M, et al. A novel behavioural fish model of nociception for testing analgesics. Pharmaceuticals 2011;4:665–80.
13. LU Sneddon. The evidence for pain in fish: The use of morphine as an analgesic. Appl Anim Behav Sci 2003;8:153–62.
14. Laitinen M, Valtonen T. Cardiovascular, ventilatory and total activity responses of brown trout to handling stress. J Fish Biol 1994;45:933–42.
15. Suski CD, Killen SS, Morrissey MB, et al. Physiological changes in largemouth bass caused by live-release angling tournaments in southeastern Ontario. N Amer J Fish. Mngt 2003;23:760–9.
16. Harms CA, Lewbart GA. Surgery in fish. Vet Clin North Am Exot Anim Pract 2000; 3:759–74.
17. Newby NC, Gamperl AK, Steven D. Cardiorespiratory effects and efficacy of morphine sulfate in winter flounder (*Pseudopleuronectes americanus*). Am J Vet Res 2007;68:592–7.
18. Fricke R, Eschmeyer WN, van der Laan R, editors. Eschmeyer's catalog of fishes: genera, species, references. 2022. Available at: http://researcharchive. calacademy.org/research/ichthyology/catalog/fishcatmain.asp.   Accessed February 28, 2022.
19. Harms CA. Anesthesia in fish. In: Fowler ME, Miller RE, editors. Zoo and Wild Animal medicine: current Therapy 4. Philadelphia: Saunders; 1999. p. 158–63.
20. Fontana BD, Alnassar N, Parker MO. Tricaine methanesulfonate (MS222) has short-term effects on young adult zebrafish (*Danio rerio*) working memory and cognitive flexibility, but not on aging fish. Front Behav Neurosci 2021;15:686102.
21. Martins T, Diniz E, Felix LM, et al. Evaluation of anaesthetic protocols for laboratory adult zebrafish (Danio rerio). PLOS One 2018;13:e0197846.
22. Baldisserotto B, Parodi TV, Stevens ED. Lack of postexposure analgesic efficacy of low concentrations of eugenol in zebrafish. Vet Anaeth Analg 2018;45:48–56.
23. Mettam JJ, Oulton LJ, McCrohan C, et al. The efficacy of three types of analgesic drugs in reducing pain in the rainbow trout, *Oncorhynchus myskiss*. Appl Anim Behav Sci 2011;133(3–4):265–74.
24. Deakin AG, Buckley J, AlZu'bi HS, et al. Automated monitoring of behaviour in zebrafish after invasive procedures. Sci Rep 2019;9–9042.
25. Lopez-Luna J, Al-Jubouri Q, Al-Nuaimy W, et al. Reduction in activity by noxious chemical stimulation is ameliorated by immersion in analgesic drugs in zebrafish. J Exp Biol 2017;220:1451–8.
26. Zaig S, Scarpellini CdS, Montandon G. Respiratory depression and analgesia by opioid drugs in freely behaving larval zebrafish. Elife 2021;10:e63407.
27. Newby NC, Wilkie MP, Stevens ED. Morphine uptake, disposition, and analgesic efficacy in the common goldfish (*Carassius auratus*). Can J Zool 2009;87:388–99.

28. Baker TR, Baker BB, Johnson SM, et al. Comparative analgesic efficacy of morphine sulfate and butorphanol tartrate in koi (*Cyprinus carpio*) undergoing unilateral gonadectomy. J Am Vet Med Assoc 2013;243:882–90.

29. Rodrigues P, Barbosa LB, Bianchinia AE, et al. Nociceptive-like behavior and analgesia in silver catfish (*Rhamdia quelen*). Physiol Behav 2019;210:112648.

30. Nordgreen J, Garner JP, Janczak AM, et al. Thermonociception in fish: Effects of two different doses of morphine on thermal threshold and post-test behaviour in goldfish (*Carassius auratus*). Appl Anim Behav Sci 2009;119(1–2):101–7.

31. Jones SG, Kamunde C, Lemke K, et al. The dose–response relation for the anti-nociceptive effect of morphine in a fish, rainbow trout. J Vet Pharmacol Ther 2012; 35:563–70.

32. Ward JL, McCartney SP, Chinnadurai SK, et al. Development of a minimum-anesthetic-concentration depression model to study the effects of various analgesics in goldfish (*Carassius auratus*). J Zoo Wildl Med 2012;43:214–22.

33. Harms CA, Lewbart GA, Swanson CR, et al. Behavioral and clinical pathology changes in koi carp (*Cyprinus carpio*) subjected to anesthesia and surgery with and without intra-operative analgesics. Comp Med 2005;55:221–6.

34. Davis MR, Mylniczenko N, Storms T, et al. Evaluation of intramuscular ketoprofen and butorphanol as analgesics in chain dogfish (*Scyliorhinus retifer*). Zoo Biol 2006;25:491–500.

35. Steenbergen PJ. Response of zebrafish larvae to mild electrical stimuli: A 96-well setup for behavioural screening. J Neurosci Methods 2018;301:52–61.

36. Curtright A, Rosser M, Goh S, et al. Modeling nociception in zebrafish: a way forward for unbiased analgesic discovery. PLoS One 2015;10:1–18.

37. Grans A, Sandblom E, Kiessling A, et al. Postsurgical analgesia in rainbow trout: is reduced cardioventilatory activity a sign of improved welfare or the adverse effects of an opioid drug? PLoS One 2014;9:1–8.

38. Chervova LS, Lapshin DN. Opioid modulation of pain threshold in fish. Dokl Biol Sci 2000;375:590–1.

39. Zhao H, Jin H, Peng H, et al. Distribution, pharmacokinetics and primary metabolism model of tramadol in zebrafish. Mol Med Rep 2016;14:5644–52.

40. Greene W, Mylniczenko ND, Storms T, et al. Pharmacokinetics of ketoprofen in Nile tilapia (*Oreochromis niloticus*) and rainbow trout (*Oncorhynchus mykiss*). Front Vet Sci 2020;7:585324.

41. Uney K, Corum DD, Terzi E, et al. Pharmacokinetics and bioavailability of carprofen in rainbow trout (*Oncorhynchus mykiss*) broodstock. Pharmaceutics 2021; 13:990.

42. Fredholm DV, Mylniczenko ND, KuKanich B. Pharmacokinetic evaluation of meloxicam after intravenous and intramuscular administration in Nile tilapia (*Oreochromis niloticus*). J Zoo Wildl Med 2016;47:736–42.

43. Martin MS. Investigation of pain and analgesic strategies in food animals. Doctoral Diss. Kansas State Univ; 2021.

44. Corum O, Terzi E, Durna Corum D, et al. Pharmacokinetics and bioavailability of meloxicam in rainbow trout (*Oncorhynchus mykiss*) broodstock following intravascular, intramuscular, and oral administrations. J Vet Pharmacol Ther 2022; 45:213–9.

45. Kane LP, O'Connor MR, Papich MG. Pharmacokinetics of a single dose of intramuscular and oral meloxicam in yellow stingrays (*Urobatis jamaicensis*). J Zoo Wildl Med 2022;53:153–8.

46. Morón-Elorza P, Cañizares-Cooz D, Rojo-Solis C, et al. Pharmacokinetics of the anti-inflammatory drug meloxicam after single 1.5 mg/kg intramuscular administration to undulate skates (*Raja undulata*). Vet Sci 2022;9:216.

47. Morón-Elorza P, Rojo-Solís C, Álvaro-Álvarez T, et al. Pharmacokinetics of meloxicam after a single 1.5 mg/kg intramuscular administration to nursehound sharks (*Scyliorhinus stellaris*) and its effects on hematology and plasma biochemistry. J Zoo Wildl Med 2022;53:393–401.

48. Raulic J, Beaudry F, Beauchamp G, et al. Pharmacokinetic, pharmacodynamic and toxicology study of robenacoxib in rainbow trout (*Oncorhynchus mykiss*). J Zoo Wildl Med 2021;52:529–37.

Pain Recognition in Reptiles

V. Latney La'Toya, DVM, CertAqV, DECZM, Dip ABVP (Reptile/Amphibian)

KEYWORDS

- Reptile • Nociception • Pain • Analgesia • Physiology • Pain assessment

KEY POINTS

- Species-specific ethograms are needed to note behavioral changes that have resulted from noxious experiences caused by potential or actual tissue damage.
- Long-term changes in behavior patterns that result in decreased interactions with the environment, decreased appetite, decreased movement, abnormal basking behaviors, and abnormal social behaviors may represent pain in reptiles.
- Future clinical pain assessment tools that are designed to evaluate changes in species-specific behaviors and individual behavioral repertoires may provide a more reliable means to guide response to analgesic interventions.

INTRODUCTION

In the last 30 years, long-awaited pharmacokinetic and pharmacodynamic analgesia studies have helped inform clinicians on how to treat pain in captive and wild reptile species, yet assessment of pain has always remained daunting. The clinical assessment of pain behavior has seen great improvements in other species, a notable example being the development of facial grimace scoring techniques currently used for rodents, rabbits, ferrets, horses, pigs, and even harbor seals.[1,2] If we aim to make similar breakthroughs for herptile species in clinical practice, critical evaluation of (1) species-specific behaviors and (2) changes in behavior, are required to recognize, quantify and treat pain. This would require a clinical appreciation of individual behavioral repertoires, and a less commonly accessible catalog of their species-specific behaviors, with insight into their adaptive cognitive capabilities. This review attempts to outline objective and subjective parameters of pain assessment in reptiles based on observational information provided by several sources. A brief review of pain physiology and a larger review of cognition are examined in the context of how it informs behavior and how tools can be developed to assess reptile pain.

The author has nothing to disclose.
Avian and Exotic Medicine & Surgery, The Animal Medical Center, 510 East 62nd Street, New York, NY 10065, USA
E-mail address: latoya.latney@amcny.org

REPTILE PAIN PHYSIOLOGY

In qualifying the basis for pain perception in reptiles, there are two main justifications that include anatomic evidence (cortex) and functional evidence of perception that is justified via cognitive parity. The *Biology of Reptilia*, a 22-volume extensive collection of sound physiology research, has three volumes specifically dedicated to reptile neurology.[3–5] Taken in conjunction with current evolutionary neurobiology studies that have generated genomic and neuroimaging data, there is still much to explore as one elucidates the neuroanatomy and its variations in a taxa that boasts more than 11,000 extant species. To date, most nociceptors studied in mammals have been demonstrated in reptiles, with the most notable difference being threshold variations to noxious stimuli. This is thought to occur due to the variation in life history and thermal ecology.[6] Comparative spinal anatomy,[4–7] brain neuroanatomy,[8–12] and physiology[13–16] have been described in chelonians,[17,18] squamates,[18–31] crocodilians,[32–34] and sphentodontids.[35] A detailed review of neurophysiology and neuroanatomy of reptile pain transmission, integration, and modulation has been previously described[36,37] and revisited in this issue for Reptile Pain Management; however, a simplified anatomic comparison of the components of comparative pain physiology is given in **Table 1** for a brief review.

BIASES AND LIMITATIONS IN REPTILE COGNITION RESEARCH

Although the discussion of the presence of reptile-based neocortical homologs has remained a pivotal area of interest in the last 30 years in comparative physiology, behavior, and anatomy journals, it has largely been accepted that the evidence of behavioral modulation in response to noxious stimuli (nocifensive behaviors, avoidance, and suspension of normal behaviors, learned avoidance) demonstrates an affective component of pain, especially when demonstrated as long-term behavioral patterns. Central processing and central nervous system modulation of an whole organism's behavior is not only attributed to survival circuits of several species.[47] The sensation of pain is perceived to possess evolutionary advantages that outweigh its immediate negative effect on welfare, it also results in behavioral changes geared to prevent future harms.[47] If this is taken in congruency with the multidimensional aspects of pain, it would suggest that our additional focus should be on identifying and validating the species-specific ethograms that monitor long-term changes in behavior patterns that have resulted from noxious experiences that caused potential or actual tissue damage.

The psychological impacts of learned experiences from noxious stimuli evade many clinical practitioners, as we are poorly equipped to medically evaluate these consequences for several reasons. First, there is a lack of ecologically relevant, species-specific behavioral ethogram tools available for use in captive herptiles. Reptile behavior research is often limited by the assumption that ectotherms only engage with their environments in the most rudimentary of ways to the near exclusion of more complex and sophisticated cognitive processes, which biases the small body of research in reptile cognition to date.[48] As reptiles inhabit extreme, rapidly changing environments, such conditions would serve to drive evolutionary processes that select for complex cognitive development and Roth provides a compelling justification to expand research in this area of focus.[48] Second, the significant negative reporting bias that exists in the field of comparative psychology prevents the development of viable ethograms. In the *Journal of Comparative Psychology* between 2000 to 2004, mammal-based research articles accounted for 74% of the studies reviewed, whereas birds accounted for 18% and reptiles 3%.[49] In a recent 100-year review of the journal's

Table 1
Comparative anatomic components of the pain pathway in mammals and reptiles[7-46]

Neural Machinery	Function	Mammals	Reptiles	References for Anatomic Evidence in Reptiles
Peripheral pain transmission				
Nociceptors[38-44]	A sensory nerve that peripheral receptors that transmit painful sensory information via afferent fibers to its cell body, which resides in the dorsal horn of the spinal cord	Aβ fibers (large, unmyelinated) Aδ fibers (small, myelinated fibers), C fibers (small, unmyelinated fibers, TRVP receptors (transient receptor potential cation channels)	Trigeminal nerve studies, crotaline studies dominate, evidence in turtles, TRVP receptors suggested in snakes	Liang 1993, Liang 1995, Terashima 1994, 1997, Williams 2019, Fowler 1999, James 2017 References[38-44]
Central pain transmission				
Spinal anatomy[7-9,19,26-28,30,32]	Transmit sensory information from cell body to brain (afferent-white matter) and back down to the spinal cord (efferent) to produce a movement-based (motor) response to a perceived noxious injury, including reflexes (involuntary motor circuits)	Ascending pathway: spinothalamic primarily, spinoreticular, spinomesenthalic, Descending motor pathway: Cortico-spinal tract (voluntary movement) Extra-pyramidal tracts, including vestibulospinal, reticulospinal, tectospinal, rubrospinal (reflexes, involuntary motor)	Ascending Pathway: Spinothalamic, Paleospinothalamic Descending pathway: interstitiospinal, vestibulospinal, reticulospinal, and reduced rubrospinal in limbless reptiles	Bagma 1982, Ebbesson 1981, Donkelaar 1982, 1983, 2000, Golby 1962, Hoogland 1981, Donkelaar 1983, Wolters 1982 References[7-9,19,26-28,30,32]
Brain anatomy	Central pain integration and modulation			

(continued on next page)

Table 1
(continued)

Neural Machinery	Function	Mammals	Reptiles	References for Anatomic Evidence in Reptiles
Thalamus[7,15,17,18]	Sensory information received by the afferents converge in the thalamus and thalamic neurons relay sensory information to the cortex (sensory-discriminative aspect of the pain experience).	Principal somatosensory nuclei are in the dorsal thalamus, thalamocortical connections are direct to the insular cortex and anterior cingulate cortex	Medialis complex in crocodiles, *N. caudalis* in turtles project to the central part of the anterior dorsal ventricular ridge (ADVR)	Donkelaar 1982, Balaban 1981, Gunturkun, 2020 References[7,15,17,18]
Midbrain[16,28,29,45]	Descending pain inhibition	Periaqueductal gray, Nucleus raphe magnus are components of serotoninergic, noradrenergic, and dopaminergic systems that centrally facilitate pain inhibition	Laminar nucleus of the torus semicircularis, nucleus raphes inferior	Wolters 1985, Donkelaar 1987, Challet 1991, Nauman 2020 Rreferences[16,28,29,45]
Limbic system[11,12,21–23,34]	Emotive-affective aspect of pain experience, memory	Amygdala	Posterior aspect of dorsal ventricular ridge (PDVR)	Lanuza 1998, Guirado 2000, Novejarque 2004, Lohman 1991, Martinez-Garcia 2009 Clark 1984 References[11,12,21–23,34]
Neocortex[13,14,16,23]	Pain processing and perception	Expansion of dorsal pallium forms the pre-frontal cortex. Controls the biopsychosocial aspects of pain and connects to the hippocampus, periaqueductal gray (PAG), thalamus, amygdala, and basal nuclei.	Nonexistent, current genetic and developmental models are conflicting for DVR homology. Calls for functional studies to demonstrate convergent DVR equivalence are prominent	Shimizu 1991, Alboitiz 1999, Novejarque 2004, Nauman 2020 References[13,14,16,23]

Anti-nociceptive targets of pain modulation

| Receptors, channels, and isoenzymes[16,38,46] | Modulation of peripheral and central nociceptive signaling | Opioid receptors (mu, delta, kappa) NMDA and AMPA-type glutamate receptor subunits, Cyclooxygenase isoenzymes, voltage-gated sodium, and potassium channels, GABA receptors | All present in studied reptiles, spinal and cortical opioid receptor distribution varies by suborder and species, NMDA in chelonians, GABA receptors present but significance in pain modulation is unknown, endogenous endorphins | Makau 2017, 2021, Fowler 1999, Naumann 2020 References[16,38,46] |

history, Burghardt notes that since 1982 only 99 articles of 8635 contained reptile-focused research, which reflects 0.01%.[50] In examining other journals, he purports that it appears that the low representation of reptile behavioral research is not peculiar to the *Journal of Comparative Psychology*, but animal behavior journals more generally. This large imbalance in the scientific understanding of reptile behavior and cognitive complexity, by implication, results in a poor understanding of their welfare as compared with other taxonomic groups. Lastly, studies that do exist that attempt to measure cognition and behavior in reptiles are inherently bias or are designed in a way that constrains the results, including limiting studies to the use of unidimensional cognitive measurements and by developing studies under the sole premise that neuroanatomy implies cognitive parity. Future studies that explore behavior and cognitive complexity should be designed with ecological relevance and this would better inform the development of valid ethograms.[48]

The development of clinical pain assessment tools for use in reptiles thus becomes inherently challenging for many reasons. Species-specific ethograms and patient-specific behaviors would need to be explored for a group of vertebrates that are arguably the most adept at thriving in complex, harsh, and dynamic environments.[48] In addition, clinicians and caretakers may only be witnessing constrained behavior, defined by living in environments that restrict the demonstration of natural behaviors. As a result, it is likely that we are missing a window of opportunity to catalog behaviors that may give us more insight on how to identify pain. All highlight challenges in deriving generalizable assessment tools, therefore an exploration into patient-based assessment may provide more of a practical measure to use in pain assessment.

PAIN RECOGNITION IN THE FIELD

There is a paucity of studies that evaluate how caretakers recognize pain in reptiles. As a result, a clinical practitioner faces the added challenges of having to make estimations about what must be painful and how to provide appropriate analgesics in several species. Most general veterinary texts and review articles consistently provide widely accepted pain behaviors that have culminated largely from clinical experience.[51–55] However, due to the lack of clinical studies in reptile behavior, each review often leads to the author's defense of the physiologic and psychological existence of nociception and pain in the taxa and a call to provide analgesia to improve welfare. All sources agree on 5 overall concepts in reptile pain behavior: changes in physiologic parameters, demonstration of nocifensive behaviors, decreased interaction within their environments, a change in mentation and/or feeding behavior, and a return to normal behaviors once the pain is alleviated.

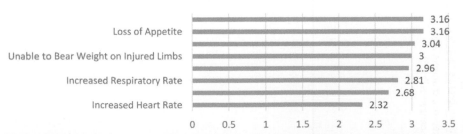

Snake Physiologic Response to Pain

Fig. 1. Most commonly ranked physiologic changes in response to pain and subjective pain behaviors by an expert panel (n).

Snake Pain Behaviors

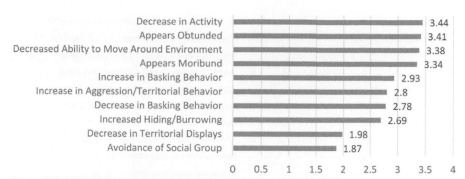

Decrease in Activity	3.44
Appears Obtunded	3.41
Decreased Ability to Move Around Environment	3.38
Appears Moribund	3.34
Increase in Basking Behavior	2.93
Increase in Aggression/Territorial Behavior	2.8
Decrease in Basking Behavior	2.78
Increased Hiding/Burrowing	2.69
Decrease in Territorial Displays	1.98
Avoidance of Social Group	1.87

Fig. 2. Most commonly ranked physiologic changes in response to pain and subjective pain behaviors by an expert panel (n).

In one study that surveyed the use of anesthesia and analgesics in reptiles by veterinarians in 2004%, 98% of the respondents indicated they believe that reptiles feel pain.[56] However, 39% of respondents in this survey reported using analgesics in more than 50% of their patients. When veterinarians were asked "How do we diagnose pain in reptiles?", 76% of the respondents said that they diagnosed pain based on the anticipated level of pain extrapolated from other species, 66% based pain on behavioral changes, 57% treated by the anticipated level of pain based on prior experience in reptiles, and 32% relied on physiologic changes to diagnose pain.[56]

A more recent study evaluated and investigated current ideas within analgesia in reptiles in 2016 via a survey while comparing veterinary care experts to animal care experts such as herpetologists and pet owners.[57] With the hopes of outlining items for the development of a behavioral ethogram, the study revealed a lack of confidence when assessing pain for both groups; however, there was a statistically significant agreement for the three top behavioral signs among three subgroups.

Crocodilian Physiologic Response to Pain

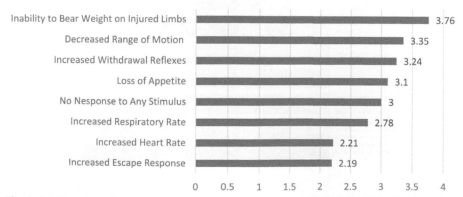

Inability to Bear Weight on Injured Limbs	3.76
Decreased Range of Motion	3.35
Increased Withdrawal Reflexes	3.24
Loss of Appetite	3.1
No Nesponse to Any Stimulus	3
Increased Respiratory Rate	2.78
Increased Heart Rate	2.21
Increased Escape Response	2.19

Fig. 3. Most commonly ranked physiologic changes in response to pain and subjective pain behaviors by an expert panel (n).

Crocodilian Pain Behaviors

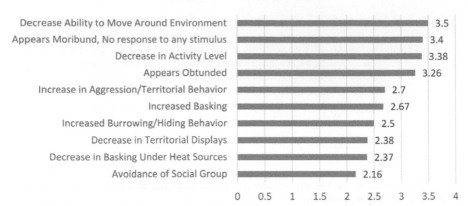

Decrease Ability to Move Around Environment — 3.5
Appears Moribund, No response to any stimulus — 3.4
Decrease in Activity Level — 3.38
Appears Obtunded — 3.26
Increase in Aggression/Territorial Behavior — 2.7
Increased Basking — 2.67
Increased Burrowing/Hiding Behavior — 2.5
Decrease in Territorial Displays — 2.38
Decrease in Basking Under Heat Sources — 2.37
Avoidance of Social Group — 2.16

0   0.5   1   1.5   2   2.5   3   3.5   4

Fig. 4. Most commonly ranked physiologic changes in response to pain and subjective pain behaviors by an expert panel (n).

In a 2010 observational study, 85 reptile veterinarians, reptile curators, and wildlife rehabilitators were surveyed as an expert panel to gather observational and physiologic criteria of pain behaviors in reptiles (Latney 2010, unpublished data).[58] Panel members were opportunistically sampled as members of the following organizations, American Association of Zoo Veterinarians, Association Reptile & Amphibian Veterinarians, American Association of Wildlife Veterinarians, and the Canadian Association of Wildlife Veterinarians.

The expert panel anonymously selected their professions and was allowed to check any and all that applied. For this response, 97.6% selected reptile veterinarian, 54.1% selected reptile owner, 12.9% selected herpetologist and wildlife rehabilitator, 17.6%

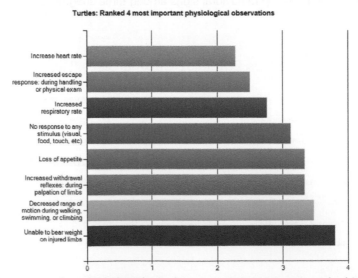

Turtles: Ranked 4 most important physiological observations

Increase heart rate
Increased escape response: during handling or physical exam
Increased respiratory rate
No response to any stimulus (visual, food, touch, etc)
Loss of appetite
Increased withdrawal reflexes: during palpation of limbs
Decreased range of motion during walking, swimming, or climbing
Unable to bear weight on injured limbs

0   1   2   3   4

Fig. 5. Most commonly ranked physiologic changes in response to pain and subjective pain behaviors by an expert panel (n).

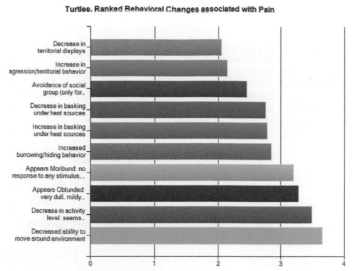

Fig. 6. Most commonly ranked physiologic changes in response to pain and subjective pain behaviors by an expert panel (n).

identified as a reptile zookeeper, and 1.2% as reptile curator. On average, 35% of the respondents claimed that they worked with more than 10 individual reptiles a week. When asked if they felt qualified to rank reptile pain behaviors, 86.1% of respondents chose "yes" for lizards, 82.7% for turtles, 78.1% for snakes, and 70.3% chose "no" for crocodilians.[57]

Participants were asked to qualify at least four of the listed eight observations as "not important, slightly important, moderately important, very important, and not

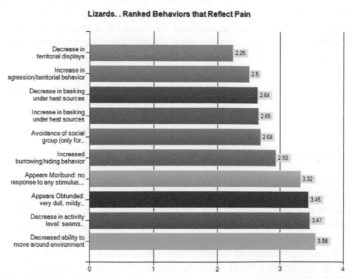

Fig. 7. Most commonly ranked physiologic changes in response to pain and subjective pain behaviors by an expert panel (n).

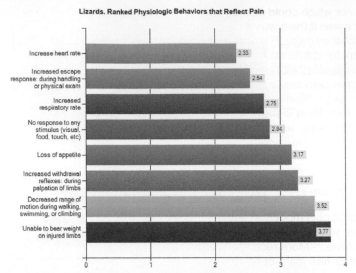

Fig. 8. Most commonly ranked physiologic changes in response to pain and subjective pain behaviors by an expert panel (n).

applicable" for physiologic changes, and at least 4 of 10 items for subjective behavioral changes. These were divided by the four major families, chelonians, snakes, lizards, and crocodilians. An open-ended response item was available for each survey so that participants could enter their own items if not listed. After evaluating their entered responses and their ranked observations, this information was presented to a focus group of 10 civilian reptile companion owners. Their observations are also included in **Figs. 1–8**.[58] Interestingly, only pet owners and those from the expert panel that worked with more than 10 reptiles weekly noted skin quality and color changes for certain lizard species as a sign of discomfort. All of the observations were ranked based on taxonomic group and by most commonly observed behaviors.

Although generalizations can be difficult to make, it appears the most common collectively ranked pain behaviors across reptile families included the following: decreased interaction with environment/mental changes, decreased appetite, decreased ability to move around enclosure, inability to bear weight on affected limbs, increased withdrawals, decreased range of motion in injured limbs, abnormal basking behaviors, social avoidance OR aggression, and skin color changes in certain lizard species (see **Fig. 1**).[58]

CLINICAL ASSESSMENT TOOLS

The responses obtained from the observational study were used to develop an inventory of items that could be tested for use in a reptile brief pain inventory, or pain scale, for use in lizards with orthopedic injury. Modeled after the human brief pain inventory, the brief pain inventory was designed to use owner observations of behaviors to classify and quantify pain-related behaviors and track resolution based on treatment responses. The self-administered questionnaire responses could be used individually or averaged to generate a pain severity score. The 18-item pain scale contained four items that asked for a description of pain/discomfort, four items that asked to quantify the severity of the animal's pain, eight items that asked how pain interferes with behavior which could also be used to develop a pain interference score, and two items that asked if there was an improvement in pain control based on treatment (Latney, unpublished data). The scales were used for each appointment during the course of treatment for lizards with orthopedic injuries. This tool does not circumvent the need for species-specific ethograms, but it attempts to close one gap clinicians struggle with in reptile pain management, it provides access to observed behaviors by one that would be an expert at knowing normal and abnormal behaviors for the individual reptile, as witnessed in their "normal" environment. The tool is still undergoing iterations of refinements, as misclassification bias, selection bias, and other unmeasured associations can influence its ability to truly discriminate between pain and other factors.

UPDATES ON PAIN BEHAVIORS FROM CLASSIC MODELS

Most adapted pain models in reptile medicine include validated thermal antinociceptive models, which have been used to elucidate opioid receptor distribution and analgesic response.[53] More recently, several inflammatory models have appeared in the literature and new pain behaviors have been reported. In one of those studies, a delayed return to normal feeding behavior was evaluated as an indicator of pain in captive ball pythons (*Python regius*).[44] Ball pythons were assigned into three treatment groups, surgical incisions, capsaicin injection, and general anesthesia. Strike time to capture rodent prey was measured and the results showed a delayed return to feeding for the surgical incision and capsaicin treatment groups while not for the anesthesia alone treatment group.[44] A decrease in return to spontaneous feeding behavior has also been documented as a post-operative observation in red-eared slider turtles (*Trachemys scripta elegans*) that underwent gonadectomy.[59]

Tachycardia has also been shown to be a repeated physiologic measure in a capsaicin-induced nociception model in ball pythons.[60] Capsaicin models and suspended formalin models have also been used in Speke's Hinge-back tortoises *Kinixys spekii*[61] and crocodiles,[62] with exposures resulting in protective behaviors after ocular exposure to capsaicin, and leg lifting, vocalization, urination, and defecation after exposure to subcutaneously administered formalin.

SUMMARY

Advances in reptile cognitive research would help to (1) better qualify behavioral responses to pain experiences, (2) monitor welfare impacts, and (3) model analgesic studies with ecologically relevant insight to better qualify interventional responses. The focus of future analgesic studies in reptiles require the continued elucidation of the opiate systems and the given variations across taxa in efficacy in nociceptive tests.[53] In addition, the development of ethograms based on ecological relevance is necessary to more appropriately identify complex behaviors as subtle perturbations that could be linked to pain responses may go unobserved. Lastly, animal models that mirror different types of clinical pain are needed for reptiles, as the most common studies are constricted to locally noxious chemo- and thermo-nociceptive models.

REFERENCES

1. MacRae AM, Makowska IJ, Fraser D. Initial evaluation of facial expressions and behaviours of harbour seal pups (Phoca vitulina) in response to tagging and microchipping. Appl Anim Behav Sci 2018;205:167–74.

2. Mogil JS, Pang DS, Dutra GG, et al. The development and use of facial grimace scales for pain measurement in animals. Neurosci Biobehav Rev 2020;116: 480–93.
3. Neurology A. In: Gans C, Northcutt RG, Ulinski P, editors. Biology of the reptilia, 9. London: Academic Press; 1979. p. 1–462.
4. Neurology B. In: Gans C, Northcutt RG, Ulinski P, editors. Biology of the reptilia, 10. London: Academic Press; 1979. p. 1–388.
5. Neurology C. Sensorimotor Integration. In: Gans C, Northcutt RG, Ulinski P, editors. Biol reptilia, 17. Chicago: The University Of Chicago Press; 1992. p. 1–781.
6. Williams CJ, James LE, Bertelsen MF, et al. Analgesia for non-mammalian vertebrates. Curr Opin Physiol 2019;11:75–84.
7. ten Donkelaar HJ. Organization of descending pathways to the spinal cord in amphibians and reptiles. Prog Brain Res 1982;57:25–67.
8. ten Donkelaar HJ. Descending pathways to the spinal cord in tetrapods: A brief outline. In: Development and regenerative capacity of descending supraspinal pathways in tetrapods- A comparative approach. Berlin: Springer; 2000. p. 9–13.
9. Bangma GC, Donkelaar HT. Afferent connections of the cerebellum in various types of reptiles. J Comp Neurol 1982;207(3):255–73.
10. Henselmans JM, Hoogland PV, Stoof JC. Differences in the regulation of acetylcholine release upon D2 dopamine and N-methyl-D-aspartate receptor activation between the striatal complex of reptiles and the neostriatum of rats. Brain Res 1991;566(1–2):8–12.
11. Martinez-Garcia F, Novejarque A, Lanuza E. The evolution of the amygdala in vertebrates. In: Kass J, Streidter GF, editors. Evolutionary neuroscience. 1st edition. Oxford: Academic Press; 2009. p. 313–92.
12. Lohman AH, Smeets WJ. The dorsal ventricular ridge and cortex of reptiles in historical and phylogenetic perspective. In: The neocortex. Boston: Springer; 1991. p. 59–74.
13. Shimizu T, Karten HJ. Multiple origins of neocortex: Contributions of the dorsal ventricular ridge. In: The neocortex 1991. Boston: Springer; 1991. p. 75–86.
14. Aboitiz F. Comparative development of the mammalian isocortex and the reptilian dorsal ventricular ridge-evolutionary considerations. Cereb Cortex 1999;9(8): 783–91.
15. Güntürkün O, Stacho M, Ströckens F. The brains of reptiles and birds. In: Kass J, editor. Evolutionary neuroscience. 2nd edition. Cambridge: Academic Press; 2020. p. 159–212.
16. Naumann RK, Laurent G. Function and evolution of the reptilian cerebral cortex. In: Kass J, editor. Evolutionary neuroscience. 2nd edition. Cambridge: Academic Press; 2020. p. 213–45.
17. Balaban CD, Ulinski PS. Organization of thalamic afferents to anterior dorsal ventricular ridge in turtles. I. Projections of thalamic nuclei. J Comp Neurol 1981; 200(1):95–129.
18. Balaban CD, Ulinski PS. Organization of thalamic afferents to anterior dorsal ventricular ridge in turtles. II. Properties of the rotundo-dorsal map. J Comp Neurol 1981;200(1):131–50.
19. Goldby F, Robinson LR. The central connections of dorsal spinal nerve roots and the ascending tracts in the spinal cord of Lacerta viridis. J Anat 1962;96:153–70.
20. Hartline JT, Smith AN, Kabelik D. Serotonergic activation during courtship and aggression in the brown anole, Anolis sagrei. Peer J 2017;5:3331. Available at. https://doi.org/10.7717/peerj.3331. Accessed December 15, 2021.

21. Lanuza E, Belekhova M, Martínez-Marcos A, et al. Identification of the reptilian basolateral amygdala: an anatomical investigation of the afferents to the posterior dorsal ventricular ridge of the lizard Podarcis hispanica. Euro J Neurosci 1998;10: 3517–34.

22. Guirado S, Dávila JC, Real MÁ, et al. Light and electron microscopic evidence for projections from the thalamic nucleus rotundus to targets in the basal ganglia, the dorsal ventricular ridge, and the amygdaloid complex in a lizard. J Comp Neurol 2000;424(2):216–32.

23. Novejarque A, Lanuza E, Martínez-García F. Amygdalostriatal projections in reptiles: A tract-tracing study in the lizard Podarcis hispanica. J Comp Neurol 2004; 479(3):287–308.

24. Díaz C, Yanes C, Medina L, et al. Golgi study of the anterior dorsal ventricular ridge in a lizard. I. Neuronal typology in the adult. J Morph 1990;203(3):293–300.

25. Díaz C, Yanes C, Medina L, et al. Golgi study of the anterior dorsal ventricular ridge in a lizard. II. Neuronal cytodifferentiation. J Morph 1990;203(3):301–10.

26. Wolters JG, De Boer-Van Huizen R, ten Donkelaar HJ. Funicular trajectories of descending brain stem pathways in a lizard (Varanus exanthematicus). Prog Brain Res 1982;57:69–78.

27. Hoogland PV. Spinothalamic projections in a lizard, Varanus exanthematicus: An HRP study. J Comp Neurol 1981;198(1):7–12.

28. Wolters JG, ten Donkelaar HJ, Steinbusch HW, et al. Distribution of serotonin in the brain stem and spinal cord of the lizard Varanus exanthematicus: an immunohistochemical study. Neurosci 1985;14(1):169–93.

29. Challet E, Pierre J, Repérant J, et al. The serotoninergic system of the brain of the viper, Vipera aspis. An immunohistochemical study. J Chem Neuroanat 1991; 4(4):233–48.

30. ten Donkelaar HJ, Bangma GC, De Boer-Van Huizen R. Reticulospinal and vestibulospinal pathways in the snake Python regius. Anat Embryol 1983;168(2): 277–89.

31. Ulinski PS. Organization of anterior dorsal ventricular ridge in snakes. J Comp Neurol 1978;178(3):411–49.

32. Ebbesson SO, Goodman DC. Organization of ascending spinal projections in Caiman crocodilus. Cell Tissue Res 1981;215(2):383–95.

33. Rodrigues SL, Maseko BC, Ihunwo AO, et al. Nuclear organization and morphology of serotonergic neurons in the brain of the Nile crocodile, Crocodylus niloticus. J Chem Neuroanat 2008;35(1):133–45.

34. Clark JM, Ulinski PS. A Golgi study of anterior dorsal ventricular ridge in the alligator, Alligator mississippiensis. J Morph 1984;179(2):153–74.

35. Reiner A, Northcutt RG. Succinic dehydrogenase histochemistry reveals the location of the putative primary visual and auditory areas within the dorsal ventricular ridge of Sphenodon punctatus. Brain Behav Evol 2000;55(1):26–36.

36. Perry SM, Nevarez JG. Pain and its control in reptiles. Vet Clin North Am Exot Anim Pract 2018;21(1):1–6.

37. Serinelli I, Soloperto S, Lai OR. Pain and Pain Management in Sea Turtle and Herpetological Medicine: State of the Art. Animals 2022;12(6):697. Available at. https://doi.org/10.3390/ani12060697. Accessed March 18,2022.

38. Fowler M, Medina L, Reiner A. Immunohistochemical localization of NMDA-and AMPA-type glutamate receptor subunits in the basal ganglia of red-eared turtles. Brain Behav Evol 1999;54(5):276–89.

39. Liang YF, Terashima SI. Physiological properties and morphological characteristics of cutaneous and mucosal mechanical nociceptive neurons with A-

δ peripheral axons in the trigeminal ganglia of crotaline snakes. J Comp Neurol 1993;328(1):88–102.

40. Liang YF, Terashima SI, Zhu AQ. Distinct morphological characteristics of touch, temperature, and mechanical nociceptive neurons in the crotaline trigeminal ganglia. J Comp Neurol 1995;360(4):621–33.

41. Terashima SI, Liang YF. Touch and vibrotactile neurons in a crotaline snake's trigeminal ganglia. Somatosens Mot Res 1994;11(2):169–81.

42. Terashima SI, Zhu AQ. Single Versus Repetitive Spiking to the Current Stimulus of A-β Mechanosensitive Neurons in the Crotaline Snake Trigeminal Ganglion. Cell Mol Neurobiol 1997 Apr;17(2):195–206.

43. Bryant BP, Kraus F. Neural basis of trigeminal chemo-and thermonociception in brown treesnakes, Boiga irregularis. J Comp Neurol A 2018;204(7):677–86.

44. James LE, Williams CJ, Bertelsen MF, et al. Evaluation of feeding behavior as an indicator of pain in snakes. J Zoo Wildl Med 2017;48(1):196–9.

45. ten Donkelaar HJ, de Boer-van Huizen R. A possible pain control system in a non-mammalian vertebrate (a lizard, Gekko gecko). Neurosci Lett 1987;83(1–2): 65–70.

46. Makau CM, Towett PK, Abelson KS, et al. Modulation of formalin-induced pain-related behaviour by clonidine and yohimbine in the Speke's hinged tortoise (Kiniskys spekii). J Vet Pharmacol Ther 2017;40(5):439–46.

47. Martínez-García F, Lanuza E. Evolution of vertebrate survival circuits. Curr Opin Behav Sci 2018;24:113–23.

48. Rothll TC, Krochmal AR, LaDage LD. Reptilian cognition- a more complex picture via integration of neurological mechanisms, behavioral constraints, and evolutionary context. BioEssays 2019;41(8):1–9, 1900033.

49. Burghardt GM. Editorial: Journal of Comparative Psychology. J Comp Psychol 2006;120(2):77–8.

50. Burghardt GM. How comparative was (is) the Journal of Comparative Psychology? A reptilian perspective. J Comp Psychol 2021;135(3):286–90.

51. Posner LP, Chinnadurai SK. Recognition and treatment of pain in reptiles, amphibians, and fish. In: Love LCM, Tom Doherty T, editors. Pain Recognition in veterinary practice. 1st edition. Ames: Blackwell Publishing; 2014. p. 417–23.

52. Schilliger L, Vergneau-Grosset C, Desmarchelier MR. Clinical Reptile Behavior. Vet Clin North Am Exot Anim Pract 2021;24(1):175–95.

53. Sladky KK, Mans C. Analgesia. In: Divers SJ, Stahl SJ, editors. Mader's reptile and Amphibian medicine and Surgery. 3rd edition. Cambridge: Elsevier Health Sciences; 2019. p. 465–74.

54. Bradbury G, Morton K. Using behavioural science to improve pain management. Practice 2017;39(7):339–41.

55. Warwick C, Arena P, Lindley S, et al. Assessing reptile welfare using behavioural criteria. Practice 2013;35(3):123–31.

56. Read MR. Evaluation of the use of anesthesia and analgesia in reptiles. J Am Vet Med Assoc 2004;224(4):547–52.

57. Ayers H. Pain recognition in reptiles and investigation of associated behavioural signs. The Vet Nurse 2016;7(5):292–300.

58. Latney LV. University of Pennsylvania Reptile Pain Behavior, An Observational Study. 2010. Unpublished data.

59. Kinney ME, Johnson SM, Sladky KK. Behavioral evaluation of red-eared slider turtles (Trachemys scripta elegans) administered either morphine or butorphanol following unilateral gonadectomy. J Herpetol Med Surg 2011;21(2–3):54–62.

60. Williams CJ, James LE, Bertelsen MF, et al. Tachycardia in response to remote capsaicin injection as a model for nociception in the ball python (Python regius). Vet Anaesth Analg 2016;43(4):429–34.
61. Makau CM, Towett PK, Abelson KS, et al. Modulation of nociception by amitriptyline hydrochloride in the Speke's hinge-back tortoise (Kiniskys spekii). Vet Med Sci 2021;7(3):1034–41.
62. Kanui TI, Hole K, Miaron JO. Nociception in crocodiles: capsaicin instillation, formalin and hot plate tests. Zool Sci 1990;7(3):537–40. Available at. http://repository.seku.ac.ke/handle/123456789/1274. Accessed December 14, 2021.

Treatment of Pain in Reptiles

Kurt K. Sladky, MS, DVM, DiplACZM, DiplECZM (Zoo Health Management & Herpetology)

KEYWORDS

• Reptile • Analgesia • Opioids • NSAIDs • Local anesthetics

KEY POINTS

- Analgesic drug administration in reptiles should be considered standard of care under clinical and research conditions, which are considered painful in other species.
- Based on current evidence, mu-opioid agonists are considered the most effective choice for analgesia in reptiles.
- Although limited data are available with respect to pharmacokinetics and/or pharmacodynamics of few non-steroidal anti-inflammatory drugs (NSAIDs) in a limited number of reptile species, we know almost nothing about NSAID efficacy. Nevertheless, we tend to use NSAIDs in reptiles for painful or inflammatory conditions with the hope that it helps the reptile return to normal behavior more rapidly.
- Preemptive administration of analgesics, and using multimodal analgesic regimes, should be considered standard of practice for excellent reptile clinical medicine, welfare, and research.

INTRODUCTION

Although I have spent much of my career trying to understand reptile pain and how to treat it, and the past 20 years have witnessed an explosion of published reptile analgesia information, there are days that I feel as though I am still learning the most effective or prudent methods to manage pain in many of my patients. "How should I manage postovariectomy pain in this Eastern indigo snake (*Drymarchon couperi*) patient? or where do I begin when considering managing chronic limb lameness due to osteoarthritis in an elderly, endangered mata mata (*Chelus fimbriata*) turtle at the zoo?" Of course, these are just hypothetical examples for illustration, but it is not uncommon for my students, residents, and colleagues to ask me similar questions, for which I, frequently, do not always have a cogent answer. The first consideration, before I answer, is what evidence-based data exist and can I apply these data directly to this patient or do I need to extrapolate and hope for the best? For example, whereas I have some evidence of analgesic efficacy of µ-opioids in red-eared slider turtles and pharmacokinetic data for meloxicam in several turtle species, do any of these published data directly translate to application for chronic pain in the mata mata? How

University of Wisconsin-Madison, School of Veterinary Medicine, 2015 Linden Drive, Madison, WI 53705 USA
E-mail address: kurt.sladky@wisc.edu

Vet Clin Exot Anim 26 (2023) 43–64
https://doi.org/10.1016/j.cvex.2022.07.004
1094-9194/23/© 2022 Elsevier Inc. All rights reserved.

confident am I in trying to manage pain in the indigo snake with so many more questions than answers with respect to managing pain in any snake species, as there is so little published information about snake analgesia? The bottom line is that, whenever possible, the choice and dosage of analgesics should be based on sound research. Unfortunately, sometimes the best we can do is extrapolate information from related, or even divergent, species. Therefore, the pursuit of clinically relevant pain and analgesia research is critical for expanding our understanding of these issues in reptiles, and for improving the welfare of reptiles under our care, and the objective of this article was to present evidence-based and clinically relevant analgesic data for use in captive reptiles. Hopefully, the information presented here will help you formulate an effective analgesia plan for your next reptile patient.

GENERAL CONSIDERATIONS
Reptile Diversity, Anatomy, and Physiology

Choosing, administering, and understanding analgesic use in reptiles presents several challenges. First, there is an enormous diversity of species across the Class *Reptilia*, one of the most phylogenetically diverse animal classes with four main orders (*Crocodylia*, *Testudines*, *Squamata*, and *Rhynchocephalia*), and greater than 7800 species worldwide. This includes massive size diversity, from a 1-g Jaragua dwarf gecko (*Sphaerodactylus ariasae*) to the 1000 kg saltwater crocodile (*Crocodylus porosus*), not to mention many venomous and large, aggressive species. Second, understanding anatomic, physiologic, and natural historical differences, especially preferred optimal body temperature ranges, are every bit as important. Third, and perhaps most important, it is necessary to continue to make progress toward more evidence-based research dedicated to advancing our understanding of effective analgesic drugs, dose-dependent effects, duration of drug efficacy, interspecies differences, and potentially deleterious drug-related adverse effects, such as cardiopulmonary depression. When considering reptile therapeutics, we have a love–hate relationship with anecdotal information that gets published and frequently becomes dogma over time because of immortalization in textbook chapter after textbook chapter. We love this information because we can read it and use it without much thought; we hate this information because it is typically a single individual's, one-time experience administering the drug to a single animal and writing that it worked. Although there is a clear need for evaluating analgesic drugs across a variety of clinical situations, particularly as they apply to acute, postsurgical pain, extrapolation of analgesic drugs and dosages across orders and species remains a necessary evil, and one that we will not overcome until we significantly expand our body of evidence-based research; but we must continue to try!

Routes of Administration

Describing the most appropriate methods for administering analgesic drugs in reptiles is challenging due to the lack of analgesic pharmacokinetic and/or pharmacodynamic data collected from reptile species across laboratory methods and clinical situations. Whether an analgesic drug is administered intravenously (IV), intramuscularly (IM), subcutaneously (SC), intracoelomically (ICe), per os (PO), or transcutaneously (TC), its effectiveness partially depends on the anatomic location of administration, the size and temperament of the individual reptile, and the environmental temperature in which the reptile is maintained (ie, preferred optimal body temperature). Anatomic location of analgesic administration is important because there is pharmacologic evidence that drug administration to the hind limbs or tail of a reptile may cause rapid clearance for drugs with tubular secretion by the renal portal system or metabolism by the hepatic first-pass effect, as in the case of opioids.[1-3] However, whether this more rapid clearance has any biological implication on the clinical effect of an analgesic drug remains unknown, as plasma concentrations may be very different than tissue concentrations of a drug. In green iguanas administered a radioactive isotope of dimercaptosuccinic acid (99mTc-DMSA) in either the hind limb or tail muscles, systemic distribution was evaluated by nuclear scintigraphy.[4] Initially, both hind limb and tail IM injections showed the distribution of 99mTc-DMSA only in the caudal half of the body and directly to the kidneys, but with time (10–30 min) there was distribution to the heart and into general circulation. Perhaps because the subject numbers were small, there was individual variability in results. Nevertheless, it must be emphasized that different drugs may be distributed differently when administered in the muscles of the hind limbs and tail, and not all drugs are eliminated rapidly from systemic circulation.[4] Although IV administration of analgesics is not common, the administration of drugs in the ventral coccygeal vein does not undergo hepatic first-pass effect, as drugs enter directly into the caudal vena cava.[3] Therefore, it is an option when using analgesics in an IV anesthetic induction combination. To date, ICe administration of analgesics is not well documented in the literature but was commonly used in early reptile analgesic research. Intramuscular and SC analgesic administration is considered much more common. Oral administration may be useful for more prolonged analgesic use, or for drugs showed to be well-absorbed and distributed after oral administration, such as tramadol.[2] Transcutaneous administration, especially with fentanyl patches may be useful in snakes and lizards for longer-term analgesia.[2]

CLINICAL ANALGESIA
Opioids and Opioid-like Analgesics

For pain management in mammals, many clinicians prefer administering either a μ-opioid agonist (eg, morphine, fentanyl, hydromorphone, etc.), a partial μ-opioid agonist (eg, buprenorphine), or a mixed-opioid, κ-agonist–μ-receptor antagonist (eg, butorphanol) (**Table 1**). Of the options for analgesics and anti-inflammatories in reptiles, opioids have been the most studied. For example, morphine sulfate, and μ-opioids in general, has been shown to be an effective analgesic in a variety of reptile species, except that snake species remain an enigma when it comes to showing μ-opioid efficacy.[1,2,5-7] In early reptile analgesia research, intraperitoneally [sic] (ICe) administered morphine (5 mg/kg) slowed the tail-flick response to a noxious thermal stimulus in anole lizards (*Anolis carolinensis*),[22] whereas young Nile crocodiles (*C niloticus*) developed significantly increased limb withdrawal latencies to a thermal noxious stimulus (hot plate) for at least 8 h with maximal effect after morphine (0.3 mg/kg and 1.0 mg/kg ICe) was administered intraperitoneally [sic].[18] In this same crocodile study, pethidine (ie, demerol) a short-acting μ-opioid agonist in humans, had a similar effect at 1.0 m/kg intraperitoneally [sic] (ICe), but for less than 3 h.[18] Using the thermal noxious stimulus limb withdrawal method (**Fig. 1**), morphine was an effective analgesic in bearded dragons (*Pogona vitticeps*; 1 and 5 mg/kg SC) and red-eared slider turtles (*Trachemys scripta elegans*; 1.5 and 6.5 mg/kg SC), but data were equivocal in corn snakes (*Elaphe guttata*), even when morphine was administered at an extremely high dose of 40 mg/kg.[7] This antinociceptive response in bearded dragons was replicated in a separate bearded dragon study after the lizards were administered morphine (10 mg/kg IM) and exposed to a femoral-based thermal noxious stimulus (see **Fig. 1**).[23] Respiratory depression is a deleterious side effect in mammals

Table 1
Evidence-based analgesics used in reptiles

Opioids	Dosage/Route	Comments	Refs.
Butorphanol	2.8 and 28 mg/kg SC	Red-eared slider turtles; no evidence of analgesic efficacy; significant respiratory depression	5,6
	2.0 and 20 mg/kg SC	Bearded dragons, corn snakes; no evidence of analgesic efficacy; significant respiratory depression	7
	1.5 and 8.0 mg/kg IM	Green iguana; antinociceptive to an electrical noxious stimulus; however, 4.0 mg/kg was ineffective	12
	1.0 mg/kg IM	Green iguanas/ineffective for analgesia; presence of observer may affect iguana response	22
	5.0 and 10.0 mg/kg IM	Black and white tegus; no antinociception to a noxious thermal stimulus	11
	5.0 mg/kg IV	Ball pythons; no physiologic changes in ball pythons administered post-operatively	24
	20.0 mg/kg SC	Red-eared sliders/ineffective for surgical analgesia	6
Buprenorphine	0.2 mg/kg SC	Red-eared slider turtles; no evidence of analgesic efficacy	16
	0.02–0.1 mg/kg IM	Green iguanas; no evidence of analgesic efficacy	12
	0.02, 0.05 mg/kg SC	Plasma concentrations equivalent to those effective for analgesia in mammals; respiratory depression not studied	21
Fentanyl	12 μg/h transdermal patch to cranial epaxial muscles	Ball pythons; high plasma concentrations (above analgesic threshold in mammals); analgesic efficacy not proven in any snake species, but anecdotal evidence from certain snake clinical cases demonstrated improved behavior after application of patch; respiratory depression	18
	12 μg/h transdermal patch to caudodorsal lumbar region	Prehensile-tailed skinks; PK, no adverse-effects reported after 24 h when skink blood levels reached human therapeutic levels; environmental temperature can significantly affect absorption	19
	0.05 mg/kg SC	Slider turtle species (Trachemys dorbigni, Trachemys scripta elegans); antinociceptive to interdigital forceps pinch	20

Drug	Dose	Comments	Ref
Hydromorphone	0.5 mg/kg SC	Red-eared slider turtles; good analgesic efficacy; respiratory depression not studied	16
	0.5, 1.0 mg/kg SC	Red-eared slider turtles, bearded dragons; PK; determined administration frequency of q24 h (bearded dragons) and q12–24h (red-eared sliders)	17
Meperidine (pethidine; demerol)	1.0 mg/kg ICe	Nile crocodiles; short-lived analgesia using hot plate test	9
	10.0, 20.0, 50.0 mg/kg ICe	Speke's hinged tortoises; analgesic at 20 & 50 mg/kg using SC formalin test	13
Morphine	1.5, 6.5 mg/kg SC	Red-eared slider turtles; good analgesic efficacy under laboratory conditions; significant respiratory depression	5,6
	1.0, 5.0, 10.0, 20.0, 40.0 mg/kg SC	Bearded dragons; analgesic efficacy under laboratory conditions; corn snakes; no evidence of analgesic efficacy even at highest doses	7
	5.0 and 10.0 mg/kg IM	Black and white tegus/antinociceptive using a thermal noxious stimulus	11
	10.0 mg/kg IM q24 h	Bearded dragons/analgesia	7
	10.0 mg/kg IM q24 h	Ball pythons/no analgesia based on no heart rate changes after capsaicin injection	14
	0.1–0.2 mg/kg IT	Red-eared slider turtles; thermal analgesia for 48 h; regional analgesia caudal body	15
	5.0 mg/kg ICe	Anole lizards; analgesia under laboratory condition using thermal noxious stimulus	8
	0.3, 1.0 mg/kg ICe	Nile crocodiles; analgesia under laboratory condition using thermal noxious stimulus	9
	2.0 mg/kg SC	Red-eared sliders; analgesia after undergoing unilateral gonadectomy	6
	2.0 mg/kg SC q24 h	Bearded dragons/antinociceptive using a thermal noxious stimulus	10
	7.5, 10.0, 20.0 mg/kg ICe	Speke's hinged tortoises; analgesic at 20 & 50 mg/kg using SC formalin tests; analgesia reversed with naloxone (5 mg/kg ICe)	13

(continued on next page)

Table 1
(continued)

Opioids	Dosage/Route	Comments	Refs.
Naloxone	0.04–5.0 mg/kg SC, IM, ICe	Various species; antagonizes mu-opioid agonists (eg, morphine)	1,2,5–7,13
Tapentadol	10.0 mg/kg IM q24–48h	Yellow-bellied slider turtles; analgesic efficacy; PK indicated 10h duration of effect	32,33
Tramadol	5.0–10.0 mg/kg PO q 48–72h	Red-eared sliders; good analgesic efficacy with relatively long duration when administered PO in chelonians; less respiratory depression than other opioids	28,31
	11.0 mg/kg PO	Bearded dragons; dampened response to noxious electrical stimulation to the tail	29
	5.0,10.0 mg/kg PO q72 h	Loggerhead sea turtles; PK; plasma concentrations consistent with efficacy for 48 h (5 mg/kg PO) or 72 h (10 mg/kg PO)	30
	10.0 mg/kg IM q48–72h	Yellow-bellied sliders; PK/PD comparing forelimb and hind limb administration; analgesia; plasma concentrations consistent with analgesia in both forelimb and hind limb	31
NSAIDS			
Carprofen	2.0, 4.0 mg/kg IM once	Bearded dragons; dampened behavioral response to noxious electrical stimulation	29
	2.0 mg/kg IM q 24h for 10d	Green iguanas; only looked at blood changes; increased ALT and AST compared with saline	36
Ketoprofen	2.0 mg/kg IV, IM once	Green iguanas; PK data indicated once daily for IM dose	43
	2.0 mg/kg IM once	Bearded dragons; dampened behavioral response to noxious electrical stimulation	29
	2.0 mg/kg IM, IV once	Loggerhead sea turtle; PK study demonstrated a single IM or IV dose had a 24 h duration	44
	2.0 mg/kg IM q24 h for up to 5 d	Loggerhead sea turtles; PK study demonstrated treatment efficacy up to 24h after a single dose. Dosage appeared safe with respect to blood clotting and other blood parameters	45
	2.0 & 20.0 mg/kg IM q 24h for 14 d (Vigneault 2022)	Bearded dragons; evaluated adverse effects; marked muscle necrosis at injection site at 20.0 mg/kg dose. No biochemical changes, no occult blood, no histopathologic lesions in kidneys, liver or gastrointestinal systems	42

Ketorolac	0.25 mg/kg IM once[70]	Eastern box turtles; PK study demonstrated a single dose had a 24 h duration	48
	0.25 mg/kg IM once	Loggerhead sea turtles; PK showed concentrations never reached those considered therapeutic in humans	47
Meloxicam	0.2 mg/kg IM q 24d for 10d	Green iguanas; blood biochemical parameters unchanged; no efficacy evaluated	36
	0.2 mg/kg PO, IV q24 h	Green iguanas; PK study; no efficacy evaluated	35
	0.2 mg/kg IM, IV; SC q24 h	Red-eared sliders; PK study; plasma concentrations consistent with therapeutic efficacy for 48 h by IM and IV administration routes;	39
	0.2 mg/kg SC once	Mojave Desert tortoises, post-surgical nonsteroidal anti-inflammatory	56,57
	0.3 mg/kg IM q24 h	Ball pythons; no physiologic changes in ball pythons administered post-operatively.	24
	0.1 mg/kg IM, IV q24 h	Loggerhead sea turtles; PK study; plasma concentrations not consistent with analgesia	37
	0.2 mg/kg PO, IM, ICe once	Red-eared slider turtles; PK study; ICe dose reached therapeutic concentrations equivalent to horse for 12h; IM dose for 8h; PO dose never reached therapeutic concentrations	38
	0.5 mg/kg PO, IM q24 h or 0.22 mg/kg IV q24 h	Red-eared sliders/PK; found better absorption IM vs PO; after IV administration, plasma levels decreased rapidly, and the elimination half-life was 7.57 h	42
	1.0 mg/kg SC	Kemp's ridley and green sea turtles/PK; q12 h for Kemp's ridley sea turtles and q48 h for green sea turtles	41
	1.0 mg/kg SC q24 h (green and Kemp's ridley sea turtles); 2.0 mg/kg SC q48 h	Kemp's ridley and green sea turtles/PK; resulted in plasma concentrations >0.5 µg/mL for 12 h for Kemp's ridley and 120 h for greens; administration of 2 mg/kg SC to loggerhead sea turtles resulted in adequate plasma concentrations for only 4 h	40

(continued on next page)

Table 1
(continued)

Opioids	Dosage/Route	Comments	Refs.
Tolfenamic acid	2.0 mg/kg IM; 2.0 & .04 mg/kg IV	Red-eared sliders; PK study; half-life longer for IM compared with IV administration; may be anti-inflammatory for 24–48h	50
	4 mg/kg IV & IM	Green sea turtles; PK study; anti-inflammatory plasma concentrations for 6-7d	49
Local Anesthetics			
Bupivacaine (0.5%)	0.5 mg/kg (keep <2.0 mg/kg) SC, IM, IT once	Red-eared sliders; excellent local nerve block and effective IT in chelonians	1,15
	1.0–2.0 mg/kg IT once	Bearded dragons; recommended 1 mg/kg for analgesia of caudal half of body; 2 mg/kg had negative systemic effects	52
Lidocaine (1% or 2%)	1.0–4.0 mg/kg (keep < 5.0 mg/kg) SC, IM, IT once	Red-eared sliders; excellent local nerve block and effective IT in chelonians	1,15
	0.2 mL/10 cm carapace length IT	Green sea turtles; cutaneous fibropapilloma excision; effective clinical analgesia	53
Lidocaine + Morphine	2.0 mg/kg + 0.1 mg/kg IT	Desert tortoises/orchiectomy analgesia	56
	2.0 mg/kg + (Mo) 0.5 mg/kg IT	Bearded dragons; neuraxial analgesia of caudal half of body for 12–24h	55
Mepivicaine (2%)	1.0 mg/kg SC once	Used as a mandibular nerve block in alligators	51
Proparacaine Ophthalmic solution (0.5%)	Topical eye drops	Blocked corneal sensitivity within 1 min of application with duration of effect at least 45 min in Kemp's ridley sea turtles; Green iguanas; bearded dragons; caiman; bearded dragons/IOP by rebound tonometry; Kemp's ridley sea turtles/one drop provided 45 min duration of action; do not exceed toxic dose 2 mg/kg; Yacare caiman/IOP by applanation tonometry	57–60

Other Anesthetics

Drug (class)	Dose	Description	Ref
Amitriptyline hydrochloride (serotonin and noradrenaline reuptake inhibitor)	3.0 mg/kg ICe	Speke's hinged-back tortoises; dampened the nociceptive response to SC formalin and capsaicin injections, but not a thermal noxious stimulus	65
Clonidine hydrochloride (α2-agonist)	40.0 μg/kg IT	Speke's hinged-back tortoises; intrathecal administration of clonidine (α2-adrenergic receptor agonist) and yohimbine (α2-adrenergic receptor antagonist) at a dose of 40 μg/kg and 37.5 μg/kg or 50 μg/kg, respectively, caused a highly significant reduction in the duration of the formalin-induced pain-related behavior.	64
Dexmedetomidine (α2-agonist)	0.1–0.2 mg/kg SC once	Ball pythons; thermal antinociception with minimal sedation	61,62
	0.2 mg/kg IM	Black and white tegus; antinociception to a thermal noxious stimulus	63
Yohimbine hydrochloride (α2-antagonist/5-HT agonist)	37.5 and 50.0 μg/kg	Speke's hinged-back tortoises; intrathecal administration of clonidine (α2-adrenergic receptor agonist) and yohimbine (α2-adrenergic receptor antagonist) at a dose of 40 μg/kg and 37.5 μg/kg or 50 μg/kg, respectively, caused a highly significant reduction in the duration of the formalin-induced pain-related behavior.	64

Abbreviations: h, hours; IM, intramuscular; IT, intrathecal; IV, intravenous; PK, pharmacokinetic; PO, oral; SC, subcutaneous; TC, transcutaneous.

administered μ-opioids, and this was replicated in the turtle data, in which we observed long-lasting respiratory depression, particularly at higher doses of morphine.[5,6] Black and white tegus (Salvator merianae) also showed antinociception to a thermal noxious stimulus after morphine administration (5 and 10 mg/kg IM),[10] and green iguanas (Iguana iguana) showed significantly reduced tail movement after an electrical stimulus was applied when morphine (1.0 mg/kg IM) was administered.[8] Similarly, morphine (5, 7.5, 10, and 20 mg/kg ICe) and pethidine (10, 20, and 50 mg/kg ICe) provided antinociception in Speke's hinged tortoises (Kinixys spekii) by dampening a limb withdrawal response after formalin was administered into the limb.[19] This antinociceptive response was abolished with the administration of the μ-antagonist, naloxone.[19] In another snake study, SC administered capsaicin was used as a noxious stimulus, which caused heart rate to elevate in ball pythons. Neither morphine (10 mg/kg IM) nor butorphanol (10 mg/kg IM) had an antinociceptive effect on the capsaicin-induced, elevated heart rate.[20] When morphine was administered intrathecally (01.–0.2 mg/kg) to red-eared slider turtles, it resulted in thermal antinociception of the hindlimbs for up to 48 h.[21]

Like morphine, hydromorphone is a μ-opioid receptor agonist, but is considered a semisynthetic ketone derivative of morphine with greater potency. Hydromorphone was shown to provide analgesia in red-eared sliders using the thermal hind limb withdrawal nociception model at 0.5 mg/kg SC for up to 24 h.[12] Hydromorphone plasma concentrations were considered analgesic, when compared with analgesic concentrations in mammals, for 12 to 24 h after bearded dragons and red-eared slider turtles were administered either 0.5 or 1.0 mg/kg but, as with morphine, respiratory depression was an adverse effect at higher doses.[17] The conclusion from this study was that an effective and relatively safe dosage of hydromorphone in both reptile species was 0.5 mg/kg SC q 24 h administered in the front half of the body.[17]

Fentanyl is a synthetic, μ-opioid receptor agonist, with 75 to 100 times the potency of morphine, which can be administered in reptiles TC as an impregnated patch (Fig. 2), SC, IM, or IV. Three separate studies have evaluated the pharmacokinetics of fentanyl in reptile species. In ball pythons (Python regius), fentanyl plasma concentrations reached 1 ng/mL (equivalent to mammalian analgesic concentration) within 4 h of application of a transdermal fentanyl patch (12.5 mcg/h).[14] In prehensile-tailed skinks (Corucia zebrata), plasma fentanyl concentrations after patch application (fentanyl dose was applied at 10% exposure of total surface area of a 25 mcg/h patch for 72 h) were detectable by 4 to 6 h and were measurable for greater than 72 h.[15] In two slider turtle species (Trachemys scripta elegans, Trachemys dorbigini), fentanyl (0.05 mg/kg SC) contributed to antinociception after a forceps-induced toe pinch.[16] A recently completed study in our laboratory evaluated the efficacy of transdermal fentanyl patch (12.5 mcg/h) administration in ball pythons exposed to the thermal noxious stimulus, and found no analgesic efficacy, even after repeating the study.[14] Our laboratory also confirmed that fentanyl was readily absorbed through the skin of the snakes and remained at very high plasma levels during patch application.[14] In the same study, we determined that fentanyl patch application decreased respiration in the snakes, so we know that fentanyl is biologically active in the snakes, even though we cannot definitively determine analgesic efficacy. However, recent anecdotal data from several snake species maintained in zoos and experiencing chronic painful conditions (eg, severe osteoarthritis/osteodystrophy) have shown that recurrent fentanyl patch application stimulates increased movement, climbing, and return to feeding (Sladky, unpublished data, 2018). Further evaluation of fentanyl analgesic efficacy using other experimental models in several snake species is currently underway. Summarizing the published μ-opioid data in reptiles provides the most consistent,

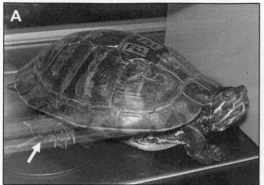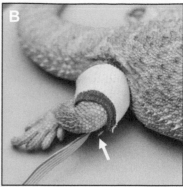

Fig. 1. Examples of noxious thermal limb withdrawal laboratory models for assessing pain and testing analgesic drugs. Red-eared slider turtle (*Trachemys scripta scripta*) with infrared heat source placed under the plantar surface of the turtle's hind limb (*white arrow*); rapid heat causes limb withdrawal measured in seconds (*A*). Bearded dragon (*Pogona vitticeps*) with heat source applied to the dorsal femoral region of the hind limb and secured with bandage material (*white arrow*); rapid heat causes limb withdrawal measured in seconds (*B*). (Bearded dragon photo courtesy of E. Couture)[23].

compelling, and convincing data in support of effective analgesics across multiple species.

Buprenorphine is an effective analgesic in many mammalian species and is used extensively because of its longer duration of action compared with other opioids. Buprenorphine has partial agonist activity at the μ-opioid receptor, partial or full agonist activity at the δ-opioid receptor, and antagonist activity at the κ-opioid receptor. Thus far, no published data have been able to substantiate the analgesic efficacy of buprenorphine in any reptile species. Buprenorphine did not alter responses to an electrical noxious stimulus in green iguanas.[8] Similarly, buprenorphine (0.1, 0.2, and 1.0 mg/kg, SC) provided no analgesic efficacy in red-eared slider turtles exposed to a noxious thermal stimulus.[12] Buprenorphine pharmacokinetics in reptiles were determined after SC administration in red-eared slider turtles, and effective dosages ranged from 0.075 to 0.1 mg/kg, which provided plasma concentrations at levels associated with analgesic efficacy in humans for approximately 24 h.[13] Interestingly, plasma concentrations of buprenorphine were reduced by approximately 70% when the drug was administered in the hind limb compared with the forelimb, supporting a significant

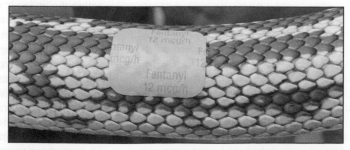

Fig. 2. Fentanyl patch (12 μg/h) placed along the lateral aspect of the dorsum of a California kingsnake (*Lampropeltis californiae*) at the anatomic level of the heart.

hepatic first-pass effect of this drug when administered SC. At present, buprenorphine is not considered to be an effective analgesic in reptiles, but more systematic research is necessary.

Butorphanol tartrate, a κ-opioid agonist/μ-opioid antagonist, was once considered the analgesic of choice in reptiles. However, most recent data support the concept that butorphanol has no clear analgesic properties in red-eared slider turtles, bearded dragons, corn snakes, ball pythons, and black and white tegus.[1,2] For example, intramuscular butorphanol (1 mg/kg) had no analgesic efficacy as determined by the use of a thermal noxious stimulus method,[9] and no isoflurane-sparing effect in green iguanas.[60] Butorphanol administered to red-eared slider turtles (2.8 and 28 mg/kg SC) and bearded dragons (2 and 20 mg/kg SC) provided no antinociception using a thermal noxious stimulus and measuring hind limb withdrawal.[5,7] In black and white tegus, butorphanol (5 and 10 mg/kg IM) had no effect on limb withdrawal to the thermal noxious stimulus.[10] In ball pythons, butorphanol administered at 5 mg/kg IM had no effect on physiologic parameters compared with saline after a surgical vertebral artery catheterization.[11] Data from the same research laboratory showed that butorphanol (10 mg/kg IM) had no antinociceptive effect on capsaicin-induced, elevated heart rate.[20] Conversely, one study showed that butorphanol (1.5 and 8 mg/kg, IM) provided antinociception in green iguanas exposed to a noxious electrical stimulus.[8] However, in the same study, butorphanol (4.0 mg/kg IM) was not statistically different from saline, so results from this study were equivocal overall, and it may speak to low subject numbers or the experimental model used. Overall, the evidence-based data on butorphanol efficacy across multiple reptile species suggest that it does not provide analgesia.

Tramadol has become a widely used analgesic alternative to other opioids in veterinary medicine, because it can be administered orally, and it has a relatively long duration of action. Tramadol and its major active metabolite, O-desmethyl-tramadol (M1), produce analgesia in mammals by activating μ-opioid receptors, but also by inhibiting central serotonin and norepinephrine reuptake.[61] Overall, tramadol binds μ-opioid receptors with 6000-times less affinity than morphine, thus having the potential for producing fewer μ-opioid-induced deleterious adverse effects, such as respiratory depression.[61] In fact, tramadol does not seem to alter breathing in humans when prescribed at typical analgesic dosages and produces significantly less respiratory depression than morphine.[61–63] In mammals, the analgesic effects of tramadol typically begin within 30 min after oral administration and have a typical duration of approximately 6 h. In red-eared slider turtles, tramadol (5.0 mg/kg; PO) significantly increased withdrawal latencies for 12 to 24 h postdrug administration, and 6 to 96 h after administration of higher tramadol dosages (10 or 25 mg/kg; PO or SC).[26] Doses of 5 mg/kg did not suppress ventilation and provided analgesia for at least 24 h in red-eared slider turtles.[63] In bearded dragons, a significant analgesic effect was observed in electrostimulation experiments at 11 mg/kg.[28] In loggerhead turtles (Caretta caretta), plasma concentrations of tramadol and M1, the primary metabolite referred to as M1, remained above the target concentration of ≥ 100 ng/mL (considered analgesic in mammals) for approximately 48 h at a dose of 5 mg/kg PO and for 72 h when tramadol was administered at 10 mg/kg PO.[29] Subjectively, appetite, swimming, and general activity level did not change after drug administration. More recently, tramadol pharmacokinetics and efficacy were evaluated in yellow-bellied slider turtles (Trachemys scripta scripta) after a single dose (10 mg/kg IM) was administered in either the hind limb or forelimb.[27] Using a thermal hind limb withdrawal latency model, antinociceptive efficacy appeared to last approximately 48 h regardless of whether the tramadol was administered in the forelimb or hind limb, and tramadol and M1 remained above a very high target plasma concentration (1 μg/mL or 1000 ng/mL) for approximately 48 h.[27] Of interest, was that the pharmacokinetic trends were similar for tramadol administration in forelimbs and hind limbs, but the concentrations of M1 were approximately 20% higher in the plasma of the group receiving tramadol in the hind limbs compared with those receiving tramadol in the forelimbs, suggesting that tramadol undergoes hepatic first-pass metabolism and the primary metabolite remains active in the systemic circulation and tissues for a longer duration. With respect to deleterious adverse effects, respiratory depression associated with tramadol administration in red-eared slider turtles (10 and 25 mg/kg SC and PO) was approximately 50% less than that measured after morphine administration.[26] Therefore, tramadol seems to be a promising analgesic alternative to traditional opioids in some reptile species, although nearly all of the current efficacy and pharmacokinetic data come from aquatic chelonian species, and there is definitely a need for more research in terrestrial reptiles.

Tapendatol, similar mechanistically to tramadol, is a human drug that shares mu-opioid receptor activation and serotonin/norepinephrine reuptake inhibition with tramadol, but tapendatol has only weak serotonergic reuptake and has more potent opioid properties without an active metabolite. Tapendatol was administered to red-eared and yellow-bellied slider turtles in order to determine analgesic efficacy using a thermal noxious stimulus model and pharmacokinetics.[24,25] After administration (5 mg/kg IM), tapendatol plasma concentrations were detectable for approximately 24 h and the duration of antinociceptive effects was approximately 10 h in both turtle species.[24,25] The shorter duration of antinociceptive efficacy, compared with tramadol, may be due to the lack of an active metabolite.

Non-steroidal Anti-inflammatory Drugs

Although not as potent as the opioids from an analgesia perspective, non-steroidal anti-inflammatory drugs (NSAIDs) are used widely in reptile clinical practice as both analgesics and for their anti-inflammatory properties (**Table 1**). NSAIDs provide analgesia in mammals by blocking the binding of arachidonic acid to cyclooxygenase enzyme (COX), preventing the conversion of thromboxane A2 to thromboxane B2 (TBX), thus preventing the production of prostaglandins (PG), potent mediators of inflammation.[64] Hence, they are commonly categorized as COX inhibitors. In addition, NSAIDs are classified based on their relative COX specificity. There are two COX enzymes, COX-1 and COX-2, which are involved in renal and gastric protection and inflammation, respectively.[64] Some NSAIDs primarily inhibit the COX-1 isoenzyme, others inhibit primarily COX-2 isoenzyme, whereas some are relatively equipotent inhibitors of COX-1 and COX-2 isoenzymes.[64] Therefore, the degree of efficacy and adverse effects may vary with each specific NSAID selected and administered.

Determining the efficacy of NSAIDs in reptiles is very difficult to measure, which is why most studies on reptiles and NSAIDs are pharmacokinetic studies. As such, it is difficult to recommend effective and safe dosing intervals as plasma concentrations of NSAIDs do not always directly correspond with clinical efficacy or tissue concentrations.[60] Although many NSAIDs seem to be relatively safe when used in reptiles, there are only a few published studies with respect to analgesic efficacy. Meloxicam, which mechanistically confers primarily COX-2 inhibition, is now widely used in clinical veterinary medicine. For example, ball pythons administered meloxicam (0.3 mg/kg, IM) before a surgical placement of an arterial catheter showed no physiologic changes (eg, heart rate, blood pressure, plasma epinephrine, and cortisol), which was similar to saline and, therefore, not indicative of any analgesic properties.[11] However, meloxicam (0.4 mg/kg IM) was effective in significantly decreasing tail movement responses in bearded dragons to electrostimulation, as was carprofen (2 mg/kg and 4 mg/kg IM) and ketoprofen (2 mg/kg IM), compared with saline.[28]

Unlike few published meloxicam efficacy data, there are several published pharmacokinetic studies of meloxicam in reptiles. Plasma concentrations of meloxicam (0.2 mg/kg, PO, IV) administered as a single dose to green iguanas were equivalent to those considered analgesic in mammals, and these concentrations were measurable out to 24 h postadministration.[37] The same study also evaluated the safety of high doses of meloxicam (1–5 mg/kg PO) administered for 12 days in a small subset of green iguanas, and observed no abnormal histologic changes to renal, hepatic, or gastric tissues.[37] Similarly, daily administration of meloxicam (0.2 mg/kg IM) or carprofen (2 mg/kg IM) for 10 days in green iguanas did not cause significant alterations to hematological or serum biochemical parameters.[30] In loggerhead sea turtles, meloxicam (0.1 mg/kg IM and IV) plasma concentrations were not consistent with analgesic plasma concentrations in humans, horses or dogs, and the half-life was short.[41] However, in a pharmacokinetic study in which meloxicam (0.2 mg/kg IM and IV) was administered to red-eared slider turtles, the IM dose, but not the IV dose, provided a therapeutic concentration range necessary for meloxicam to provide analgesic and anti-inflammatory effects equivalent to those in mammals for approximately 48 h.[42] In a separate study evaluating the pharmacokinetics of meloxicam (0.2 mg/kg PO, ICe, and IM) in red-eared slider turtles, only the ICe and IM routes, but not the PO route, provided mean plasma concentrations of meloxicam that were above those considered effective to induce anti-inflammatory effects in mammals for approximately 8 h (IM) or 12 h (ICe).[38] In a comparative sea turtle study, administration of meloxicam (1 mg/kg SC) in Kemp's ridley (*Lepidochelys kempii*) and green sea turtles (*Chelonia mydas*) resulted in plasma concentrations greater than those considered effective in mammals for 12 and 120 h, respectively, whereas the administration of meloxicam (2 mg/kg SC) to loggerhead sea turtles resulted in plasma concentrations greater than those considered effective in mammals for only 4 h.[45] The same research group used a follow-up, multidose pharmacokinetic study to show that meloxicam (1 mg/kg SC) should be administered to Kemp's ridley sea turtles every 12 h and in green sea turtles every 48 h.[44] In red-eared slider turtles, IM administration of meloxicam (0.5 mg/kg) provided the most consistent clinical pharmacokinetic profile compared with IV (0.22 mg/kg) or PO (0.5 mg/kg), with a terminal half-life of 7.57 h, whereas oral bioavailability was only 37%.[43] With recent increased interest in determining the efficacy and pharmacokinetics of meloxicam in a variety of reptile species, the resulting data look promising, but efficacy data continue to lag behind the pharmacokinetic data.

Ketoprofen is relatively equipotent in the inhibition of both COX-1 and COX-2 isoenzymes. Many veterinarians who work with sea turtle species subjectively feel that it has been a good choice in terms of improving behavior, particularly of injured free-ranging turtles that end up in rehabilitation facilities. Ketoprofen (2 mg/kg, IV), administered to green iguanas, had a long half-life (31 h) compared with ketoprofen pharmacokinetics in mammals, but the bioavailability after IM (2 mg/kg) administration was 78% with a relatively short half-life (8.3 h).[31] In loggerhead sea turtles, a ketoprofen dose (2 mg/kg IM or IV q24 h) is likely appropriate based on therapeutic plasma concentrations equivalent to mammals.[32] Regarding safety, ketoprofen (2 mg/kg IM) administered q24 hr for up to 5 days in loggerhead sea turtles appeared to be safe with respect to blood clotting and other blood alterations.[33] Recently, the safety of ketoprofen was evaluated in bearded dragons.[34] Bearded dragons were administered ketoprofen at 2 doses (2.0 and 20.0 mg/kg IM in triceps muscle), and several parameters were measured including; serum biochemical changes, presence of occult blood, and histopathology of the triceps muscle, gastrointestinal, hepatic, and renal systems. The only significant adverse reaction was severe triceps muscle necrosis in the 20.0 mg/kg group. Otherwise, there were no other measured adverse changes.[34] The group evaluating ketoprofen safety in loggerhead sea turtles also evaluated the pharmacokinetics of a single dose of ketorolac (0.25 mg/kg IM), a COX-1 and COX-2 inhibitor, in loggerhead sea turtles, and determined that therapeutic plasma concentrations equivalent to humans were never achieved, so they could not recommend its use in this species.[36] However, the same dose of ketorolac (0.25 mg/kg IM) administered to eastern box turtles (*Terrapene carolina carolina*) provided plasma concentrations above a therapeutic target level for 24-h analgesia, suggesting once-daily dosing.[35]

Recently, tolfenamic acid, which has relatively equipotent COX-1 and COX-2 inhibition, was evaluated pharmacokinetically in two species of chelonians. Tolfenamic acid is traditionally used in humans, primarily for relieving migraine headaches. In green sea turtles, plasma concentrations after a single dose of tolfenamic acid (4 mg/kg IM) achieved levels considered anti-inflammatory for up to 7 days.[47] The results in red-eared slider turtles administered tolfenamic acid (2 and 4 mg/kg IV and 2 mg/kg IM) were less convincing and may have been therapeutic for less than 24 h.[46]

Local Anesthetics

Local anesthetics can be used alone or as part of a multimodal anesthetic/analgesic regimen. These include lidocaine, bupivacaine, and mepivacaine, or topical ocular proparacaine, which block peripheral nerve transmission to the dorsal horn by inhibiting sodium influx into the neurons and therefore blocking the nociceptive signal from traveling along the nerve fibers. For all local anesthetics, the pain transmission is blocked as long as the local anesthetic nerve block lasts, but inflammation and pain will still develop at the site of injury and will be transmitted to the central nervous system after the effect of the block has ceased. Because of its significant analgesic effect, any local block that is correctly executed will significantly decrease the required amount of other anesthetic agents, but additional analgesia is warranted for postoperative pain management in many cases. With respect to the local effects of these anesthetics, there is only one published reptile study, in which mepivacaine was used as a mandibular nerve block in an American alligator (*Alligator mississippiensis*).[51] In this study, a nerve locator was used to facilitate the procedure. Lidocaine (2%) (up to 5 mg/kg total dose) can be used for local ring blocks or line blocks. Lidocaine may be diluted with bicarbonate or sterile water at a 1:1 ratio or greater to decrease the pain of injection and allow the increased volume to be infused without reaching a toxic dose. In addition, topical lidocaine (4%) is commonly administered directly to wounds before and after debridement for local analgesia, particularly in the chelonian species. Intrathecal administration of local anesthetics is useful for surgical procedures of the tail, phallus, cloaca, and hind limbs.[20] Intrathecal administration of lidocaine (4 mg/kg) or bupivacaine (1 mg/kg) in red-eared sliders resulted in a motor block of the hindlimbs for approximately 1 h and 2 h, respectively (**Fig. 3**).[21] Lidocaine (4 mg/kg; <1 h duration), bupivacaine (1 mg/kg; 1–2 h duration) or preservative-free morphine sulfate (0.1–0.2 mg/kg; duration of up to 48 h) can be administered intrathecally between the coccygeal vertebrae of turtles and bearded dragons (see **Fig. 3**).[21,48] For example, bupivacaine (0.1 mL for each 10 cm of the carapace) was administered intrathecally in order to facilitate surgical excision of fibropapillomas from the posterior flippers of a green sea turtle.[49] In a different study, lidocaine (1 mL/20–25 kg) was administered intrathecally in hybrid Galapagos tortoises (*Chelonoidis niger*) before phallectomy surgery.[65] Lidocaine can be combined with morphine for intrathecal administration as

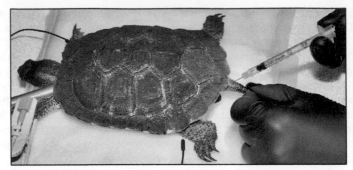

Fig. 3. Needle placement for administering neuraxial analgesia/anesthesia in a red-eared slider turtle (*Trachemys scripta scripta*) (see technique description under **Fig. 4**). (Photo courtesy of Christoph Mans.).[3].

well. In bearded dragons, lidocaine (2 mg/kg) + morphine (0.5 mg/kg) IT was effective for providing analgesia to the caudal half of the body for 12 to 24 h (**Fig. 4**).[50] In desert tortoises (*Gopherus agassizii*) undergoing orchiectomy, lidocaine (2 mg/kg) + morphine (0.1 mg/kg) IT was effective in providing analgesia in the caudal half of the body.[39,40] For topical ocular administration, proparacaine hydrochloride (0.5%) has been used clinically in reptiles during eye exams, especially to measure intraocular pressure. Proparacaine was shown to be effective in blocking corneal sensitivity in Kemp's ridley turtles for up to 45 min, with a 1-min onset to effect.[52] Similar proparacaine results were determined in bearded dragons[40] and Yacare caiman (*Caiman yacare*).[54] Although no efficacy data exist for liposome-encapsulated bupivacaine (Nocita; approved for use in dogs and cats), this locally administered adjunct to multimodal analgesia has been used in several reptile species during surgical closure at the mammalian dose (5.3 mg/kg or 0.4 mL/kg) (Sladky, unpublished data). The duration of action in mammals is approximately 72 h, but we have no idea about the duration of action in reptiles. However, of importance is that this formulation is significantly more expensive than simply instilling the surgical wound with standard bupivacaine.

Other Drug Classes

There are few published data showing analgesic efficacy associated with the administration of anesthetic drugs, such as dissociative anesthetics, α2-adrenergic receptor agonists, benzodiazepines, serotonin, and noradrenaline reuptake inhibitors, or calcium-channel blockers in reptiles (**Table 1**). Although α2-adrenergic drugs are commonly used, in combination with ketamine or midazolam for sedation and anesthetic induction in reptiles, few data exist with respect to the analgesic effects of these drugs. Dexmedetomidine (0.1–0.2 mg/kg SC) produced antinociception to a thermal noxious stimulus for up to 24 h in ball pythons.[57,58] Similarly, in black and white tegu lizards exposed to a thermal noxious stimulus, dexmedetomidine (0.2 mg/kg, IM) provided antinociception without sedation, whereas midazolam (1.0 mg/kg, IM) provided no antinociception, but caused sedation.[59] In Speke's hinged tortoises, intrathecal administration of clonidine (40 μg/kg; an α2-adrenergic receptor agonist) and yohimbine (37.5 μg/kg or 50 μg/kg; an α2-adrenergic receptor antagonist) caused a significant reduction in the duration of formalin-induced hind limb withdrawal.[56] The same laboratory also showed that amitriptyline hydrochloride (3.0 mg/kg ICe), a serotonin and noradrenaline reuptake inhibitor used for neuropathic pain and as an

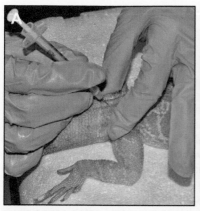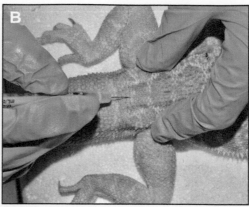

Fig. 4. Needle placement for administering neuraxial analgesia/anesthesia in a bearded dragon (*Pogona vitticeps*). The neuraxial technique is accomplished using the following guidelines[3]: identify the sacrococcygeal junction by lateral movement of the tail base; following sterile preparation and using an insulin syringe, insert needle at approximately 75-degree angle midline at the level of the sacrococcygeal junction with the bevel facing cranially (*A*); slowly advance needle until a twitch of a pelvic limb or tail occurs (this may or may not happen) (*B*); aspirate before drug administration, to check for the presence of blood; if blood is aspirated, abort the injection and restart process with new needle/syringe; administer drug(s) slowly over 2 to 5 s, depending on volume. If there is no obvious motor block of the pelvic limbs or if cloacal tone is not lost within 5 to 10 min, another injection at the same dose can be performed. (Photo courtesy of Christoph Mans.).[3]

antidepressant in humans, was antinociceptive as measured by limb withdrawal after limb injection of both formalin or capsaicin in Speke's hinge-back tortoises.[55] A quick word about other commonly used anesthetic drugs in reptiles without evidence-based data to support analgesia. Although there is interest in, and compelling data to support the idea that low-dose ketamine, a dissociative anesthetic, provides analgesia in mammals, there are no efficacy data in reptiles, even though it is used widely for sedation. Similarly, although many veterinarians are administering alfaxalone, a neurosteroid, for sedation in a variety of reptile species, there is no evidence of any analgesic activity in reptiles or mammals. Along these same lines, gabapentin, a calcium-channel blocker used in humans for control of neuropathic pain, is being widely used as a broad-spectrum analgesic in veterinary medicine, however, there are no published data supporting efficacy in reptiles. In sum, the α2-agonists may show great promise for providing analgesia with minimal sedation in reptiles.

Multimodal Analgesic Approaches

In reptiles, like mammals, multimodal drug paradigms may be the best approach for managing pain. Multimodal analgesia refers to the administration of multiple drugs and/or drug types, which have analgesic efficacy at different levels of the central and peripheral nervous system. For example, opioids will have the greatest efficacy at opioid receptors in the central and peripheral nervous system, whereas NSAIDs administered at the same time as the opioid will have the greatest efficacy as anti-inflammatory agents in the peripheral tissues. Local anesthetics can enhance multimodal analgesic protocols by blocking the initial pain cascade at the peripheral level. In concert, all of these drugs have the potential to minimize the transmission of pain signals to the brain, especially when administered preemptively, before a potentially painful procedure is established.

SUMMARY

The field of reptile analgesia has dramatically expanded during the last 20 years, affording us some sense of what might work and what likely does not work. Perhaps more importantly is the fact that many veterinarians are more aware than ever before, that reptiles experience pain in ways similar to mammals, and that conditions deemed painful in mammals should be addressed through the use of multimodal analgesics in reptile patients. On the basis of our current knowledge, when considering opioids, μ-opioid receptor agonists, such as morphine and hydromorphone, are the preferred choice. Tramadol (5–10 mg/kg PO) is a good choice for long-acting analgesia in some reptile species. Personally, I like using hydromorphone in most reptile species (0.5 mg/kg SC or IM in the cranial half of the body), or a fentanyl patch especially in snakes (empirically, 12 μg/h patch in snakes < 5 kg; 25 μg/h patch in snakes 5–10 kg). Although administering NSAIDs to reptiles may make us feel better than the patient because we have few methods for measuring efficacy, I tend to add meloxicam (0.5–1.0 mg/kg SC) or ketoprofen (2 mg/kg SC) to my analgesic mix. Local anesthetic blocks are excellent and complementary drugs to add to combinations. Instilling lidocaine or bupivacaine directly SC for a local block or into a nerve bundle for a regional block can facilitate a more normal recovery. In addition, administering these local anesthetics directly into the tissues of a surgical wound (standard bupivacaine or liposome-encapsulated bupivacaine) may help with postsurgical recovery. If a neuraxial block is warranted for invasive procedures in the caudal half of the body of lizards and chelonians, consider a combination of lidocaine (2 mg/kg) $\pm$ morphine (0.5 mg/kg). Extrapolation of analgesic efficacy across orders and species remains a major limitation, and there is a clear need for evaluating analgesic drugs across a variety of clinical situations, particularly as they apply to postsurgical pain. Developing objectively derived methods for evaluation of pain in animals is critical, but these methods must be species- and context-specific. In addition, determining pharmacokinetic parameters, duration of drug efficacy, species-specific requirements, and deleterious adverse effects of opioid drugs in different reptile species remains critical to continue to advance the field of reptile analgesia.

DISCLOSURE

Nothing to disclose.

REFERENCES

1. Sladky KK, Mans C. Analgesia. In: Mader DR, Divers S, editors. Current therapy in reptile medicine and surgery. 3rd edition. St Louis (MO): Elsevier-Saunders; 2014. p. 217–28.

2. Sladky KK. Reptile and Amphibian Analgesia. In: Miller ER, Calle PP, Lamberski N, editors. Fowler's zoo and wild animal medicine, vol. 9. St Louis (MO): Elsevier-Saunders; 2019. p. 421–39.

3. Ferreira TH, Mans C. Sedation and anesthesia of lizards. Vet Clin NA Exot Anim Pract 2022;25:73–95.

4. Burgos-Rodriguez AG, Hoover JP, Zollinger TJ, et al. Distribution of 99mTc-dimercaptosuccinic Acid after Intramuscular Injection in the Caudal Limb and Tail of

Green Iguanas, *Iguana iguana*, Using Nuclear Scintigraphy. J Herp Med Surg 2008;18:37–44.

5. Sladky KK, Miletic V, Paul-Murphy J, et al. Analgesic efficacy and respiratory effects of butorphanol and morphine in turtles. J Am Vet Med Assoc 2007;230: 1356–62.

6. Kinney M, Johnson SM, Sladky KK. Behavioral evaluation of red-eared slider turtles (*Trachemys scripta*) administered either morphine or butorphanol following unilateral gonadectomy. J Herp Med Surg 2011;21:54–62.

7. Sladky KK, Kinney ME, Johnson SM. Analgesic efficacy of butorphanol and morphine in bearded dragons and corn snakes. J Am Vet Med Assoc 2008; 233:267–73.

8. Greenacre CB, Schumacher JP, Tacke G, et al. Comparative antinociception of morphine, butorphanol, and buprenorphine versus saline in the green iguana, *Iguana iguana*, using electrostimulation. J Herp Med Surg 2006;16:88–92.

9. Fleming GJ, Robertson SA. Assessments of thermal antinociceptive effects of butorphanol and human observer effect on quantitative evaluation of analgesia in green iguanas (*Iguana iguana*). Am J Vet Res 2012;73:1507–11.

10. Leal WP, Carregaro AB, Bressan TF, et al. Antinociceptive efficacy of intramuscular administration of morphine sulfate and butorphanol tartrate in tegus (*Salvator merianae*). Am J Vet Res 2016;78:1019–24.

11. Olesen MG, Bertelsen MF, Perry SF, et al. Effects of preoperative administration of butorphanol or meloxicam on physiologic responses to surgery in ball pythons. J Am Vet Med Assoc 2008;233:1883–8.

12. Mans C, Lahner LL, Baker BB, et al. Antinociceptive efficacy of buprenorphine and hydromorphone in red-eared slider turtles (*Trachemys scripta elegans*). J Zoo Wildl Med 2012;43:662–5.

13. Kummrow MS, Tseng F, Hesse L, et al. Pharmacokinetics of buprenorphine after single-dose subcutaneous administration in red-eared sliders (*Trachemys scripta elegans*). J Zoo Wildl Med 2008;39:590–5.

14. Kharbush R, Gutwillig A, Hartzler K, et al. Antinociceptive and respiratory effects following application of transdermal fentanyl patches and assessment of brain μ-opioid receptor mRNA expression in ball pythons. Am J Vet Res 2017;78:785–95.

15. Gamble KC. Plasma fentanyl concentrations achieved after transdermal fentanyl patch application in prehensile-tailed skinks, *Corucia zebrata*. J Herp Med Surg 2008;18:81–5.

16. Kaminishi APS, de Freitas AC, Henderson R, et al. Antinociceptive and physiological effects of subcutaneously administration of fentanyl in *Trachemys* spp. (Testudines: Emydidae). Intl J Adv Engineer Res Sci 2019;6:311–6.

17. Hawkins SJ, Cox S, Yaw TJ, et al. Pharmacokinetics of subcutaneous administered hydromorphone in bearded dragons (*Pogona vitticeps*) and red-eared slider turtles (*Trachemys scripta elegans*). Vet Anaesth Analg 2019;46(3):352–9.

18. Kanui TI, Hole K. Morphine and pethidine antinociception in the crocodile. J Vet Pharmacol Ther 1992;15:101–3.

19. Wambugu SN, Towett PK, Kiama SG, et al. Effects of opioids in the formalin test in the Speke's hinged tortoise (*Kinixy's spekii*). J Vet Pharmacol Ther 2010;33: 347–51.

20. Williams CJA, James LE, Bertelsen MF, et al. Tachycardia in response to remote capsaicin injection as a model for nociception in the ball python (*Python regius*). Vet Anaesth Analg 2015;43:429–34.

21. Mans C. Clinical technique: Intrathecal drug administration in turtles and tortoises. J Exot Pet Med 2014;23:67–70.

22. Mauk MD, Olson RD, Lahoste GJ, et al. Tonic immobility produces hyperalgesia and antagonizes morphine analgesia. Science 1981;13:353–4.
23. Couture EL, Monteirob BP, Aymen J, et al. Validation of a thermal threshold nociceptive model in bearded dragons (*Pogona vitticeps*). Vet Anaesth Analg 2017; 44:676–83.
24. Giorgi M, Lee H-K, Rota S, et al. Pharmacokinetic and pharmacodynamics assessments of tapentadol in yellow-bellied slider turtles (*Trachemys scripta scripta*) after a single intramuscular injection. J Exot Pet Med 2015;24:317–25.
25. Giorgi M, De Vito V, Owen H, et al. PK/PD evaluations of the novel atypical opioid tapentadol in red-eared slider turtles. Med Weter 2014;70:530–5.
26. Baker BB, Sladky KK, Johnson SM. Evaluation of the analgesic effects of oral and subcutaneous tramadol administration in red-eared slider turtles. J Am Vet Med Assoc 2011;238:220–7.
27. Giorgi M, Salvadori M, De Vito V, et al. Pharmacokinetic/pharmacodynamics assessments of 10 mg/kg tramadol intramuscular injection in yellow-bellied slider turtles (*Trachemys scripta scripta*). J Vet Pharmacol Ther 2015;38:488–96.
28. Greenacre CB, Massi K, Schumacher JP, et al. Comparative antinociception of various opioids and non-steroidal anti-inflammatory medications versus saline in the bearded dragon (*Pogona vitticeps)* using electrostimulation. Proc Annu Conf Rept Amph Vet 2008;87–8.
29. Norton TM, Cox S, Nelson S, et al. Pharmacokinetics of tramadol and o-desmethyltramadol in loggerhead sea turtles (*Caretta caretta*). J Zoo Wildife Med 2015;46:262–5.
30. Trnková S, Knotková Z, Hrdá A, et al. Effect of non-steroidal anti-inflammatory drugs on the blood profile in the green iguana (*Iguana iguana*). Vet Med (Czech) 2007;52:507–11.
31. Tuttle AD, Papich M, Lewbart GA, et al. Pharmacokinetics of ketoprofen in the green iguana (*Iguana iguana*) following single intravenous and intramuscular injections. J Zoo Wildl Med 2006;37:567–70.
32. Thompson KA, Papich MG, Higgins B, et al. Ketoprofen pharmacokinetics of R-and S-isomers in juvenile loggerhead sea turtles (*Caretta caretta*) after single intravenous and single-and multidose intramuscular administration. J Vet Pharmacol Ther 2018;41:340–8.
33. Harms CA, Ruterbories LK, Stacy NI, et al. Safety of multiple-dose intramuscular ketoprofen treatment in loggerhead turtles (*Caretta caretta*). J Zoo Wildl Med 2021;52(1):126–32.
34. Vigneault A, Lair S, Gara-Boivin C, et al. Evaluation of the Safety of Multiple Intramuscular Doses of Ketoprofen in Bearded Dragons (*Pogona vitticeps*) ketoprofen in bearded dragons. J Herp Med Surg 2022;32. preprint.
35. Cerreta AJ, Masterson CA, Lewbart GA, et al. Pharmacokinetics of ketorolac in wild Eastern box turtles (*Terrapene carolina carolina*) after single intramuscular administration. Vet Pharm Therap 2019;42:154–9.
36. Gregory TM, Harms CA, Gorges MA, et al. Pharmacokinetics of ketorolac in juvenile loggerhead sea turtles (*Caretta caretta*) after a single intramuscular injection. J Vet Pharmacol Ther 2021;44:583–9.
37. Divers SJ, Papich M, McBride M, et al. Pharmacokinetics of meloxicam following intravenous and oral administration in green iguanas (*Iguana iguana*). Am J Vet Res 2010;71:1277–83.
38. Uney K, Altan F, Aboubakr M, et al. Pharmacokinetics of meloxicam in red-eared slider turtles (*Trachemys scripta elegans*) after single intravenous and intramuscular injections. Am J Vet Res 2016;77:439–44.

39. Proenca LM, Fowler S, Kleine S, et al. Coelioscopic-assisted sterilization of female Mojave desert tortoises (*Gopherus agassizii*). J Herp Med Surg 2014;24: 95–100.

40. Proenca LM, Fowler S, Kleine S, et al. Single surgeon coelioscopic orchiectomy of desert tortoises (*Gopherus agassizii*) for population management. Vet Rec 2014; 175:404–9.

41. Lai OR, Di Bello A, Soloperto S, et al. Pharmacokinetic behavior of meloxicam in loggerhead sea turtles (*Caretta caretta*) after intramuscular and intravenous administration. J Wildl Dis 2015;51:509–12.

42. Di Salvo A, Giorgi M, Catanzaro A, et al. Pharmacokinetic profiles of meloxicam in turtles (*Trachemys scripta scripta*) after single oral, intracoelomic and intramuscular administrations. Vet Pharmacol Therap 2015;39:102–5.

43. Rojo-Solís C, Ros-Rodriguez JM, Valls M. Pharmacokinetics of meloxicam (Metacam) after intravenous, intramuscular, and oral administration in red-eared slider turtles (*Trachemys scripta elegans*). Proc Conf Am Assoc Zoo Vet 2009;228.

44. Norton TM, Clauss T, Overmeyer R. Multi-injection pharmacokinetics of meloxicam in Kemp's ridley (*Lepidochelys kempii*) and green (*Chelonia mydas*) sea turtles after subcutaneous administration. Animals 2021;11:3522.

45. Norton TM, Clauss T, Sommer R, et al. Pharmacokinetic behavior of meloxicam in loggerhead (*Caretta caretta*), Kemp's ridley (*Lepidochelys kempii*), and green (*Chelonia mydas*) sea turtles after subcutaneous administration. J Zoo Wildl Med 2021;52(1):295–9.

46. Coruma O, Atikb O, Coruma DD, et al. Pharmacokinetics of tolfenamic acid in red-eared slider turtles (*Trachemys scripta elegans*). Vet Anaesth Analg 2019; 46:699–706.

47. Raweewan N, Chomcheun T, Laovechprasit W, et al. Pharmacokinetics of tolfenamic acid in green sea turtles (*Chelonia mydas*) after intravenous and intramuscular administration. J Vet Pharmacol Ther 2020;43:527–31.

48. Ferreira T, Fink DM, Mans C. Evaluation of neuraxial administration of bupivacaine in bearded dragons (*Pogona vitticeps*). Vet Anaesth Analg 2021;48:798–803.

49. Futema F, de Carvalho FM, Werneck MR. Spinal anesthesia in green sea turtles (*Chelonia mydas*) undergoing surgical removal of cutaneous fibropapillomas. J Zoo Wildl Med 2020;51:357–62.

50. Fink DM, Ferreira TH, Mans C. Neuraxial administration of morphine combined with lidocaine induces regional antinociception in inland bearded dragons (*Pogona vitticeps*). Am J Vet Res 2022;83:212–7.

51. Wellehan JFX, Gunkel CI, Kledzik D, et al. Use of a nerve locator to facilitate administration of mandibular nerve blocks in crocodilians. J Zoo Wildl Med 2006;37:405–8.

52. Gornik KR, Pirie CG, Marrion RM, et al. Baseline corneal sensitivity and duration of action of proparacaine in rehabilitated juvenile Kemp's Ridley sea turtles (*Lepidochelys kempii*). J Herp Med Surg 2015;25:116–21.

53. Schuster EJ, Strueve J, Fehr MJ, et al. Measurement of intraocular pressure in healthy unanesthetized inland bearded dragons (*Pogona vitticeps*). Am J Vet Res 2015;76:494–9.

54. Ruiz T, Campos WNS, Peres TPS, et al. Intraocular pressure, ultrasonographic and echobiometric findings of juvenile Yacare caiman (*Caiman yacare*) eye. Vet Ophtalmol 2015;18:40–5.

55. Makau CM, Towett PK, Abelson KSP, et al. Modulation of nociception by amitriptyline hydrochloride in the Speke's hinge-back tortoise (*Kiniskys spekii*). Vet Med Sci 2021;7:1034–41.

56. Makau CM, Towett PK, Abelson KSP, et al. Modulation of formalin-induced pain-related behaviour by clonidine and yohimbine in the Speke's hinged tortoise (*Kiniskys spekii*). J Vet Pharmacol Ther 2017;40:439–46.
57. Bunke L, Sladky KK, Johnson SM. Antinociceptive efficacy and respiratory effects of dexmedetomidine in ball pythons (*Python regius*). Am J Vet Res 2018; 79:718–26.
58. Karklus AA, Sladky KK, Johnson SM. Respiratory and antinociceptive effects of dexmedetomidine and doxapram in ball pythons (*Python regius*). Am J Vet Res 2021;82:11.
59. Bisetto SP, Melo CF, Carregaro AB. Evaluation of sedative and antinociceptive effects of dexmedetomidine, midazolam and dexmedetomidine-midazolam in tegus (*Salvator merianae*). Vet Anaesth Analg 2018;45:320–8.
60. Mosley CA, Dyson D, Smith DA. Minimum alveolar concentration of isoflurane in green iguanas and the effect of butorphanol on minimum alveolar concentration. J Am Vet Med Assoc 2003;222:1559–64.
61. Lewis KS, Han NH. Tramadol: A new centrally acting analgesic. Am J Health Syst Pharm 1997;54:643–52.
62. Scott LJ, Perry CM. Tramadol: A review of its use in perioperative pain. Drugs 2000;60:139–76.
63. Mastrocinque S, Fantoni DT. A comparison of preoperative tramadol and morphine for the control of early postoperative pain in canine ovariohysterectomy. Vet Anaesth Analg 2003;30:220–8.
64. Budsberg SC. Nonsteroidal anti-inflammatory drugs. In: Gaynor J, Muir WW, editors. Handbook of veterinary pain management. 2nd edition. Toronto: Mosby; 2009. p. 183–239.
65. Rivera S, Divers SJ, Knafo SE, et al. Sterilisation of hybrid Galapagos tortoises (*Geochelone nigra*) for island restoration. Part 2: phallectomy of males under intrathecal anaesthesia with lidocaine. Vet Rec 2011;168:78.

Pain Recognition and Assessment in Birds

Nicole A. Mikoni, DVM[a],

David Sanchez-Migallon Guzman, LV, MS, Dipl, ECZM (Avian, Small Mammal), Dipl, ACZM[b],*,

Joanne Paul-Murphy, DVM, Dipl, ACZM, Dipl, ACAW[b]

KEYWORDS

- Pain recognition • Pain assessment • Avian • Acute pain • Chronic pain
- Visceral pain • Somatic pain • Pain-related behaviors

KEY POINTS

- Avian species display a variety of physiologic and behavioral alterations that can be used to recognize and assess pain and discomfort.
- Differences in the source (visceral, somatic, neuropathic), chronicity (acute vs chronic), and degree (mild, moderate, severe) of pain can lead to differences in pain response in birds.
- Stress even in the absence of pain can significantly alter behavior and therefore should be accounted for when evaluating avian patients suspected to be in discomfort.
- In addition to evaluating for abnormal behaviors suggestive of being associated with noxious stimuli, a decrease or lack of normal behavioral displays can also signify pain in avian species.
- Given the overall reduction in ability to express pain via facial expression in birds, in contrast to mammals, evaluation of the avian patient should instead focus on the whole individual, and variations in positioning of the tail, wings, and crest may provide useful information.

INTRODUCTION

The recognition and assessment of behavioral changes associated with pain in birds are crucial tools in providing adequate pain management and supportive care in clinical, laboratory, zoologic, rehabilitation, and even companion animal settings.[1–3] Despite birds being a highly diverse class of vertebrates, comprising almost 10,000 different species, there is still much to be determined regarding how to create specific

[a] William R. Pritchard Veterinary Medical Teaching Hospital, University of California, Davis School of Veterinary Medicine, 944 Garrod Drive, Davis, CA 95616, USA; [b] Department of Medicine and Epidemiology, University of California, Davis School of Veterinary Medicine, Davis, CA 95616, USA

* Corresponding author.

E-mail address: guzman@ucdavis.edu

Vet Clin Exot Anim 26 (2023) 65–81
https://doi.org/10.1016/j.cvex.2022.09.002
1094-9194/23/© 2022 Elsevier Inc. All rights reserved.

criteria to recognize and assess pain in these animals.[4,5] In addition to being familiar with the normal, unaltered behavior of a given avian species, one must also recognize that different species may respond to pain in unique manners. However, current information regarding species-specific behaviors of birds in pain is limited, and although it is known that birds have the anatomic and physiologic components to respond to painful stimuli, a validated way of measuring these responses has yet to be determined. A pain scale or other assessment created for one avian species would ideally need to be validated for that given species, and extrapolations made to other avian species may not be accurate.

THE PHYSIOLOGY OF PAIN IN BIRDS

For the purposes of this article, a brief overview of the physiology of pain in avian species is provided; for a more in-depth discussion of this aspect of avian medicine, please refer to "Pain in Birds: The Anatomical and Physiological Basis" in *Veterinary Clinics: Exotic Animal Practice*.[6] In response to introduction of a noxious stimulus (one that may damage tissues), there are 2 physiologic processes involved: a peripheral process involving detection and transmission of information concerning potential tissue damage, and a central process governing cerebral response to this information.[4] The peripheral nervous system in birds can be further classified into 3 specific types of nociceptors: high-threshold mechanothermal nociceptors, mechanical nociceptors, and thermal nociceptors.[4,5,7,8] These nociceptive fibers synapse onto the spinal cord neurons in the outermost layers of the dorsal horn in birds, where the release of neurotransmitters then actives neurons up the spinal cord to the brainstem.[9,10] High-threshold mechanothermal nociceptors respond to temperatures above 40°C as well as mechanical stimulation, with impulse conduction generally being very slow and requiring increasing the magnitude of a stimulus to increase the number of responses. Mechanical nociceptors respond to alterations in pressure or mechanical deformation, such as the creation of an incision along a skin surface.[4,7] Thermal nociceptors respond to both hot and cold variations in temperature without the requirement of associated mechanical changes, with birds typically being more sensitive to hot noxious stimuli than cold.[11]

As a noxious stimulus induces these peripheral receptors, it is then transmitted to several areas of the midbrain and forebrain to prompt the central nervous system response.[5,6] More specifically, identification of μ-opioid, κ-opioid, and δ-opioid receptors has been identified in the midbrain and forebrain of several avian species.[12–14] When a noxious stimulus is encountered, birds are capable of responding via central processing of nociceptive information, with the endogenous opioid system releasing endogenous opioids, such as β-endorphin, Met-enkephalin, and Leu-enkephalin, and dynorphin.[15,16] These endogenous opioid peptides then act in a neuromodulatory, hormonal, and paracrine fashion to mediate analgesic and other physiologic functions in response to a noxious stimulus. β-Endorphin has been appreciated to be present in a wide variety of avian species and maintains its structure between different birds, indicating its shared importance in response to noxious stimuli or stress.[16] In studies performed in chickens (*Gallus gallus*)[17,18] and pigeons (*Columba livia*),[17] the distribution of neurons associated with central nervous system response to pain has been found to be similar to that seen in the nociceptive tracts of monkeys, cats, and other mammals, thereby indicating a complex and structured anatomic mechanism for detecting and reacting to noxious stimuli. These reactions are what caretakers must then interpret in their behavioral and physiologic assessment of pain in an avian patient.

BEHAVIORAL AND PHYSIOLOGIC ALTERATIONS WITH PAIN IN BIRDS

It is critical to be familiar with the normal, unstressed behaviors of an avian species of interest, as these are unique from both a species and an individual standpoint. Differences in age, gender, and species all have the capacity to alter behavioral variability from a physiologic standpoint.[19,20] Environmentally, disparities can be seen depending on the social dynamics of a given species, whether a species is naturally a prey or a predatory one, and the upbringing of an individual captive bird, particularly in terms of being socially raised versus individually raised.[1,3,20] The effects of stress in an individual, even in the absence of pain, also significantly alters behavior, as has been reported in studies with cockatiels (*Nymphicus hollandicus*),[21] European starlings (*Sturnus vulgaris*),[22] and trumpeter swans (*Cygnus buccinator*).[23] If references are available, an observer studying pain responses in a bird should ideally be familiar with how the bird's species generally responds to stress to not confound any behavioral alterations, such as those ethograms previously published for cockatiels.[21]

Although behavioral indicators of pain are complex in nature, an advantage of using behavioral indicators of pain is that these changes are often more immediate and can be appreciated externally, in comparison to physiologic indicators (described in later discussion in this article) that take time and processing to quantify.[24] These changes may include fight-or-flight responses (struggling, vocalizing, aggression), conservation or withdrawal responses (immobility, laxity of extremities, lack of vocalizations), reduction or absence of normal behaviors, addition of abnormal behaviors, alterations in response to motivational tasks, and changes with interactions between conspecifics or handlers (the lattermost being in relation to companion and other captive birds). Situations in which pain in avian species has been observed and reported in the literature include changes in behavior associated with beak trimming, buccal injection, comb and wattle trimming, feather plucking, fractured bones (both naturally occurring and surgically induced), developmental limb abnormalities, toe trimming, osteotomy, pododermatitis, arthritis (both naturally occurring and induced), chronic wounds/neuropathic pain, venipuncture and subcutaneous PIT tag placement, degenerative joint disease, electrical stimuli, thermal stimuli, mechanical stimuli, and absence of brachial plexus nerve blockage in the face of wing-clamping and pectoral muscle pinpricks (**Table 1**).

Of those species studied, there were several behavioral changes noted that aided in the recognition of pain in relation to a noxious situation/stimulus. Pigeons experiencing pelvic limb fracture were found to place considerably less weight on the affected limb and appear lame, spent less time exploring their environment, spent less time preening themselves, and spent more time lying on the bottom of their enclosure as opposed to perching.[25,26] In similar studies of musculoskeletal-related pain, psittacines (Hispaniolan Amazon parrots, *Amazona ventralis*,[27] and green-cheeked conures, *Pyrrhura molinae*[28]) with induced arthritis were found to bear less weight and ambulate less on their affected limb, had increased ruffling and an unkempt appearance to their feathers, groomed the affected limb more frequently than would be considered general maintenance grooming, and took both more attempts and a longer timeframe to reach a grape reward compared with these activities before induction of arthritis. Chickens suffering from keel bone fractures exhibited an overall decrease in mobility and confidence with ambulation, took a greater amount of time both to navigate off of perches when placed and to reach a food reward when prompted, and used available perches less when given the option to rest on this or the bottom of their

Table 1
Selected pain-related behavioral changes observed in avian species experiencing various noxious stimuli

Species	Pain Stimulus	Collective Observations for Pain-Related Changes in Behavior
Chickens	Beak trimming (I)	*Decreased behaviors:* Appetite and feed consumption, general activity (walking, running, environmental exploration), dust bathing, ground-scratching, egg production, weight gain ± additional weight loss, drinking, preening, pecking (both environmental and at novel objects), environmental exploration using beak, head shaking, beak wiping, agonistic behaviors, pecking speed/frequency/force, pulling on novel objects *Increased behaviors:* Resting (standing or laying down), response time investigating novel environmental object
	Buccal injection (I)	Largely motionless crouch following injection, head tucked into body, fewer alert head movements, ruffled feathers, ocular changes (closing eyes, pupil changes)
	Comb/wattle trimming (I)	Decreased food intake and standing, increased resting
	Feather plucking (I)	Jumping, wing-flapping, vocalizations, immobility, lowered head and tail, withdrawal from handlers
	Induced arthritis (I)	*Decreased behaviors:* Head movements, dust bathing, preening, oral behaviors (eating, drinking, pecking) *General behavioral observations:* One-legged standing, limping/severe lameness, increased resting (standing and sitting), drooping head and tail, ruffled feathers, ocular changes (closing eyes), lying with affected limb outstretched, "pain-coping behaviors" (one-legged standing, limping)
	Mechanothermal (I)	Suddenly rising, shuffling, pecking at probe, twitching
	Thermal (I)	Immobility, ocular changes (closing eyes), crouched and drawn in posture
	Wing clamp & pectoral pinprick (I)	Vocalizations, feather-picking/pecking, agitation
	Keel bone fracture (N)	*Decreased behaviors:* Pop hole use, egg production, perch use, mobility (obstacle course and flying down from perch), drinking, periods of standing, vertical locomotion (decreased perch/nest box use), general activity (walking, running), perch transitions, feeding (plus weight loss)

(continued on next page)

Species	Pain Stimulus	Collective Observations for Pain-Related Changes in Behavior
Table 1 (*continued*)		
	Limb abnormalities (N)	*Increased behaviors:* Latency/hesitancy to land/jump from perch, time sleeping on floor, self-selection to return to an area where analgesics were previously provided, hesitancy and time needed to fly down from perch (especially higher perches), time immobile on perch once perched, sitting, and resting *Decreased behaviors:* Walking ability (some = complete inability to walk), ability to complete motivational obstacle course, walking speed, lameness, dust bathing, vertical wing shakes, time standing, number of trips to feeder, foot impact force when walking, short stride length and duration, completion of obstacle course, latency to lie *Increased behaviors:* Self-selection of food containing an analgesic, tonic immobility, time spent laying down (including while eating), time in "double support phase" (standing on both limbs), time to cross obstacle course
	Pododermatitis (N)	Increased tonic immobility
Turkeys (domestic)	Beak trimming (I)	*Decreased behaviors:* Feed intake, weight gain ± weight loss, ± changes in social pecking frequency, general activity, eating/drinking, agonistic behaviors, preening, environmental exploration *Increased behaviors:* Vocalizations during beak-trimming procedures, struggling during handling, resting
	Toe trimming (I)	Decreased feeding, standing, walking (acute and chronic), and running
	Degenerative hip disease (N)	Less standing, activity, eating/drinking, and less sexual activity (males)
	Pododermatitis (N)	*Decreased behaviors:* Walking, walking speed, "normal" behaviors (eating, drinking), preening, standing, group resting *Increased behaviors:* Sleeping, time spent in "double support phase" (standing on both legs)
Psittacines	Thermal/electrical (I)	Vigorously flinching wings
	Induced arthritis (I)	*Decreased behaviors:* Weight-bearing on affected limb, motor behaviors, hanging time from cage, standing, ambulation, perching, locomotion/ability to stay on a rotating perch *Increased behaviors:* Changes in motivated behavior, number of

(*continued on next page*)

Table 1 (continued)		
Species	Pain Stimulus	Collective Observations for Pain-Related Changes in Behavior
		attempts to grab grape reward, feather ruffling, overgrooming of affected limb
Pigeons (domestic)	Femoral fracture (I)	Changes in posture, standing, exploration, preening, decreased weight-bearing and perching, more time laying on the floor/not moving, decreased exploratory behavior
	Induced arthritis (I)	Increased one-legged standing
	Chronic wound, neuropathic pain (N)	Dull, lean body condition, repeated self-mutilation
Raptors	Pododermatitis (N)	Lameness, atypical body posture, limb withdrawal, vocalizations
	Chronic wound, neuropathic pain (N)	Self-mutilation
	Orthopedic pain (N)	Changes in appetite, lameness, changes in activity/agility, decreased head movements and beak clacks
Ducks	Bill trimming (I)	Decreased preening, eating, drinking, exploratory pecking, weight gain, bill-related behaviors, and activity; increased resting
Emu	Declawing (I)	Decreased conspecific aggression
Blue tits	Venipuncture & subcutaneous PIT tag placement (I)	Opening of beak, erection of crown feathers, twitching/flinching body

Abbreviations: I, induced painful stimulus; N, naturally occurring painful stimulus.

(Nicole A. Mikoni, David Sanchez-Migallon Guzman, Erik Fausak, Joanne Paul-Murphy "Recognition and Assessment of Pain-Related Behaviors in Avian Species: An Integrative Review," Journal of Avian Medicine and Surgery, 36(2), 153–172, [9 August 2022].)

enclosure.[29,30] As a particular example of the importance of recognizing normal behaviors in a given species and how these may change with pain, observation of red-tailed hawks (*Buteo jamaicensis*) recovering from orthopedic trauma had behaviors such as movement around the enclosure, head motions and environmental monitoring, and beak clacks to all be significantly decreased in birds recovering from orthopedic injury.[31]

Physiologic variables have also been used as objective indicators of pain in avian species, although variations between species and individuals must again be considered. Changes in vital signs (heart rate and respiratory rate), blood pressure, plasma corticosterone, fecal corticosterone, leukograms, and electroencephalogram readings have been evaluated when assessing pain in birds, but some have proven to be more reliable than others. Plasma corticosterone, for example, increased significantly in birds simply being handled for venipuncture for sample collection,[21,32] so may not be useful when assessing pain in situations in which stress is inherent. Conversely, fecal corticosterone is a noninvasive and nonstressful sample to collect from avian subjects and is similarly increased compared with plasma corticosterone in birds experiencing adverse scenarios.[33]

TYPES OF PAIN
Acute versus Chronic Pain

In addition to the species-specific considerations of pain recognition and assessment in avian species, the differences in a patient experiencing acute versus chronic pain deserves consideration. With acute pain, sensations typically last for the duration of the healing process of an injury and are generally accompanied by autonomic changes that often respond to analgesic treatment. Chronic pain, conversely, may persist beyond the expected healing time of a disease or injury, or involve an alternation in the nervous system that hinders return to normal sensation.[24] Given these differences, behavioral signs of acute versus chronic pain may differ in a studied individual, especially depending on the overall severity of an injury or illness. Signs of severe, acute pain in birds may involve changes in eye expression (pupil size, palpebral fissure size, tear production, and so forth), restlessness, lameness, changes in temperament, changes in appetite, changes in physical activity, hunched body posture, vocalizations, and overgrooming/self-mutilation[3,5,34] (**Fig. 1**). If conditions progress to chronic pain, or if a bird is experiencing visceral, musculoskeletal, neuropathic, or other internal conditions that can result in chronic pain development, then behavioral shifts may present themselves as well. Signs of chronic pain may include increased guarding behavior of a chronically painful area, avoidance of previously performed behaviors that have been recognized by the individual to exacerbate pain, self-isolation, feather destructive behaviors and self-mutilation of painful areas (or, in opposition, a lack of grooming altogether), inappetence/anorexia, weight loss, and, in producing animals, absence or decrease in weight gain or egg production.[4,5,24,34–36]

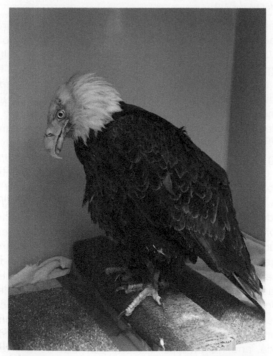

Fig. 1. Bald eagle (*Haliaeetus leucocephalus*) following a traumatic mandibular fracture showing abnormal mentation, pupil dilation, and head posture consistent with acute pain. (*Courtesy of* David Sanchez-Migallon Guzman, LV, MS, DECZM (Avian, Small mammal), DACZM, Davis, CA.)

Few studies have been dedicated to the assessment of chronic pain in birds given the prolonged period of time needed to perform these studies; however, behavioral responses of chronic musculoskeletal and neuropathic conditions have been described. An assessment of behavioral changes by adult male turkeys (*Meleagris gallopavo*) with variable degrees of degenerative hip disorders found that, in affected birds that did not receive an analgesic steroid (betamethasone), the amount of time spent standing, ambulating, preening, and dust bathing decreased. More time was spent feeding, but untreated birds took fewer trips to feeding stations compared with the treated birds and were more prone to self-isolation and refraining from strutting and sexual activity.[37] Studies assessing the long-term behavioral consequences of partial beak amputation in chickens found that chickens demonstrated adverse behavioral changes indicative of pain for as long as 6 weeks postamputation. Signs appreciated in these studies included a decrease in exploratory pecking of the chickens' environment, reduction in beak wiping and head shaking, increased guarding behavior of the affected area (head/beak), and decreased drinking of water.[7,36,38] Commercial turkeys with extensive foot pad dermatitis spent reduced periods of time standing or ambulating, resting with group members, exploratory and general pecking, and preening and considerably more time resting in an isolated fashion compared with their healthier counterparts.[39] Similarly, owners of companion avian species often notice changes in their birds with chronic disease or pain, often commenting on aspects such as inappetence/anorexia, decreased interactions with the handler and/or environmental stimuli, weight loss, and changes in grooming behaviors.[20]

Somatic Versus Visceral Pain

Somatic pain refers to pain caused by noxious stimuli, such as force, temperature, or swelling, that activate receptors in the skin, muscle, skeleton, joints, and/or connective tissues. Visceral pain, conversely, is associated with insult to or inflammation of hollow organs. Common presentations of somatic insults include spinal or musculoskeletal trauma, postsurgical orthopedic conditions, external wounds, and chronic conditions, such as osteoarthritis. Visceral pain may involve instances of ischemia, pulmonary thrombosis, inflammation of any coelomic organ (pancreatitis, nephritis, pleuritis, and so forth), and postsurgical procedures involving any coelomic organ.[40] From a clinical perspective, somatic pain may be more easily recognized owing to the underlying cause being more easily appreciated via general observation or physical examination. As an example, geriatric raptors used for hunting purposes that develop osteoarthritis are reported to display signs of pain, including a decrease in appetite with weight loss, lethargy, reluctance to walk and/or fly, difficulties or inability to use a perch, and/or reactivity to motion or manipulation of an arthritic joint.[41] Given the position of the keel and its involvement in locomotion, production chickens with keel bone fractures often display behavioral changes associated with changes in mobility, including increased hesitancy and time needed to fly down from perches (especially higher perches), hesitancy to jump back up onto perches or elevated nest boxes once on the ground, and a decrease in standing and walking behaviors.[29,30,42–46] Indicators of visceral pain are less easily described, as the behavioral changes secondary to visceral pain are often nonspecific and involve clinical signs, such as generalized lethargy, hyporexia/anorexia, and weight loss. Visceral pain additionally tends to be more diffuse in nature, although can sometimes be localized to an area within the coelom in birds when external pressure is applied to the area causing discomfort.[40] Although certain changes in body positioning have been associated with underlying visceral pain in mammals, such as the "pray position" in dogs with underlying pancreatitis and a hunched posture with reluctance to move in rabbits with gastrointestinal stasis, similar postural reactions have yet to be described for visceral pain in avian species.

Neuropathic Pain

Neuropathic pain is defined as pain initiated or caused by a primary lesion, dysfunction, or transitory perturbation of the peripheral or central nervous system.[47] Oftentimes, neuropathic pain can also be a concurrent component of primary issues, such as orthopedic conditions or trauma (**Fig. 2**). Although a clinician may be doing an exceptional job at managing the somatic sources of pain, certain behavioral signs of discomfort may persist if neuropathic pain is not addressed. Reports of neuropathic pain in avian species are limited; however, cases have been reported in raptors, pigeons, and chickens. An adult male prairie falcon (*Falco mexicanus*) was observed continuously self-mutilating an area of historic injury along its right proximal patagium despite complete healing of the prior fracture and associated surface wounds, and this behavior ceased following a regional nerve block to address the neuropathic pain.[35] Neuropathic pain was also described by Cowan and colleagues[48] in a case study of a male fantail domestic pigeon (*Columba livia domestica*) that developed a granuloma along the right inguinal region following administration of an inactivated Newcastle disease vaccine. Compared with the aviary mates, the affected pigeon had a dull and depressed mentation with decreased feed intake and lean body

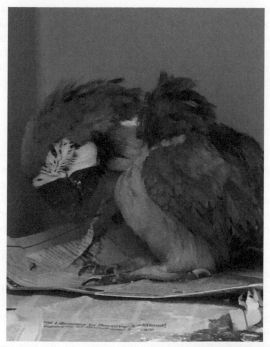

Fig. 2. Blue and gold macaw (*Ara ararauna*) following surgical amputation of tail due to an invasive uropygial gland adenocarcinoma showing abnormal mentation, and head and body posture consistent with neuropathic pain. These clinical signs markedly improved following administration of analgesics. (*Courtesy of* David Sanchez-Migallon Guzman, LV, MS, DECZM (Avian, Small mammal), DACZM, Davis, CA.)

condition. Although the granuloma was initially treated with debridement and supportive antibiotic and anti-inflammatory care, the pigeon continued to display self-
mutilation of the affected area for greater than 1.5 months. It was not until gabapentin
was added to the treatment plan to alleviate potential underlying neuropathic pain
stimuli that the pigeon ceased overgrooming the wound, and the wound was able
to fully heal.[48] Agitation, vocalizations, and pecking at the source of the stimuli
when clamping the wings and pricking the pectoralis muscles were elicited in
chickens, and all behaviors ceased following administration of a brachial plexus nerve
block despite repeat stimulation.[49]

Severity of Pain

During assessment of the behavioral changes thought to be due to pain, the expected
severity of pain should be taken into account when both evaluating these behaviors
and designing a pain management plan. Pain can be classified as mild, moderate,
or severe. The pain caused by something such as an accidental truncation of the
nail during a nail trim, as an example, is much milder compared with that caused by
a major orthopedic procedure. However, even routine procedures such as venipuncture and placement of monitoring tags have been associated with behavioral indicators of discomfort in birds. A study performed by Schlicht and Kempenaers[50]
evaluated the effects of ringing, blood sampling, and transponder tag placement in
blue tits (*Cyanistes caeruleus*). Although the birds' reactions to placement of leg rings
was minimal, 8 of 10 blue tits exhibited behavioral displays in response to venipuncture and subcutaneous tag placement. These behaviors included instantaneous
defensive displays, such as beak-opening and erection of the crown feathers, rapid
blinking of the eyes, and sharp twitching away from the painful stimulus being administered.[50] Paying close attention to aberrant behaviors (or the absence of normally present behaviors) can help in assessing a bird's severity of pain. Likewise, observing
how a patient behaves both preoperatively (both in health and when presented for
illness before surgery) and postoperatively can help monitor for signs of discomfort
and assist in tailoring effective analgesic plans.

CLINICAL CONSIDERATIONS

The recognition and assessment of pain in avian species presented in clinical settings
have, at this point in time, significant limitations. In many instances, evaluation of a bird
suspected to be in pain is based on indirect assessment rather than direct physiologic
measurements or clear behavioral indicators. Nonetheless, assumptions can be made
regarding the underlying disease or associated procedure for an affected bird, such as
the sound reasoning that a bird undergoing orthopedic surgery will be in pain postoperatively. Concurrently, generalized methods of quantifying pain, such as visual analog
or numeric rating pain scales, can be applied to provide clinicians a tool for evaluation
of an avian patients' pain status on a daily basis.

Aspects of clinical practice that could confound accurate assessment of avian pain
include effect of the observer on the bird's behavior (especially in terms of wildlife species), effects of some analgesics or sedatives that can alter behavior, and concurrent
physiologic conditions (anesthetic recovery, hypothermia, and so forth) that could
make a bird appear painful despite adequate analgesia. As has been established in
some avian species, the presence of stress can alter observed behaviors.[21] Similarly,
certain prey species have been noted to alter their behaviors when in the presence of
an observer versus when observed remotely.[20,51] Thus, when possible, it may be
best to evaluate avian patients via remote means, such as external monitoring devices,

Table 2
Behavioral scoring system used to assess Hispaniolan parrots with experimentally induced arthritis and receiving various analgesic treatments

Behavior	Score
Voluntary	Voluntary
Activity	0 = Moving around cage, 1 = moving on perch, 2 = no activity
Inactive time	0 to 15 = No. of minutes parrot was inactive
Locomotion	0 = Both pelvic limbs, 1 = only 1 pelvic limb, 2 = no movement
Perching posture	0 = 2 limbs visible, 1 = 1 limb visible, 2 = hock-sitting, 3 = unilateral hock-sitting
Perching grasp	0 = Both feet, 1 = only 1 foot
Stand and ambulate with arthritic limb	0 = No, 1 = yes
Hang from top of cage	0 to infinity = No. of times parrot hung for >10 s
Appearance	0 = Smooth feather, 1 = slightly fluffed, 2 = very fluffed; feathers sticking out,
Feathers ruffled	0 = no, 1 = yes
Feather ruffling	0 to infinity = No. of times parrot ruffled feathers
Preening	1 = With beak and feet, 2 = with beak only, 3 = none
Grooming	0 to infinity = No. of times parrot groomed
Rub beak on metal perches	0 = No, 1 = yes
Rub beak on wood	0 = No, 1 = yes
Attitude	0 = Alert, 1 = signs of slight depression, 2 = signs of depression
Use injected limb to hold food reward while eating it	0 = No, 1 = yes
Use noninjected limb to hold food reward while eating it	0 = No, 1 = yes
Visits to food dish	0 to infinity = No. of times to food and water
Time spent eating food	0 to 15 = No. of minutes
Picking at arthritic limb with beak	0 = No, 1 = yes
Motivated (associated with obtaining grape food reward)	
Attempts made to get food reward	0 to infinity = No. of attempts
Time from introduction of food reward to first contact with reward	0 to 15 = No. of minutes
First contact with food reward	0 to 15 = No. of minutes
Time spend eating food reward	0 to 15 = No. of minutes

(Paul-Murphy, J. R., Sladky, K. K., Krugner-Higby, L. A., Stading, B. R., Klauer, J. M., Keuler, N. S., Brown, C. S., & Heath, T. D. (2009). Analgesic effects of carprofen and liposome-encapsulated butorphanol tartrate in Hispaniolan parrots (Amazona ventralis) with experimentally induced arthritis, American Journal of Veterinary Research, 70(10), 1201–1210. Retrieved Sep 23, 2022, https://avmajournals.avma.org/view/journals/ajvr/70/10/ajvr.70.10.1201.xml[2].)

to gain more accurate evaluations of behaviors and any discomfort present. Medications, such as opioids, can at times result in agitation or other behavioral alterations in avian species.[52] Assessing a patient both before and after drug administration can help to evaluate the effectiveness of analgesics provided and determine if any new or altered behaviors are more likely to be a consequence of the drug administered. Evaluation of physiologic parameters, such as body temperature, is not as commonly

Table 3
Numeric rating pain scales evaluated to assess severity of pain after surgical induction of lameness in pigeons

Score	Behavioral Observation
Pigeon's attitude in the presence of the observer	
0	Alert and attentive; tries to escape and fly with insistence
1	A little curious; still tries to escape but with only mild effort
2	Stays quiet on perch with little reaction to presence of observer
3	Stands on floor and displays little reaction to presence of observer
4	Stands on floor and displays no reaction to presence of observer
5	Lies on floor and displays no reaction to presence of observer
Fractured limb position in the presence of observer:	
0	Appears to bear equal weight on both limbs
1	Bears weight on both limbs but less weight on fractured limb
2	Bears weight on both limbs but obviously less weight on fractured limb
3	Able to bear weight on both limbs but reluctant to do on fractured limb
4	Does not bear weight on fractured limb but stands on nonfractured limb
5	Lies on the floor
Subjective observer evaluation of degree of pain overall:	
0	No signs of pain; pigeon appears as it did before surgery
1	Appears uncomfortable on 1 limb but discomfort not always obvious
2	Evidence of discomfort on 1 limb but no other obvious signs of pain
3	Overall, appears moderately disturbed by pain in its fractured limb
4	Overall, appears highly disturbed by pain in its fractured limb
5	Lies on the floor; does not appear able to stand
Pigeon's motor activity during 10 min of video recording:	
0	Highly active; perches, moves around, explores, preens, or eats
1	Moderately active; moves a little, but mainly stays quiet on its perch
2	Awake but quiet; stays quiet on its perch, does not preen, looks around
3	Very quiet; sleeps on its perch or stands on the floor; does not preen
4	Obvious decreased reaction; stands or lies on the floor and appears asleep
5	No reaction; lies on the floor and does not react to any stimuli

(Desmarchelier, M., Troncy, E., Beauchamp, G., Paul-Murphy, J. R., Fitzgerald, G., & Lair, S. (2012). Evaluation of a fracture pain model in domestic pigeons (Columba livia), American Journal of Veterinary Research, 73(3), 353–360. Retrieved Sep 23, 2022, from https://avmajournals.avma.org/view/journals/ajvr/73/3/ajvr.73.3.353.xml.)[26]

performed in conscious avian patients, and the presence of hypothermia has been documented to interfere with accurate pain assessment in mammalian species, such as rats,[53] and is therefore worth being cognizant of when monitoring avian species.

FUTURE DIRECTIONS FOR IMPROVING ASSESSMENT OF AVIAN PAIN

Integrating behavioral components into avian patient monitoring and care could provide improvement in the overall welfare of that patient. If caretakers are more aware of behaviors commonly displayed by healthy animals, then alterations from or absence of these behaviors can help to assess if an animal is in pain or otherwise disturbed. Incorporating behavioral questions in the history-taking process for client-owned animals

> **Box 1**
> **Behavioral and postural parameters to consider when evaluating pain in birds. Parameters should be evaluated in context to appropriateness for avian species being evaluated. Please note that the parameters presented in this box are summarized based on historic studies performed on birds in pain but have not been validated. For each category, expected normal behavior is listed at the top, with the changes being progressive with increased levels of pain.**
>
> Mentation
> - Alert and attentive
> - Quiet
> - Depressed
>
> Environmental interaction
> - Engaged and interactive with environment (toys, conspecifics, food/water dishes, observers/caregivers)
> - Reserved and interacts with less with environment than expected
> - Largely inactive/resting and not engaging with surroundings
>
> Perching
> - Easily maneuvers onto perch and is able to traverse along it without difficulty
> - Able to initially maneuver onto perch, but then remains largely within the same spot once perched
> - Unable to or does not perch and remains on floor of enclosure
>
> Maintenance behaviors
> - Performs maintenance behaviors (preening, shaking plumage, scratching, stretching, wiping beak, and so forth) readily
> - Performs maintenance behaviors at a decreased frequency than expected
> - Does not perform any noticeable maintenance behaviors when observed
>
> Locomotion
> - Moving frequently and easily around enclosure, either horizontally or, where appropriate, vertically
> - Will occasionally move self to different locations within cage, but slowly
> - Largely immobile during the observation period
>
> Focal preening of singular area
> - Minimal to no increase in attention in regards to one spot repeatedly (grooms all body parts similarly when preening body)
> - Occasional pecking/biting at one spot repeatedly
> - Significant overgrooming/biting at one spot repeatedly
>
> Body posture
> - Body and neck held erect and engaged
> - Body erect, but with neck and head lowered and held closer to chest
> - Body held low or against vertical surface (wall, enclosure side, and so forth), or body lying fully on the floor
>
> Appetite
> - Visits feeder/food dish readily while awake
> - Visits feeder at a reduced frequency compared with patient's normal
> - Does not visit feeder at all during observed period while awake

could provide valuable insight into both the normal behaviors observed at home in a familiar environment and changes that accompany a presenting complaint. Behavioral evaluations of wild avian species and birds under human care within zoo or rehabilitation settings can help assess a bird's pain status on presentation and subsequently compare any changes indicative of improvement as treatment is implemented.

As behavioral indicators of pain hopefully become more recognized in avian species through future research, the development of accurate and reliable avian pain scales should be at the forefront of concurrent development. When considering the possible variations between different avian species and individuals within a species, an ideal avian pain scale should encompass specific details, such as species, environment (prey vs predatory species, captive/companion vs wild, and so forth), rearing conditions, age, and sex.[1,24] The type of pain (acute vs chronic, location, underlying cause) also affects behavioral changes noted in birds. Specific pain behaviors should be clearly defined and consistent as well, given the use of tools such as these among a wide variety of evaluators, such as veterinary students, clinicians throughout divergent settings (clinical, zoologic, laboratory, and so forth), wildlife rehabilitators, and others. Behavioral indicators of pain can vary drastically between avian species, making species-specific algorithms essential, as well as recognizing that extrapolations to different avian species not specifically studied for a used pain scale may not be accurate. Behavioral (**Table 2**)[2] and numeric (**Table 3**)[26] pain scales have been used in prior avian studies, but their application to scenarios outside of those evaluated in a research setting remains limited.

Future avian pain scales will consider the value of assessing the whole individual versus solely the region of the head or face (**Box 1**). Many mammalian species are evaluated clinically using a grimace scale; however, avian species lack many of the distinct facial expressions often associated with pain in mammals. Apart from potential changes in ocular expression and body positioning as a response to pain,[36] avian species lack the ability to use aural, nasal, or facial muscle positioning changes to express discomfort. However, additional facial aspects, such as blinking frequency and facial region/beak temperature, have been shown to be useful in evaluating response to stressors in poultry chicks[54] and may similarly prove useful in evaluating painful avian patients as well. Evaluation of crown feather height, pupil area, and angle of throat feathers in Japanese quail (*Coturnix japonica*) has also shown variation in response to various environmental settings.[55] Thus, there may be several parts of a bird apart from the face that can become altered with behavioral changes, such as the tail, carriage of the wings, and head crests in those species that have them, and these areas are worth further investigation.

SUMMARY

Although advancements continue to be made as time progresses, there is still much to be discovered regarding the recognition and assessment of pain in avian species. Accurate pain evaluation is essential for provision of supportive care and analgesia and aids in the improvement of an animal's quality of life. Among birds, considerable species-specific and individual-specific differences in behavioral response exist despite exposure to similar noxious stimuli. Variations in the type and severity of pain experienced can additionally alter an individual's behavioral pain response. The development of ethograms describing both normal and stressed (without pain) avian behaviors can help distinguish behavioral changes associated with pain, and care should be taken to observe a bird's whole body in addition to evaluating facial features. Implementation of behavioral questionnaires for client-owned birds in clinical settings would also clarify individual behavioral responses that may be indicators of pain. A thorough understanding of these behavioral and postural alterations can help tailor the development of accurate avian pain scales and subsequent provision of adequate pain relief in the future.

CLINICS CARE POINTS

- When assessing for pain in avian species, the absence of normal behaviors can be as important as the presence of abnormal behaviors in response to painful stimuli.

- Indirect behavioral observations can provide heightened evaluation of overall level of pain when assessed in conjunction with physiologic alterations.

- Generalized methods of quantifying pain, such as visual analog or numeric rating pain scales, can be applied to provide clinicians a tool for evaluation of an avian patient's pain while awaiting development of more species-specific pain scales.

DISCLOSURE

The authors of this article do not have any commercial or financial conflicts of interest. All authors are currently employed by University of California, Davis.

REFERENCES

1. Paul-Murphy J, Ludders J, Robertson S, et al. The need for a cross-species approach to the study of pain in animals. J Am Vet Med Assoc 2004;224(5): 692–7.
2. Paul-Murphy J, Sladky K, Krugner-Higby L, et al. Analgesic effects of carprofen and liposome-encapsulated butorphanol tartrate in Hispaniolan parrots (Amazona ventralis) with experimentally induced arthritis. Am J Vet Res 2009;70(10):1201–10.
3. Malik A, Valentine A. Pain in birds: a review for veterinary nurses. Vet Nurs J 2018; 33(1):11–25.
4. Machin KL. Avian pain: physiology and evaluation. Compend Contin Educ Pract Vet 2005;27(2):98–109.
5. Machin KL. Recognition and treatment of pain in birds. Pain Management in Veterinary Practice 2013;407–15. Wiley-Blackwell, Hoboken, New Jersey.
6. Douglas JM, Guzman DSM, Paul-Murphy J. Pain in birds: the anatomical and physiological basis. Vet Clinics: Exot Anim Pract 2018;21(1):17–31.
7. Gentle MJ. Pain in birds. Anim Welf 1992;1(4):235–47.
8. LU Sneddon, Elwood RW, Adamo SA, et al. Defining and assessing animal pain. Anim Behav 2014;97:201–12.
9. Beausoleil NJ, Holdsworth SE, Lehmann H. Avian nociception and pain. Sturkie's avian physiology. Cambridge, MA: Academic Press; 2022. p. 223–31.
10. Cortelli P, Giannini G, Favoni V, et al. Nociception and autonomic nervous system. Neurol Sci 2013;34(1):41–6.
11. Necker R, Reiner B. Temperature-sensitive mechanoreceptors, thermoreceptors and heat nociceptors in the feathered skin of pigeons. J Comp Physiol 1980;135:201–7.
12. Bardo MT, Bhatnagar RK, Gebhard GF, et al. Opiate receptor development in midbrain and forebrain of posthatch chicks. Devel Brain Res 1982;3(4):668–73.
13. Reiner A, Brauth SE, Kitt CA, et al. Distribution of mu, delta, and kappa opiate receptor types in the forebrain and midbrain of pigeons. J Comput Neurosci 1989; 280(3):359–82.
14. Csillag A, Bourne RC, Stewart MG. Distribution of mu, delta, and kappa opioid receptor binding sites in the brain of the one-day-old domestic chick (Gallus domesticus): an in vitro quantitative autoradiographic study. J Comput Neurosci 1990;302(3):543–51.
15. Reiner A, Davis BM, Brecha NC, et al. The distribution of enkephalinlike immunoreactivity in the telencephalon of the adult and developing domestic chicken. J Comput Neurosci 1984;228(2):245–62.
16. Scanes CG, Pierzchala-Koziec K. Perspectives on endogenous opioids in birds. Front Physio 2018;9:1842.

17. Fernandez-Lopez A, Revilla V, Candelas MA. A comparative study of alpha2- and beta-adrenoceptor distribution in pigeon and chick brain. Eur J Neurosci 1997;9(5):871–83.
18. Zhai S-Y, Atsumi S. Large dorsal horn neurons which receive inputs from numerous substance P–like immunoreactive axon terminals in the laminae I and II of the chicken spinal cord. Neurosci Res 1997;28:147–54.
19. Hawkins MG. The use of analgesics in birds, reptiles, and small exotic mammals. J Exot Pet Med 2006;15(3):177–92.
20. Paul-Murphy J, Hawkins MG. Bird specific considerations: Recognizing pain behaviour in pet birds. In: Gaynor JS, Muir WW, editors. Handbook of veterinary pain management. 3rd ed. St. Louis, MO: Elsevier; 2014. p. 536–54. Ch. 26.
21. Turpen KK, Welle KR, Trail JL, et al. Establishing stress behaviors in response to manual restraint in cockatiels (Nymphicus hollandicus). J Avian Med Surg 2019; 33(1):38–45.
22. Remage-Healey L, Romero LM. Daily and seasonal variation in response to stress in captive starlings (Sturnus vulgaris): glucose. Gen Comp Endo 2000;119(1):60–8.
23. Henson P, Grant TA. The effects of human disturbance on trumpeter swan breeding behavior. Wildl Soc Bull 1991;19(3):248–57.
24. Anil SS, Anil L, Deen J. Challenges of pain assessment in domestic animals. J Am Vet Med Assoc 2002;220(3):313–9.
25. Desmarchelier M, Troncy E, Fitzgerald G, et al. Analgesic effects of meloxicam administration on postoperative orthopedic pain in domestic pigeons (Columba livia). Am J Vet Res 2012;73(3):361–7.
26. Desmarchelier M, Troncy E, Beauchamp G, et al. Evaluation of a fracture pain model in domestic pigeons (Columba livia). Am J Vet Res 2012;73(3):353–60.
27. Cole GA, Paul-Murphy J, Kruger-Higby L, et al. Analgesic effects of intramuscular administration of meloxicam in Hispaniolan parrots (Amazona ventralis) with experimentally induced arthritis. Am J Vet Res 2009;70(12):1471–6.
28. Paul-Murphy J, Kruger-Higby L, Tourdot RL, et al. Evaluation of liposome-encapsulated butorphanol tartrate for alleviation of experimentally induced arthritic pain in green-cheeked conures (Pyrrhura molinae). Am J Vet Res 2009; 70(10):1211–9.
29. Nasr MAF, Nicol CJ, Murrell JC. Do laying hens with keel bone fractures experience pain? PLoS One 2012;7(8):e42420.
30. Nasr MAF, Murrell J, Wilkins LJ, et al. The effect of keel fractures on egg-production parameters, mobility and behaviour in individual laying hens. Anim Welf 2012;21(1):127–35.
31. Mazor-Thomas JE, Mann PE, Karas AZ, et al. Pain-suppressed behaviors in the red-tailed hawk (Buteo jamaicensis). Appl Anim Behav Sci 2014;152:83–91.
32. Heatley JJ, Oliver JW, Hosgood G, et al. Serum corticosterone concentrations in response to restraint, anesthesia, and skin testing in Hispaniolan Amazon parrots (Amazona ventralis). J Avian Med Surg 2000;14:172–6.
33. Ludders JW, Langenberg JA, Czekala NM, et al. Fecal corticosterone reflects serum corticosterone in Florida sandhill cranes. J Wildl Dis 2001;37:646–52.
34. Hawkins MG, Paul-Murphy J, Guzman DSM. Recognition, assessment, and management of pain in birds. Current therapy in avian medicine and surgery. Philadelphia, PA: WB Saunders; 2016. p. 616–30.
35. Shaver SL, Robinson NG, Wright BD, et al. A multimodal approach to management of suspected neuropathic pain in a prairie falcon (Falco mexicanus). J Avian Med Surg 2009;23(3):209–13.
36. Duncan IJH, Slee GS, Seawright E. Behavioural consequences of partial beak amputation (beak trimming) in poultry. Br Poult Sci 1989;30:479–88.

37. Duncan IJH, Beatty ER, Hocking PM, et al. Assessment of pain associated with degenerative hip disorders in adult male turkeys. Res Vet Sci 1991;50(2):200–3.
38. Gentle MJ, Waddington D, Hunter LN, et al. Behavioural evidence for persistent pain following partial beak amputation in chickens. Appl Anim Behav Sci 1990; 27(1–2):149–57.
39. Sinclair A, Wyneken CW, Veldkamp T, et al. Behavioural assessment of pain in commercial turkeys (Meleagris gallopavo) with foot pad dermatitis. Br Poult Sci 2015;56(5):511–21.
40. Mathews K, Kronen PW, Lascelles D, et al. Guidelines for recognition, assessment and treatment of pain: WSAVA Global Pain Council. J Small Anim Pract 2014;55:E10–68.
41. Chitty J. Care of the geriatric raptor. Veterinary Clin North Am Exot Anim Pract 2020;23(3):503–23.
42. Armstrong EA, Rufener C, Toscano MJ, et al. Keel bone fractures induce a depressive-like state in laying hens. Sci Rep 2020;10(1):1–14.
43. Casey-Trott TM, Widowski TM. Behavioral differences of laying hens with fractured keel bones within furnished cages. Front Vet Sci 2016;3:42.
44. Casey-Trott TM, Widowski TM. Validation of an accelerometer to quantify inactivity in laying hens with or without keel-bone fractures. Anim Welf 2018;27(2):103–14.
45. Rentsch AK, Rufener CB, Spadavecchia C, et al. Laying hen's mobility is impaired by keel bone fractures and does not improve with paracetamol treatment. Appl Anim Behav Sci 2019;216:19–25.
46. Wei H, Bi Y, Xin H, et al. Keel fracture changed the behavior and reduced the welfare, production performance, and egg quality in laying hens housed individually in furnished cages. Poult Sci 2020;99(7):3334–42.
47. Jensen TS, Baron R, Haanpaa M, et al. A new definition of neuropathic pain. Pain 2011;152(10):2204–5.
48. Cowan ML, Monks DJ, Raidal SR. Granuloma formation and suspected neuropathic pain in a domestic pigeon (Columba livia) secondary to an oil-based, inactivated Newcastle disease vaccine administered for protection against pigeon paramyxovirus-1. Aust Vet J 2014;92(5):171–6.
49. Figueiredo JP, Cruz ML, Mendes GM, et al. Assessment of brachial plexus blockade in chickens by an axillary approach. Vet Anaesth Analg 2008;35(6):511–8.
50. Schlicht E, Kempenaers B. The immediate impact of ringing, blood sampling and PIT-Tag implanting on the behaviour of blue tits cyanistes caeruleus. Ardea 2018; 106(1):39–98.
51. Pinho RH, Leach MC, Minto BW, et al. Postoperative pain behaviours in rabbits following orthopaedic surgery and effect of observer presence. PLoS One 2020;15(10):e0240605.
52. Guzman DSM, Douglas JM, Beaufrere H, et al. Evaluation of the thermal antinociceptive effects of hydromorphone hydrochloride after intramuscular administration to orange-winged Amazon parrots (Amazona amazonica). Am J Vet Res 2020;81(10):775–82.
53. Klune CB, Robbins HNK, Leung VSY, et al. Hypothermia during general anesthesia interferes with pain assessment in laboratory rats (Rattus norvegicus). J Amer Asso Lab Anim Sci 2020;59(6):719–25.
54. Pijpers N, van den Heuvel H, Duncan IH, et al. Understanding chicks' emotions: are eye blinks & facial temperatures reliable indicators? bioRxiv 2022;1–21.
55. Bertin A, Cornilleau F, Lemarchand J, et al. Are there facial indicators of positive emotions in birds? A first exploration in Japanese quail. Behav Processes 2018; 157:470–3.

Treatment of Pain in Birds

David Sanchez- Migallon Guzman, LV, MS, Dipl. ECZM (Avian, Small Mammal), Dipl. ACZM*, Michelle G. Hawkins, VMD, Diplomate ABVP (Avian Practice)

KEYWORDS

- Avian • Analgesia • Opioid • Multimodal • Nonsteroidal anti-inflammatory
- Locoregional analgesia

KEY POINTS

- Species differences in pharmacokinetics and pharmacodynamics of analgesic drugs in birds warrants careful extrapolation of drug doses and frequency of administration.
- New studies are encouraging the use of opioid drugs like hydromorphone or buprenorphine (including high-concentrated and sustained-release formulations) in some avian species, and also revealing a more complex picture in regard to efficacy, duration of action, and adverse effects of opioid drugs.
- Although there are a growing number of nonsteroidal anti-inflammatory drug (NSAID) options for birds, with newer drugs like mavacoxib offering longer action or grapiprant offering COX-sparing alternatives, meloxicam remains the most studied NSAID with a large number of studies and scarce reports of adverse effects when used at the recommended dosages.
- The pharmacokinetics and safety of local anesthetics like lidocaine and bupivacaine have been evaluated and are used for locoregional techniques like brachial plexus block, ischiatic-femoral nerve block, and spinal (intrathecal) anesthesia.
- Other drugs like gabapentin, amantadine, and cannabinoids provide additional treatment options to consider in the management of chronic pain. Dietary supplementation, like eicosapentaenoic acid, docosahexaenoic acid, glucosamine, chondroitin sulfate, as well as polysulfate glycosaminoglycans, and physical rehabilitation are important treatment modalities to consider in many cases, especially for chronic pain management.

INTRODUCTION

Effective pain management involves addressing the underlying process or injury that induced pain, as well as use of pharmacologic and nonpharmacologic methods to reduce the activation of nociceptors and transmission of the nociceptor signals and their modulation, projection, and further processing in the central nervous systems. Because these mechanisms involve multiple pathways and a variety of neurotransmitters, balanced or multimodal analgesia acting at different stages of the pain pathways with

Department of Medicine and Epidemiology, School of Veterinary Medicine, University of California Davis, One Shields Avenue, Davis, CA 95616, USA
* Corresponding author.
E-mail address: guzman@ucdavis.edu

Vet Clin Exot Anim 26 (2023) 83–120
https://doi.org/10.1016/j.cvex.2022.09.003
1094-9194/23/© 2022 Elsevier Inc. All rights reserved.

vetexotic.theclinics.com

different mechanisms of action is highly recommended. Such strategies are based also on the type and severity of pain and might include the combination of drugs like opioids, nonsteroidal anti-inflammatory drugs (NSAIDs), local anesthetics, and/or other drugs like gabapentin, amantadine, and cannabinoids acting at different points in the nociceptive system, thereby helping to provide greater pain relief while reducing the risk of adverse effects when combined.

GENERAL CONSIDERATIONS

Treatment of pain in birds presents many challenges. With more than 10,400 species identified, there are a wide range of anatomic and physiologic differences that warrant a species-specific approach. In practice, the number of species that a clinician might be presented with is more limited, but still can be several hundred species. With only a few species in which a limited number of analgesic drugs have been studied, the clinician is often obligated to extrapolate from published studies. In these instances, caution is advised because significant differences have been already identified even in birds within the same order (eg, psittaciformes). Some of these differences are illustrated later in this article. Even when an analgesic drug has been studied in a specific species, a basic understanding of the studies and clinical judgment is required to appropriately use the evidence-based information available from pharmacokinetic or pharmacodynamic studies. If a recommended general dose and frequency of administration is used, this should only be considered a starting point of a process that requires further evaluation of the patient before and after administration. It is even more important for drugs that are administered multiple times, either during a few days of a postoperative period or long-term administration for chronic pain, where continuous evaluation of the pain and patient are needed to optimize the choice of drugs, doses, and frequency of administration in the protocol.

OPIOIDS AND OPIOIDLIKE DRUGS

Opioids are used for moderate to severe pain, such as traumatic or surgical pain. Opioids reversibly bind to specific receptors in the central and peripheral nervous system. These drugs are categorized as agonists, partial agonists, mixed agonist/antagonists, or antagonists based on their ability to induce an analgesic response once bound to a specific receptor. The most common adverse effects reported with opioids are sedation, cardiac and/or respiratory depression, vomiting, and diarrhea/constipation. In many cases, these drugs may be reversed with antagonists, which will also terminate analgesia. There are a growing number of opioid drugs, including different doses and formulations in some cases, which have been evaluated in avian species (**Table 1**).

Few studies have been conducted regarding the distribution, quantity, structure, and function of each opioid receptor type in birds. In an earlier study in pigeons, the regional distribution of μ, κ, and δ receptors in the forebrain and midbrain were similar to that in mammals but the κ and δ receptors were more prominent in the pigeon forebrain and midbrain than μ receptors and 76% of opioid receptors in the forebrain were determined to be κ-type.[1] These findings, together with earlier studies in opioids in birds, led to a paradigm in which kappa agonist opioids like butorphanol were considered the drugs of choice for pain management in birds. More recent studies looking at opioid receptor in chicks (*Gallus gallus domesticus*),[2] pigeons, and cockatiels (*Nymphicus hollandicus*),[3] together with a large number of recent studies on opioids in birds, are challenging this paradigm and finding that in some species mu agonist opioid drugs might actually be better choices when treating pain in some species. The results of these studies are described in the following paragraphs. When looking

Table 1
Selected opioid and opioidlike analgesics evaluated in avian species by either pharmacokinetic or pharmacodynamic studies

Drug	Dose (mg/kg)	Route of Administration	Frequency (h)	Species	Comments	Type of Study	Reference
Hydromorphone	0.1, 0.3, 0.6	IM, IV	Single dose	Cockatiels	Failed to increase thermal nociception thresholds despite achieving plasma concentrations considered therapeutic in other species. Some birds showed mild sedation at the highest doses	PK/PD	Houck et al,[28] 2018
	0.1, 1, 2	IM, IV	Single dose	Orange-winged Amazon parrot	Increased thermal nociceptive threshold at 1 and 2 mg/kg for 3 and 6 h, respectively. Agitation, nausealike behavior at the highest doses. Maintained above 1 ng/mL plasma concentrations for 6 h following 1 mg/kg IM with an elimination half-life of 1.74 h	PK/PD	Sanchez-Migallon et al,[29] 2020, Sanchez-Migallon et al,[30] 2020
	0.1, 0.3, 0.6	IM, IV	Single dose	American kestrels	Increased the thermal nociception threshold for 3–6 h. Some birds moderate sedation at the highest doses	PK/PD	Guzman et al,[26] 2014, Guzman et al,[27] 2013
Fentanyl	Targeted controlled infusions 240–480 µg/kg/h	IV	Constant-rate infusion	Hispaniolan Amazon parrot	Reduced isoflurane MAC% in a dose-related manner, with significant effects on heart rate, blood pressure at the highest rate	PK/PD	Pascoe et al,[38] 2018; Hawkins et al,[43] 2018

(continued on next page)

Table 1
(continued)

Drug	Dose (mg/kg)	Route of Administration	Frequency (h)	Species	Comments	Type of Study	Reference
	0.02, 0.2	IM SC	Single dose	White cockatoos	0.02 mg/kg did not affect thermal and electrical nociceptive threshold; 0.2 mg/kg did affect both withdrawal thresholds but only in some birds and hyperactivity in first 15–30 min	PK/PD	Hoppes et al,[37] 2013
	10–30 µg/kg/h	IV	Constant-rate infusion	Red-tailed hawks	Reduced isoflurane MAC 31%–55% in a dose-related manner, without significant effects on heart rate, blood pressure, $Paco_2$, Pao_2.	PK/PD	Pascoe et al,[38] 2018, Pavez et al,[39] 2011
	25 µg/h	TD patch	Single dose	Chicken	Large interindividual variability. Maintained plasma concentrations above 0.2–1.2 ng/mL for 72 h	PK	Delaski et al,[41] 2017
Buprenorphine	0.6, 1.2, 1.8	IM, IV	Single dose	Cockatiels	Failed to increased thermal nociceptive thresholds despite achieving plasma concentrations considered therapeutic in other species. Some birds mild sedation at the highest doses	PK/PD	Guzman et al,[48] 2018
	0.1	IM	Single dose	Gray parrots	No change in withdrawal response to noxious stimulus despite achieving plasma concentrations considered therapeutic in other species	PK/PD	Paul-Murphy et al,[5] 1999, Paul-Murphy et al,[47] 2004

Drug	Dose (mg/kg)	Route	Species	Dosing	Effect	PK/PD	References
	0.1, 0.3, 0.6	IM, IV	American kestrels	Single dose	Increased withdrawal thermal thresholds for at least 6 h and maintained plasma concentration over 1 ng/mL for 9 h	PK/PD	Gustersen et al,[53] 2014; Ceulemans et al,[54] 2014
	0.25 0.5	IM	Domestic pigeons	Single dose	Increased latency period for withdrawal from a noxious electrical stimulus of 2 h at 0.25 mg/kg and for 5 h for 0.5 mg/kg	PD	Gaggermeier et al,[6] 2001
Buprenorphine sustained-release formulation	1.8	IM, SC	American kestrels	Single dose	Increased thermal threshold for almost 24 h and maintained plasma concentration over 1 ng/mL for 48 h	PK/PD	Guzman et al,[49] 2018, Guzman et al,[51] 2017
Buprenorphine high-concentration	0.3, 1.8	SC	Red-tailed hawk	Single dose	Plasma concentrations were maintained above 1 ng/mL for at least 24 and 48 h, with an elimination half-life of elimination half-life was 6.23 and 7.84 h for the low and high doses, respectively	PK	Gleeson et al,[52] 2018
Butorphanol	5	IM	Hispaniolan Amazon parrots	Single dose	Increased thermal nociceptive threshold for 30 min	PD	Laniesse et al,[8] 2020
	5	PO	Hispaniolan Amazon parrots	Single dose	Oral bioavailability< 10%; do not recommend this route of administration	PK	Sanchez-Migallon et al,[10] 2011
	2	IM	Hispaniolan Amazon parrots	Single dose	No cardiopulmonary negative effects with sevoflurane anesthesia for endoscopy	PD	Klaphake et al,[12] 2016

(continued on next page)

Table 1
(continued)

Drug	Dose (mg/kg)	Route of Administration	Frequency (h)	Species	Comments	Type of Study	Reference
	2	IM	Single dose	Hispaniolan Amazon parrots	Failed to increase foot withdrawal thermal and electrical thresholds at 2 mg/kg	PD	Sladky et al,[11] 2006
	1	IM	Single dose	Cockatoos, gray parrots, blue-fronted Amazon parrots	Isoflurane-sparing study showed significant reduction in MAC in the cockatoos and gray parrots, but not Amazon parrots	PD	Curro[17] 1994, Curro[18] 1994
	1–2	IM	Single dose	Gray parrots	Increased electrical withdrawal threshold at 2 mg/kg	PD	Paul-Murphy et al,[5] 1999
	1, 3, 6	IM	Single dose	American kestrel	Failed to increase foot withdrawal thermal thresholds, but instead caused hyperaesthesia or hyperalgesia and agitation in males receiving 6 mg/kg; not recommended in American kestrels	PK/PD	Guzman et al,[19] 2014
	2	IV	Single dose	Domestic chickens	Remained above minimum effective concentration for analgesia in mammals for ~2 h	PK	Singh et al,[15] 2015
	2	IV	Single dose	Chicken	Decreased time to finish the obstacle course	PD	Singh et al[14] 2017; Hawkins et al,[175] 2016
	2,4	IV	Single dose	Guinea fowl	4 mg/kg resulted in arrhythmias and hypotension; one bird died	PD	Escobar et al,[176] 2012

Drug	Doses	Route	Species		Effect	PK/PD	Reference
Nalbuphine	12.5, 25, 50	IM	Hispaniolan Amazon parrots	Single dose	12.5 mg/kg resulted in increased thermal withdrawal thresholds for 3 h; higher doses did not increase duration of effect	PK/PD	Keller et al,[22] 2011; Sanchez-Migallon et al,[23] 2011
Tramadol	10, 20, 30	PO	Hispaniolan Amazon parrots	Single and multiple dose	30 mg/kg maintained above target plasma concentrations for ~8 h and increased thermal withdrawal response for ~6–8 h	PK, PD	Souza et al,[58] 2013; Souza et al,[60] 2012; Sanchez-Migallon et al,[61] 2012
	5, 15, 30	PO	American kestrel	Single dose	5 mg/kg significantly increased thermal withdrawal thresholds; higher doses resulted in less antinociceptive effects	PD	Guzman, et al,[62] 2014
	11	PO	Red-tailed hawks	Single dose	Maintained human plasma therapeutic concentrations for ~4 h 15 mg/kg q 12 h suggested based on the study	PK	Souza et al,[57] 2011
	11	PO	American bald eagles	Single dose	5 mg/kg q 12 h suggested based on study	PK	Souza et al,[55] 2009
	7.5	PO	Indian peafowl	Single dose	Maintained plasma human therapeutic concentrations for 12–24 h	PK	Black et al,[56] 2010

(continued on next page)

Table 1
(continued)

Drug	Dose (mg/kg)	Route of Administration	Frequency (h)	Species	Comments	Type of Study	Reference
	30	PO	Single dose	Muscovy ducks	Improved several variables in induced acute arthritis model as measured by ground reactive forces. Maintained above plasma target concentrations for at least 12 h	PK,PD	Bailey et al,[64] 2019, Bailey et al[177] 2019
	10	PO	Single dose	African penguin	Dose once daily seems adequate	PK	Kilburn et al,[63] 2014

Abbreviations: CRI, constant rate infusion; IM, intramuscular; IV, intravenous; MAC, minimum anesthetic concentration; PD, pharmacodynamic; PK, pharmacokinetic; PO, orally; q/h, every hour; SC, subcutaneously; t(1/2) = half-life; TD, transdermal.

at the structure of opioid receptors (μ, κ, and δ) in the peregrine falcon (*Falco peregrinus*), snowy owl (*Bubo scandiacus*), and blue-fronted Amazon parrot (*Amazona aestiva*), nucleotide homologies with humans only ranged from 77% to 82%, which might account for some of the differences seen in the efficacy of these drugs.[4]

Butorphanol

Butorphanol formulations have been studied in gray parrots and Timneh parrots (*Psittacus erithacus* and *Psittacus timneh*),[5] domestic pigeons,[6] red-tailed hawks (*Buteo jamaicensis*),[7] great horned owls (*Bubo virginianus*),[7] Hispaniolan Amazon parrots (*Amazona ventralis*),[8-13] broiler chickens (*G gallus domesticus*),[14,15] Indian peafowls (*Pavo cristatus*),[16] sulfur-crested cockatoos and yellow-crested cockatoos (*Cacatua galerita, Cacatua sulphurea cintrinocristata,* and *Cacatua sulphurea sulphurea*),[17] blue-fronted Amazon parrots (*Amazona aestiva aestiva*),[18] green-cheeked conures (*Pyrrhura molinae*),[13] American kestrels (*Falco sparverius*),[19] and orange-winged Amazon parrots (*Amazona amazonica*).[8,20] Most of these studies have evaluated the pharmacokinetics of the standard butorphanol tartrate formulation and there are some studies on sustained-release formulations, but only a few have evaluated the analgesic effects. Pharmacokinetic studies have shown that butorphanol has an excellent parenteral but poor oral bioavailability (less than 10%), is quickly absorbed both subcutaneously (SC) and intramuscular (IM), and has a very short half-life (eg, Hispaniolan Amazon parrots 0.51 hours, red-tailed hawks 0.93 hours, great horned owls 1.78 hours, American kestrels 1.48 hours, chickens 1.19 hours), which makes frequent administration (q 2–3 h) or continuous rate infusion (CRI) needed.[7,10,15,19] Pharmacodynamic studies have shown that relatively high doses are required in psittacines (eg, 1 mg/kg in gray parrots when using electrical antinociception and 5 mg/kg in Amazon parrots when using thermal antinociception) with a very short duration of action and relatively small effect (between 20 minutes and 1.5 hours in the aforementioned examples), but studies are lacking to evaluate the effect of different doses.[5,8,11] A study involving gray parrots, white cockatoos (*Cacatua alba*), and blue-fronted Amazon parrots using the minimum anesthetic concentration (MAC) sparing effect technique to determine the analgesic properties of butorphanol (1 mg/kg IM) resulted in a reduction of isoflurane MAC in cockatoos and gray parrots but not in blue-fronted Amazon parrots, indicating species variability to either the dose or the drug itself.[18] In white cockatoos, butorphanol significantly reduced isoflurane MAC from 1.44% ± 0.07% to 1.08% ± 0.05%.[17,18] Based on these studies, doses of 1 to 5 mg/kg have been recommended in psittacines.[21] In raptors, the results of the only pharmacodynamic study have been very different from those in psittacines. American kestrels receiving 1, 3, and 6 mg/kg IM had no thermal antinociceptive effects and even showed hyperalgesia in the males at the higher dose. These results discourage the use of butorphanol for analgesia in American kestrels and other birds of the *Falco* genus, but it is unknown if these findings can be extrapolated to other raptors. In chickens, lame broilers receiving 2 mg/kg intravenous (IV) finished an obstacle course faster than the controls, and together with the latency-to-lie results reported in the same study, may be analgesic for up to 2 hours. The butorphanol sustained-release formulations and osmotic pumps, although promising, unfortunately are not readily available to the clinicians and thus not frequently used.

Nalbuphine

Nalbuphine has been studied in Hispaniolan Amazon parrots, including standard and sustained-release formulations. Pharmacokinetic studies have shown that the standard nalbuphine hydrochloride has a similar pharmacokinetic profile as butorphanol, with a slightly shorter half-life.[22] The pharmacodynamic studies using thermal antinociception resulted in significant results at 12.5 mg/kg for up to 3 hours, whereas higher doses of 25 and 50 mg/kg were not different from control.[23] The nalbuphine sustained-release formulation, although promising because it resulted in a longer half-life[24] and duration of effect up to 12 hours,[25] is unfortunately not readily available to the clinician.

Hydromorphone

Hydromorphone has been studied in American kestrels,[26,27] cockatiels,[28] and orange-winged Amazons.[29,30] The pharmacokinetic studies have shown that hydromorphone has a good parenteral IM bioavailability, is quickly absorbed, and has a longer half-life (eg, 1.26 hours in American kestrels, 0.99 hours in cockatiels and 1.74 hours in orange-winged Amazon parrots) than butorphanol in the species evaluated but still requires administration every 3 to 6 hours commonly. Analgesiometry studies have shown that relatively high doses are required in psittacines when compared with raptors. In raptors, the studies in American kestrels have shown that hydromorphone at 0.1, 0.3, and 0.6 mg/kg IM had a dose-dependent effect using the thermal antinociception model.[27] In psittacines, in contrast, studies in cockatiels using the same antinociceptive dose in kestrels showed no significant effect.[28] In orange-winged Amazon parrots, higher doses of hydromorphone at 1 and 2 mg/kg showed thermal antinociception for 3 to 6 hours, respectively.[30] Agitation, nausealike behavior (including vomiting in one bird), ataxia, and pupillary constriction were observed following administration of the 1 and 2 mg/kg hydromorphone doses and warrant consideration for lower doses for clinical use in this species.

Morphine

Morphine has been studied in chickens in multiple studies (G gallus domesticus). The only pharmacokinetic study followed IV administration of 2 mg/kg and resulted in a half-life of 68 minutes, with a large volume of distribution and clearance.[31] The pharmacodynamic results from earlier studies have been conflicting and difficult to interpret likely due to the high doses evaluated, but more recent studies suggest that morphine might have analgesic and MAC-sparing effect in this species. In an early study, 200 mg/kg IM of morphine was required to produce antinociception in chicks using the toe pinch test,[32] but in a later study using noxious electrical stimulation, morphine produced analgesia in chicks at 30 mg/kg.[33] Further investigations using noxious thermal stimulation reported strain-dependent analgesic effects of morphine, requiring doses of 15, 30, and 100 mg/kg for 2 different White Leghorns lines and a cross of Rhode Island Red × Light Sussex, respectively,[34] and analgesia and hyperalgesic effects at 30 mg/kg, for Rhode Island Red cross, and White Leghorn and Cal-White strains, respectively.[35] In a MAC reduction study in chickens, 3 doses of morphine injected IV caused a dose-dependent decrease in isoflurane MAC in all birds.[36] The baseline isoflurane MAC of 1.24% ± 0.05% was reduced to 15.1% ± 2.7%, 39.7 ± 3.1%, and 52.4 ± 4.0% at doses of 0.1, 1.0, and 3.0 mg/kg, respectively.[36] In a recent study evaluating the analgesic efficacy of morphine, lame broiler chickens underwent an obstacle course (OC) and latency-to-lie (LTL) test before injection. The administration of 2 mg/kg IV morphine resulted in an increased time to finish the OC because sedation occurred, resulting in the chicks tending to sit down rather than walk and confounding assessment of its analgesic effects.[14]

Fentanyl

Fentanyl has been studied in white cockatoos,[37] red-tailed hawks,[38,39] helmeted guineafowl (Numida meleagris),[40] chickens,[41,42] and Hispaniolan Amazon parrots.[38,43] Pharmacokinetic studies have shown significant differences in the half-life, ranging from 30 to 90 minutes, discouraging extrapolation between species. In chickens, 25 μg/h transdermal fentanyl patches have shown a large variability in plasma concentrations,[41] but all chickens reached the human target plasma concentrations of 0.2 to 1.2 ng/mL within 2 to 4 hours and maintained above target for 72 hours with a rapid decrease in plasma concentrations following removal of the patch. The transdermal veterinary formulation evaluated in helmeted guineafowl was discontinued.[40] The pharmacodynamic studies have shown in psittacines that significantly higher doses or rates than other species are needed to see the desired analgesic or MAC-sparing effects, and that at these doses or rates other adverse effects occur, like agitation in awake white cockatoos receiving 0.2 mg/kg IM[37] or decrease in the heart rate and blood pressure in anesthetized Hispaniolan Amazon parrots in a dose-dependent manner.[43] In raptors, the findings have been very different and the rates required to see the same MAC-sparing effects have been 17 times lower than in psittacines and without any significant negative effect in heart rate or blood pressure. After a loading dose, rates of 10 to 30 μg/kg/h IV CRI were needed in red-tailed hawks to achieve MAC decreases ranging from 31% to 55% in a dose-dependent manner.[39,44]

Methadone

Methadone has been studied in orange-winged Amazon parrots (Guzman DS-M, Knych H, Douglas J, et al. Pharmacokinetics of methadone after intravenous and intramuscular administration of a single dose to orange-winged Amazon parrots (*Amazona amazonica*), unpublished, 2020; Guzman DS-M, Douglas J, Beaufrère H, et al. Evaluation of thermal antinociceptive effects after intramuscular administration of methadone to orange-winged Amazon parrots (*Amazona amazonica*), unpublished, 2020) and chickens.[45,46] The pharmacokinetic studies have shown a longer half-life than other opioid drugs but with differences between species (eg, orange-winged Amazon parrots 2.3 hours, chickens under anesthesia 3 hours). The pharmacodynamic study with thermal antinociception has shown that relatively high doses are required in orange-winged Amazon parrots (eg, 6 mg/kg IM). Agitation, ataxia, and nausealike behavior were observed following administration and warrant consideration for lower doses for clinical use in this species. In chickens, MAC-sparing effects were found at 6 mg/kg IM, but not at 3 mg/kg, with a reduction of 29%, 27%, and 10% at 15, 30, and 45 minutes after methadone administration, respectively.[46]

Buprenorphine

Buprenorphine has been studies in gray parrots,[5,47] domestic pigeons (*Columba livia*),[6] American kestrels,[48–51] red-tailed hawks,[52] cockatiels,[48] and orange-winged Amazon parrots.(Guzman DS-M, Douglas J, Beaufrère H, et al. Evaluation of thermal antinociceptive effects after intramuscular administration of concentrated buprenorphine to orange-winged Amazon parrots (*Amazona amazonica*), unpublished, 2020.) The pharmacokinetic studies have been performed in standard, sustained-released (Buprenorphine SR LAB) and concentrated formulations (1.8 mg/mL; Simbadol) Those studies have shown major differences in the half-life between species (eg, 1.5 hours in American kestrels[53] and 6.23 hours in red-tailed hawks[52]). In red-tailed hawks, 0.3 mg/kg and 1.8 mg/kg doses using concentrated buprenorphine resulted in plasma concentrations maintained above 1 ng/mL for at least 24 and 48 hours, respectively.[52] The pharmacodynamic studies in psittacines have been discouraging because of the lack of significant effect with electrical or thermal antinociception in the species and doses evaluated (eg, 0.1 mg/kg IM in gray parrots[5] and 0.6, 1.2, and 1.8 mg/kg IM in cockatiels[48]). Recent unpublished studies have shown a small but significant effect in orange-winged Amazon parrots following 2 mg/kg IM, but not at 1 and 0.1 mg/kg doses. In contrast, the pharmacodynamic studies in raptors have shown a longer duration of action than other opioids (eg, could last 6–9 hours in American kestrels following 0.6 mg/kg IM[54]) with mild sedation. High doses have been shown to be well tolerated and provide longer analgesic effects with moderate sedation. Sustained-release formulations are commercially available (eg, Buprenorphine SR LAB), which have shown also to be well tolerated and prolonged the effects (eg, 24 hours following 1.8 mg/kg SC in American kestrels) minimizing handling and the need for repeated injections.[49]

Tramadol

Tramadol has been evaluated in bald eagles (*Haliaeetus leucocephalus*),[55] peafowl (*P cristatus*),[56] red-tailed hawks,[57] Hispaniolan Amazon parrots,[58–61] American kestrels,[62] African penguins (*Spheniscus demersus*),[63] and Muscovy ducks (*Cairina moschata domestica*).[64] The pharmacokinetics of tramadol has shown variability in half-life between species (eg, red-tailed hawks 1.3 hours and African penguins 7.3 hours). In all the species in which the metabolites have been evaluated in pharmacokinetic studies, the primary active metabolite O-desmethyltramadol (M1) has also been measured confirming concentrations that would be analgesic in other species and a longer half-life than the parent drug in most cases. There have also been large differences in the oral bioavailability between species, which was found to be 24% in Hispaniolan Amazon parrots[60] but almost 98% in bald eagles[55] and needs to be taken into consideration when extrapolating doses between studies and routes of administration. The pharmacodynamic studies have shown large differences in the doses required for thermal antinociception between the psittacines and raptors species studied following oral administration, which could be explained by the differences in the pharmacokinetics alone. For example, Hispaniolan Amazon parrots showed thermal antinociception at 30 mg/kg administered orally and at 5 mg/kg IV, but not at 10 or 20 mg/kg administered orally, whereas American kestrels at 5 mg/kg orally had already a significant effect and higher doses of 15 and 30 mg/kg resulted in a shorter duration of action and gastrointestinal adverse effects in a few birds. No sedation or agitation was seen in these psittacine and raptor studies. In Muscovy ducks 30 mg/kg orally was effective in improving several variables in a temporary arthritis model in the intertarsal joint and assessed by ground-reactive forces measured by a pressure-sensitive walkway system.[64]

NONSTEROIDAL ANTI-INFLAMMATORY DRUGS

NSAIDs are used to relieve musculoskeletal and visceral pain, acute pain, and chronic pain such as in osteoarthritis. The pharmacologic activity of NSAIDs has been reviewed elsewhere, and the mechanism of action is similar when administered to birds.[65,66] A broad tissue distribution of cyclo-oxygenase (COX) has been demonstrated in chickens.[67] The relative expression of COX-1 and COX-2 enzymes varies between species, and both enzymes are important in pain and inflammation. The application and dosages of NSAID formulations continues to be scientifically evaluated and clinically applied in birds (**Table 2**). The intention of recently developed NSAIDs has been to spare COX-1 and emphasize COX-2 inhibition with the goal of providing analgesia and suppressing inflammation without inhibiting the physiologically important prostaglandins. The common NSAIDs used in avian medicine include meloxicam, carprofen, celecoxib, robenacoxib, and piroxicam, each with a distinct COX-1/COX-2 ratio and differing reports of effectiveness and toxicity in birds.

The most common adverse effects of NSAIDs include effects on the gastrointestinal system, renal system, and coagulation. NSAIDs have been implicated in humans and mammals with an increased risk of myocardial infarction and delays in bone healing,[68,69] but these effects have not been substantiated to date in birds. It is prudent to remember these adverse effects are often dose dependent and are associated with chronic administration. The kidney uses both COX-1 and COX-2 for prostaglandin synthesis, and injury occurs when renal prostaglandin synthesis is inhibited. Originally it was hypothesized that the adverse renal effects of NSAIDs were linked primarily to COX-1 inhibition, but COX-2 metabolites have been implicated in the maintenance of renal blood flow, mediation of renin release, and regulation of sodium excretion. Therefore, in conditions of relative intravascular volume depletion and/or renal hypoperfusion such as dehydration, hemorrhage, hemodynamic compromise, heart failure, and renal disease, interference with COX-2 activity can have significant deleterious effects on renal blood flow and glomerular filtration rate.

The pharmacokinetics of NSAIDs are typically measured from plasma samples, but it is important to remember that tissue kinetics may differ significantly, with drugs that have short plasma half-lives being active in the tissue long after the drug has disappeared from the plasma. In mammals, this has been evaluated using tissue cages where it is possible to measure the effect and duration of the NSAID by quantitating the effect on prostaglandins in the tissue. With robenacoxib in cats, for example, the mean plasma residence time (MRT) following oral administration was 3.3 hours, whereas the MRT in tissue was 24 hours.[70] To the authors' knowledge, only a single report describes the use of this model in turkeys for evaluation of sodium salicylate,[71] but the researchers did not include plasma concentrations.

Meloxicam

Meloxicam is the most widely used anti-inflammatory medication today in avian practice (see Table 2). Meloxicam is a COX-2-selective NSAID that demonstrates COX-1 selectivity at higher doses.[72–74] Meloxicam is currently available in the United States as an oral tablet, oral suspension, and injectable formulation. Pharmacokinetic studies of meloxicam in chickens,[72,75,76] ostriches (Struthio camelus),[77] emus (Dromaius novaehollandiae),[74,78] mallard ducks,[73] Bilgorajska geese (Anser anser domesticus),[79] brown pelicans (Pelecanus occidentalis),[80] turkeys (Meleagris spp),[73] Japanese quail (Coturnix japonica),[81] chukar partridge (Alectoris chukar),[82] domestic pigeons,[73] zebra finches (Taeniopygia guttata),[83] ring-necked parakeets (Psittacula krameria),[84] Hispaniolan Amazon parrots,[85] gray parrots,[86] cockatiels,[87] flamingos (Phoeniconaias minor, Phoenicopterus ruber),[88–90] African penguins (S demersus),[91] red-tailed hawks and great-horned owls,[92] and multiple vulture species (Gyps africanus, Gyps coprotheres, Torgos tracheliotos, and Neophron pernopterus)[93] have been published.

Differences in dosage, bioavailability, clearance, and elimination half-lives most likely contribute to the clinical differences seen with the use of this NSAID. For example, the elimination half-life of meloxicam in chickens and pigeons is 3 times as long as that in ducks, ostriches, and turkeys.[73] Meloxicam in Wyandotte hens had greater area under the plasma concentration versus time curve, a smaller elimination rate constant, and a longer terminal half-life, and the drug persisted longer in their egg yolks compared with White Leghorn hens suggesting the dosing interval of meloxicam administered orally may be every 24 hours as opposed to every 12 hours in White Leghorn chickens. Following 1 mg/kg oral administration of meloxicam, the elimination half-life and bioavailability of meloxicam in Hispaniolan Amazon parrots was

Table 2
Selected nonsteroidal anti-inflammatory drugs evaluated in avian species by pharmacokinetic, pharmacodynamic evaluations, toxicologic, or clinical studies

Drug	Dose (mg/kg)	Route	Frequency	Species	Comments	Type of Study	Reference
Meloxicam	1	IV, PO	Single dose	Cockatiel	Very low (11%) oral bioavailability and shorter half-life than other psittacines	PK	Dhondt et al,[87] 2017
	1 / 0.5	IM, IV, PO / IM	Single dose / Multiple dose q 12 h for 14 d	Gray parrots	1 mg/kg would maintain target plasma concentrations for 24 h; 0.5 mg/kg IM q 12 h did not cause renal lesions	PK/TOX	Montesinos et al,[86] 2017; Montesinos et al,[101] 2015
	1 / 1, 1.6	IM / PO	q 24	Gray parrot	Moderate bioaccumulation. Elevation of the renal marker NAG at highest dose	PK	Montesinos et al,[94] 2019
	1 / 1 / 1.6	IM, IV / IM / PO	Single dose / Multiple dose q 12 h / Multiple dose q 12 h	Hispaniolan Amazon parrots	1 mg/kg IM maintains above plasma concentration for 12 h; Oral bioavailability (49%–75%) suggests higher oral doses of 1.6 mg/kg q 12 h needed; Effective in arthritis model; No adverse effects in multiple-dose study	PK, PK, PD, TOX	Molter et al,[85] 2013; Dijkstra et al,[105] 2015; Cole et al,[178] 2009
	0.1	IM	24 for 7 d	Budgerigars	Glomerular congestion	TOX	Pereira and Werther,[100] 2007
		IM	Single dose	Ring-necked parakeets		PK	Wilson et al,[84] 2004
	0.5	IV, PO	Single dose	Red-tailed hawks and great-horned owls		PK	Lacasse et al,[92] 2013
	2	IM, PO	Single dose	Cape Griffon vultures	Short $t_{1/2}$ <45 min	PK	Naidoo et al,[93] 2008

Dose	Route	Frequency	Species	Comments	Type	Reference
1	PO	Multiple dose q 12 h for 5 d	Chicken	2-wk withdrawal time should be adequate to avoid drug residues in eggs	PD	Souza et al,[75] 2018
0.5	IV	Single dose	Chickens, ostrich, ducks, turkeys, pigeons	Variable distribution, slow clearance except ostrich	PK	Baert and De Backer[73] 2003
2	IM	Multiple dose	Japanese quail	2 mg/kg IM q 12 h for 14 d did not cause significant renal lesions but resulted in muscle necrosis	TOX	Sinclair et al,[103] 2012
2	IM	Multiple dose	Japanese quail	2 mg/kg IM q 12 h for 14 d did not cause significant renal lesions but resulted in muscle necrosis	TOX	Sinclair et al,[103] 2012
0.5, 2	IM-PO	Multiple dose	Pigeon	2 mg/kg was needed for significant analgesia in orthopedic pain	PD	Desmarchelier et al,[102] 2012
0.2	PO	Single dose	Brown pelican	Longest half-life of any avian species to date of 36.3 h. Caution in frequency of administration required	PK	Horgan et al,[80] 2020
0.5, 1	IM PO	Single dose	African penguin	Based on plasma concentrations, recommended 1 mg/kg orally every 48 h and 0.5 mg/kg IM every 24 h	PK	Morrison et al,[91] 2018
Sustained-release meloxicam						
3	SC	Single dose	Hispaniolan Amazon parrot	Very high interindividual variability. Remained above target plasma concentrations for 12–96 h	PK	Guzman et al,[96] 2017
3	SC	Single dose	American flamingos	Remained above target plasma concentrations for 0.5–4 h	PK	Sim and Cox,[97] 2018

(continued on next page)

Table 2
(continued)

Drug	Dose (mg/kg)	Route	Frequency	Species	Comments	Type of Study	Reference
Celecoxib	10	IV, PO	Single dose	Cockatiel		PK	Dhondt et al,[87] 2017
Mavacoxib	4	IV, PO	Single dose	Cockatiel	Very long half life	PK	Dhondt et al,[87] 2017
	6	PO	Single dose	Caribbean flamingos	Very high interindividual variability	PK	Huckins et al,[117] 2020
Carprofen	3	IM	12	Hispaniolan Amazon parrots	Insufficient to restore weight-bearing in arthritis model	PD	Cox et al,[122] 2011
	5	IV, IM, PO	Single dose	White-backed vultures		PK, PD	Naido124 2018
	30	IM	Single dose	Chickens	Arthritis painful behaviors reduced 1 h after treatment	PD	Hocking et al,[179] 2005
	1	IM	Single dose	Chickens	Improved locomotion of lame birds 1 h after treatment	PD	McGeowen et al,[119] 1999
Ketoprofen	2.0	IV,IM,PO	Single dose	Quail	Low bioavailability IM, PO. Short IV elimination half-life	PK	Graham et al,[125] 2005
	12	IM	Single dose	Chickens	Arthritis painful behaviors reduced 1 h after treatment	PD	Hocking et al,[179] 2005
	2.5	IM	24 for 7 d	Budgerigars	Tubular necrosis	TOX	Pereira and Werther,[100] 2007
	5	IM	Single dose	Mallard ducks	12 h activity	PD	Machin et al,[126] 2001
	2.0 5.0	PO IM, IV	12–24	King eiders	Mortality associated with drakes	CS	Mulcahy et al,[180] 2003

Drug	Dose	Route	Frequency	Species	Comments	Type	Reference
Flunixin meglumine	5	IV	Single dose	Budgerigars and Patagonian conures			Musser et al,[181] 2013
	5.0	IM	Single dose	Mallard ducks	12-h activity but muscle necrosis injection site	PD	Machin et al,[126] 2001
	5.5	IM	24: 7 d	Budgerigars	Severe renal lesions	TOX	Pereira and Werther,[100] 2007
	1.1	IV	Single dose	Chickens, ostrich, ducks, turkeys, pigeons	Chickens had long half-life but 10 min half-life in ostrich	PK	Baert and De Backer,[73] 2003
	3	IM	Single dose	Chickens	Arthritis painful behaviors reduced 1 h after treatment	PD	Hocking et al,[179] 2005
Piroxicam	0.5–0.8	PO	12	Whooping cranes	Used for acute myopathy and chronic arthritis	CS	Hanley et al,[182] 2005
	0.5	PO	Single dose	Brolgascranes		PK	Keiper et al,[130] 2017
Grapiprant	30	PO	Single dose	Red-tailed hawks	Based on plasma concentrations, q 12 h with food suggested; concentrations without food 88% higher	PK	Rodriguez et al,[147] 2021; Rodriguez et al,[148] 2022

Abbreviations: CS, care report or case series; NAG, *N*-acetyl beta glucosaminidase; PD, pharmacodynamic; PK, pharmacokinetic; PO, orally; q/h, every hour; TOX, toxicity.

15.8 ± 8.6 hours and 49% to 75%, respectively.[85] However, in gray parrots following 1 mg/kg meloxicam orally, the elimination half-life was more than twice that of Hispaniolan Amazon parrots with significantly lower oral bioavailability (38.1% ± 3.6%).[86] In cockatiels, following oral administration of 1 mg/kg meloxicam of the commercial formulation, it was found to have only 11% oral bioavailability and an elimination half-life of less than 1 hour.[87] The highly variable bioavailability in avian species[85,86,92] is quite different from that in mammals where it is usually 85% or greater.[87] A possible explanation could be variability in proventricular pH among species.[86] In a multiple-dose pharmacokinetic study performed in gray parrots evaluating 3 different dosages (1 mg/kg, IM, every 24 hours; 1 mg/kg, orally, every 24 hours; and 1.6 mg/kg, orally, every 24 hours) plasma concentrations were maintained at values greater than effective analgesic concentrations described for other avian species and evidence of moderate drug accumulation was found with both IM and oral routes of administration.[94] In White Leghorn chickens, dosing of meloxicam 1 mg/kg orally every 12 hours for 5 days resulted in the presence of meloxicam residues in eggs in the yolks and whites after 8 and 3 days, respectively,[75] whereas Wyandotte chickens administered a single 1 mg/kg dose showed residues after 4 and 9 days, respectively.[76] Based on these results, a 2-week withdrawal time should be adequate to avoid drug residues in eggs meant for consumption.[75,76] Meloxicam was also identified in two-thirds of unfertilized eggs of captive bearded vultures after breeding failure, but the implication is unclear.[95] The large variability in pharmacokinetics between avian species is one of the main issues with analgesic therapy in birds, because cross-species allometric scaling is not reliable and therefore pharmacokinetic/pharmacodynamic analysis is required in every species.[73]

A sustained-release formulation of meloxicam (Meloxicam SR) has been evaluated in 2 species: Hispaniolan Amazon parrots[96] and American flamingos.[97] Based on the results of these studies its use cannot be recommended due to the huge pharmacokinetic variability (parrots) and lack of difference from standard meloxicam (flamingos).

There are very few studies evaluating the pharmacodynamics of meloxicam to date. In an experimental trial in lame chickens, meloxicam significantly increased the thermal threshold compared with saline.[98] Administration of meloxicam at 0.5 mg/kg IM or 2 mg/kg IM reduced clinical signs associated with experimental systemic inflammation induced by *Escherichia coli* lipopolysaccharide in broiler chickens, but dexamethasone was ultimately preferred by the investigators for its clinical effects of reducing the acute inflammation.[99]

Because higher doses of meloxicam can block COX-1 enzyme activity, this drug has the potential to induce the adverse effects of gastrointestinal, renal, and cardiac toxicity seen in mammals, yet reports of intoxication at doses used in avian practice are minimal. In several studies evaluating the adverse effects of meloxicam in budgerigars (*Melopsittacus undulatus*; 0.1 mg/kg IM),[100] gray parrots (0.5 mg/kg IM),[101] zebra finches (1–2 mg/kg orally),[83] domestic pigeons (2 mg/kg IM),[102] Japanese quail (2 mg/kg IM),[103] American kestrels (2–20 mg/kg orally),[104] and Hispaniolan Amazon parrots (1.6 mg/kg orally)[105] no significant renal, gastrointestinal, or hemostatic adverse effects were reported at doses in the therapeutic range. However, 2 of 9 American kestrels had gastric ulceration after a dose of 20 mg/kg.[106] Plasma and urine N-acetyl-β-D-glucosaminidase activities were significantly increased in gray parrots at 1.6 mg/kg meloxicam administered orally every 24 hours for 7 days.[94] Elimination half-lives of meloxicam are highly variable, as indicated earlier, and those species with rapid elimination[87] are less likely to have adverse effects. Anecdotal reports of visceral gout and gastrointestinal ulceration in brown pelicans, using dosages commonly used in mammalian species, prompted a pharmacokinetic study using a single dose of 0.2 mg/kg orally. The elimination half-life was 36 hours, the highest reported to date in any species, heightening suspicion that adverse effects, including renal toxicity, may be attributed to this.[80] The renal effects of NSAIDs have been of particular concern in the Asian vultures (*Gyps bengalensis*, *Gyps indicus*, and *Gyps tenuirostris*),[107,108] but meloxicam may be the exception because of its short elimination half-life (<1 hour) in those birds.[109] However, recently meloxicam was detected in eggs of captive bearded vultures (*Gypaetus barbatus*).[95] Despite meloxicam's large therapeutic range and relative safety compared with other NSAIDs, these new data demonstrate that dose extrapolation is not a suitable method for meloxicam dose determination in avian species. Species-specific pharmacokinetic, efficacy, and toxicity studies are necessary to determine appropriate dosages for different species.

Celecoxib, Mavacoxib, Robenacoxib

The newer NSAID coxibs celecoxib, mavacoxib, and robenacoxib are COX-2 selective as opposed to meloxicam, which is COX-2 preferential, inhibiting both COX-1 and COX-2. Celecoxib in humans is used for acute pain, osteoarthritis, rheumatoid arthritis, and spondylitis (see Table 2). Its use in veterinary medicine is off label in the United States; it is not approved for use in any veterinary species. Celecoxib 10 mg/kg administered orally every 24 hours has been used to reduce inflammation associated with avian bornavirus.[110] A recent study in cockatiels using this dose did not alter the clinical presentation, viral shedding, gross lesions, histopathology, or viral distribution in cockatiels experimentally inoculated with Parrot bornavirus-2,[111] but the birds were infected with a large viral load inducing severe disease, so it is difficult to determine whether this drug has any efficacy against natural inflammation induced by this disease. Anecdotally, there are suggestions of very high doses of 30 to 40 mg/kg divided orally every 12 hours, then long term 15 to 20 mg/kg orally every 12 hours for gastrointestinal signs, and 60 to 80 mg/kg divided orally every 12 hours for central nervous system involvement with avian bornavirus.[112] Mavacoxib administered orally has a long mean half-life of 15.5 days in dogs, allowing for monthly dosing after 2 loading doses administered 1 week apart.[113]

The single-dose pharmacokinetics and oral bioavailability of celecoxib 10 mg/kg orally and mavacoxib 4 mg/kg orally were evaluated in the cockatiel.[87] Mavacoxib was completely absorbed (bioavailability = 111%), but celecoxib only had a mean oral bioavailability of 56%.[87] Bioavailability of the coxibs is often directly associated with feeding status; the presence of food has been shown to increase absorption of both NSAIDs.[114] The cockatiels in this study were fed ad libitum. A further study in cockatiels with ad libitum feeding and additional gavage feedings during the study showed that changes in body temperature, mentation, and posture were less pronounced with a single dose of mavacoxib 4 mg/kg administered orally compared with celecoxib 10 mg/kg at the tested dosages[115]; this is likely associated with the higher oral bioavailability of mavacoxib in cockatiels compared with celecoxib and meloxicam. Plasma concentrations of 0.4 μg/mL mavacoxib, found to be effective in osteoarthritic dogs,[116] were maintained for 1000 hours (41.6 days) in the cockatiels in the aforementioned studies,[87,115] and Caribbean flamingos maintained plasma concentrations greater than 0.4 μg/mL for 120 hours after a single dose of 6 mg/kg.[117] Elimination half-lives in cockatiels (135 hours)[87] and Caribbean flamingos (*P ruber*; 74.5 hours)[117] were not as long as in dogs but are still much longer than most NSAID elimination half-lives in birds and prompt additional studies to determine dosing regimens.[117]

No studies have been published to date on the use of robenacoxib, also a long-acting COX NSAID; however, it is being used anecdotally at 2 to 10 mg/kg IM[118] weekly initially, and then monthly in birds with clinical avian bornavirus.[112] Robenacoxib is available as tablets and in an injectable formulation currently in the United States.

Carprofen

The oral bioavailability of carprofen was reported to be 61% in Japanese quail.[81] Carprofen given SC improved the locomotion of lame domestic fowl, significantly, in a dose-dependent manner,[119] and lame birds self-selected food containing carprofen.[120] When carprofen was administered at 3 to 4 mg/kg in drinking water, 15% of birds died on day 10 of treatment, so short-term (<7 days) therapy for lameness was recommended.[121] Carprofen administered at 3 mg/kg IM every 12 hours was insufficient to restore weight-bearing in induced arthritis in Hispaniolan parrots.[122] In pigeons, doses of 2, 5, and 10 mg/kg given IM once daily over 7 days resulted in significant increases in alanine transaminase and aspartate aminotransferase and a mild decrease in total protein (primarily globulin).[123] In addition, small intestinal vascular congestion was noted grossly and hepatic necrosis, renal congestion, and myodegeneration of the pectoral muscles were noted histologically. These effects were significantly associated with dosing.[123] Although not significant, hepatic lipidosis was also noted and the frequency increased with dose. The investigators speculated that this may be secondary to decreased food consumption noted in pigeons within the highest dosing group.[123]

Even though it is thought that carprofen ingested by *Gyps* vultures does not pose a toxic risk like diclofenac, there are still concerns about its safety in these birds. In a recent pharmacokinetic and toxicoloigc study in white-backed vultures (*G africanus*) of 5 mg/kg were administered IV, IM, and orally for the pharmacokinetic study and a subset of birds were administered the dosage found at injection sites in cattle (64 mg/kg) for the toxicology study. Carprofen was well tolerated at 5 mg/kg via all routes of administration, but oral bioavailability was only 42%.[124] One vulture died in the toxicology study with elevations of uric acid and potassium levels identified, like toxicity found with diclofenac and ketoprofen in *Gyps* vultures. The investigators suggested that carprofen should not be used in domesticated ungulates in areas where carcasses are accessible or provided to vultures at supplementary feeding sites.[124]

Ketoprofen and Piroxicam

Ketoprofen is commonly used parenterally because of limited oral pharmacokinetic data and difficulty in accurately dosing in small species. In Japanese quail (*C japonica*) ketoprofen (2 mg/kg orally, IM, IV) showed very low oral (24%) and IM (54%) bioavailability and the shortest half-life reported for any species.[125] Additional studies are needed to determine whether drug formulation or interspecies physiologic contrasts account for these differences. In mallard ducks ketoprofen (5 mg/kg IM) decreased blood thromboxane B_2 levels for approximately 12 hours.[126]

Ketoprofen and meloxicam were detected in the eggs of captive-reared bearded vultures.[95] Two studies evaluating the effects of an extraordinarily high single dose (50 mg/kg IM) of ketoprofen, as a premedication to ketamine and midazolam in pigeons, found no significant clinical differences, biochemistry analytes, or histopathology between the groups.[127,128] Regardless of their findings, the extremely high dosing of this drug should be reviewed in multidose studies and with the utmost caution before considering it for clinical use.

Piroxicam is a nonselective NSAID used for its anti-inflammatory properties and its value as a chemopreventative and antitumor agent; it has a much higher potency against COX-1 than COX-2. In chickens, IM administration of 1 to 2 mg/kg of piroxicam twice daily for 4 days failed to result in gastrointestinal lesions consistent with toxicity.[129] Piroxicam has been used in cranes for more than 20 years to treat a variety of conditions including trauma, inflammation, and postoperative pain with minimal observed side effects.[130] A pharmacokinetic study in brolga cranes *(Grus rubicunda)* evaluated 2 single doses of 0.5 mg/kg and 1 mg/kg administered orally, finding that daily administration might be appropriate for this species based on plasma concentrations.[130]

Scavenging bird species such as vultures and eagles may be exposed to NSAIDs when they feed on livestock carcasses.[131,132] The NSAID diclofenac played the major role in the catastrophic decline in vulture populations on the Indian subcontinent.[133] Subsequently, other NSAIDs have also been identified as toxic to vultures. Ketoprofen and nimesulfide, a sulfonamide NSAID, caused visceral gout and death in vultures, whereas meloxicam and tolfenamic acid (TA) were reported to be safe.[108,134–139]

Tolfenamic Acid

Other NSAIDs must be identified to reduce the use of those toxic to vultures and other scavengers. TA is an NSAID belonging to the fenamates group.[140] This NSAID inhibits both COX-1 and COX-2 receptor activity and exerts potent antitumor activity by both COX-dependent and -independent pathways.[141] TA was detected in 20% Eurasian griffon vulture *(Gyps fulvus)* nestling samples,[142] suggesting it is being used more frequently by veterinarians in the region. A study evaluated the safety of TA in 3 *Gyps* species, all of which are susceptible to diclofenac poisoning. Two birds administered 3.5 mg/kg TA orally via gavage died with elevated uric acid levels and severe visceral gout, yet the remainder showed no adverse clinical or biochemical signs at the same or even higher doses, suggesting the deaths may have been an anomaly due to the high dose used and the high ambient temperatures at the time of the experiment.[135] Tolfenamic acid is likely to be safe to *Gyps* vultures at concentrations encountered by wild birds and could therefore be promoted as a safe alternative to toxic NSAIDs.[135]

To date only the pharmacokinetics of TA are reported in chukar partridge,[143] Japanese quail,[143] and geese *(Anser cygnoides)*.[144] The elimination half-lives of TA administered orally in chukar partridges, Japanese quail, and geese were 1.25, 1.95, and 2.31 hours, quite similar to meloxicam.[143,144] This short half-life is important in preventing drug accumulation and delaying toxic effects in repeated administrations in birds.[93] Bioavailability after a 2 mg/kg dose was 87.91%, 77.87%, and 76.03% for the IM, SC, and oral routes, respectively, in geese, and 57.32% via the oral route in Japanese quail suggesting good absorption in these species.

At present, there are no specific dosing recommendations for TA in birds, but it is recommended at doses of 2 to 4 mg/kg in mammals and reptiles.[145,146] Although the few studies to date are promising, additional studies evaluating clinical efficacy, multiple-dose pharmacokinetics, safety, and residue data of TA should be conducted before widespread use of TA in birds at mammalian doses.

Grapiprant

Grapiprant is a prostaglandin E_2 (PGE_2) receptor antagonist approved for use in dogs in the United States (see Table 2). Grapiprant binds to the EP4 receptor, blocking the sensitization of sensory neurons and stimulation of inflammation mediated by the PGE_2 receptor; it does not rely on inhibition of COX enzymes and preserves functions associated with COX enzyme pathways. Oral administration of a single dose of grapiprant at 30 approximately 30 mg/kg to fasted red-tailed hawks reached plasma concentrations 19 to 32 times the canine therapeutic concentrations within 2 hours approximately and with no adverse effects identified.[147] Grapiprant administered at the same dose to the same red-tailed hawks with food had lower plasma concentrations by 88%, with delayed absorption and a similar half-life.[148] Grapiprant plasma concentrations were achieved above the canine therapeutic concentrations within 16 hours postmedication. Mean concentrations were maintained for approximately 20 hours. Simulations support a dosing frequency of 12-hour intervals with food reaching minimum effective concentrations established for canines, although it is unknown whether these plasma concentrations are therapeutic for birds.[148] Further studies to evaluate grapiprant pharmacokinetics, efficacy, and safety in red-tailed hawks and other avian species are needed.

OTHER DRUGS
Gabapentin

Gabapentin is an analogue of the neurotransmitter γ-aminobutyric acid that binds to voltage-gated calcium channels acting presynaptically to decrease the release of excitatory neurotransmitters, especially glutamate (**Table 3**). In humans and animals, it is best used as an adjunct to other analgesics and seems to be most effective for neuropathic pain. Some formulations of gabapentin contain xylitol, and these should not be used in birds until further safety evidence is available. The pharmacokinetics of gabapentin have been evaluated in several species, including Hispaniolan Amazon parrots,[149] great horned owls,[150] and Caribbean flamingos.[151] The oral bioavailability was found to be high (>80%) in Hispaniolan Amazon parrots,[149] and the peak plasma concentration occurred between 0.5 and 2.5 hours.[149,150] The half-life has been in the range of 3 to 5 hours, and so gabapentin should be administered 2 to 3 times per day to maintain adequate plasma concentrations. In great horned owls following oral administration of 11 mg/kg orally, plasma gabapentin concentrations were maintained above 2 µg/mL for 9.6 hours.[150] In Caribbean flamingos, gabapentin dosed at 25 mg/kg orally in most birds maintained plasma concentrations above the therapeutic range established for humans for approximately 12 hours; however, dosages as high as 37 mg/kg orally every 12 hour may be needed in some individuals.

Amantadine

Amantadine is an antiviral medication that increases dopamine in the central nervous system and weakly inhibits the N-methyl-D-aspartate receptors that contribute to chronic pain (see Table 3).[152] Amantadine is synergistic with NSAIDs, opioids, and gabapentin/pregabalin. In humans, amantadine has been shown to decrease opioid use in postoperative patients, decrease pain in postherpetic neuralgia, and aid in neuropathic analgesia.[153,154] Amantadine orally administered to dogs at 3 to 5 mg/kg every 24 hours in conjunction with meloxicam showed significant improvement in the management of osteoarthritis pain refractory to meloxicam alone.[155] In orange-winged Amazon parrots, single- and multiple-dose pharmacokinetic profiles were evaluated following 10 mg/kg orally once and 5 mg/kg orally every 24 hours for 7 days.[156] The heart rate, respiratory rate, behavior, and urofeces were monitored. Half-life was 23.2 and 21.5 hours for the single- and multiple-dose studies, respectively. No obvious adverse effects were observed. Based on these results, once-daily administration of amantadine at 5 mg/kg orally in orange-winged Amazon parrots can maintain above-target plasma concentration with weak accumulation. For long-

Table 3
Local anesthetic evaluated in avian species by either pharmacokinetic or pharmacodynamic evaluations

Drug	Dose (mg/kg)	Route	Frequency Q~hr	Species	Comments	Type of Study	Reference
Lidocaine	2	PN	Single dose	Hispaniolan Amazon parrot	No effect on motor function, muscle relaxation, or wing droop was observed	PD	da Cunha et al,[168] 2013
	6	IV	Single dose	Chicken	6 mg/kg did not cause clinically relevant effects on HR or MAP	PD	Brandao et al,[159] 2015
	20	PN	Single dose	Chickens	High failure rate	PD	da Cunha et al,[167] 2013
	2.5	IV	Single dose	Chicken		PK	Da Cunha et al,[161] 2012
	0.5, 1, 2	IT	Single administration	Chicken	Onset of pericloacal anesthesia 1–2 min, and duration of effect 4.5, 11.3, and 21.3 min, respectively	PD	Kazemi-Darabadi[170] 2019
	15	PN	Single dose	Mallard ducks	Ineffective in producing local analgesia	PD	Brenner et al,[160] 2010
Bupivacaine	5	PN	Single dose	Chickens	High failure rate	PD	Figueiredo[167] 2008
	3	IA	Single dose	Chickens	Effective in treating arthritic pain	PD	Hocking et al,[165] 1997
	1.33, 1.96	IV	Single administration	Chicken	1.96 mg/kg IV bupivacaine associated with a 50% probability of a clinically relevant change in MAP and HR, whereas 1.33 mg/kg IV bupivacaine is associated with a 1% probability of causing the same effect	PD	DiGeronimo et al,[164] 2015
	0.1, 0.25, 0.5	IT	Single administration	Chicken	Onset of pericloacal anesthesia 9, 4.33, and 3.33 min, and duration of effect was 11.18 and 54 min, respectively	PD	Khamisabadi et al,[162] 2021
	2	SC	Single dose	Mallard ducks		PK	Machin and Livingstone,[163] 2001
	2, 8	PN	Single dose	Mallard ducks	Ineffective in producing local analgesia	PD	Brenner et al,[160] 2010

Abbreviations: HR, heart rate; IA, intra-articular; IT, intrathecal; MAP, mean arterial pressure; PN, perineural.

term administration, especially for other species, it is recommended to check plasma concentrations over time. Further studies evaluating safety and efficacy of amantadine in orange-winged Amazon parrots and other avian species are warranted. It is also important to remember that the use of amantadine in chickens, ducks, and turkeys is prohibited in the United States by the US Food and Drug Administration.

Cannabinoids

Cannabinoids have been evaluated in other species for their multiple effects including pain relief and anti-inflammatory properties, making it an attractive therapeutic option in birds with chronic pain. Cannabidiol (CBD) is the primary nonpsychoactive cannabinoid derived from the cannabis plant (*Cannabis sativa*) that can interact with the endocannabinoid system, but other cannabionoids like cannabidiolic acid (CBDA) have gained more recent interest. The single-dose pharmacokinetics of a CBD oral formulation (50 mg/mL; Canna Companion) have been evaluated in Hispaniolan Amazon parrots.[157] The C_{max} were 213 and 562 ng/mL at 0.5 and 4 hours, respectively, with an elimination half-life of 1.28 hours for the 120 mg/kg dose. The highly variable results and short half-life of the drug in Hispaniolan Amazon parrots, even at high doses, suggests that this formulation would have to be administered at least 3 to 4 times daily. More recently a commercial hemp (*C sativa*) extract (100 mg/mL; Ellevet) that contains CBD, CBDA, Δ -tetrahydrocannabinol 9, tetrahydrocannabinolic acid, cannabigerol, cannabigerolic acid, and cannabichromene (45.2, 49, 1.86, 0.56, 0.69. 1.21, 1.53 mg/mL respectively) was evaluated in orange-winged Amazon parrots in a single- and multiple-dose pharmacokinetic and safety study at a dose of 30/ 32.5 mg/kg administered orally of CBD/CBDA.[158] The half-life in the multiple-dose study was 8.6 and 6.3 hours for CBD and CBDA, respectively. Interesting differences in the metabolism of some of the cannabinoids when compared with other species studied were found. The results from that study were encouraging for an every 12-hour administration, based on plasma concentrations and limited safety data in the 7 days multiple-dose study. Evaluation of other formulations and also in other species is recommended to further characterize the analgesic potential of CBD, CBDA, and other cannabinoids in birds.

LOCAL ANESTHETICS AND REGIONAL TECHNIQUES

Local anesthetics reversibly bind to Na^+ channels and block impulse conduction. The duration of action depends on the molecular properties and lipid solubility of the drug. Following local application, the anesthetic will be quickly absorbed into the bloodstream, increasing the potential for toxic reactions. Typically, local anesthetics are administered via topical application, local injection, or splash blocks.

Lidocaine

Lidocaine is an amide local anesthetic that decreases neuronal excitability by blocking voltage-dependent sodium channels thus preventing the conduction of action potentials that mediate nociception (**Table 4**). Empirically, doses of 2 to 3 mg/kg have been recommended, although previous studies in chickens and mallard ducks showed no toxic effects following IV administration of 6 mg/kg[159] or 15 mg/kg[160] for brachial plexus block, respectively. The pharmacokinetics of lidocaine following 2.5 mg/kg IV administration in anesthetized chickens showed a rapid half-life and seems to share similar mechanisms of metabolism and elimination to mammalian species reported.[161] The effects of lidocaine were evaluated in 2-kg broiler chickens during spinal anesthesia.[162] During this study, lidocaine was administered in doses of 0.5, 1, and

Table 4
Other drugs evaluated in avian species by either pharmacokinetic or pharmacodynamic studies

Drug	Dose (mg/kg)	Route	Frequency (Q/h)	Species	Comments	Type of Study	Reference
Gabapentin	11	PO	Single dose	Great horned owl	Plasma concentrations maintained above 2 µg/mL for 9.6 h. Suggests q 8 h administration	PK	Yaw et al,[150] 2015
	30 10, 30	IV PO	Single dose	Hispaniolan Amazon parrot	Elimination half-life was 5.41 and 3.74 h, respectively. Suggests 15 mg/kg q 8 h	PK	Baine et al,[149] 2015
	15, 25	PO	Single dose	Caribbean flamingos	Elimination half-life of 3.39 and 4.46 h, respectively. Suggests administration of 25 mg/kg q 12 h, but some individuals could need higher doses	PK	Browning et al,[151] 2018
Amantadine	10, 5	PO	Single (10) dose and multiple (5) doses	Orange-winged Amazon parrots	Half-life of 21.5 h in multiple doses. Reached plasma concentrations associated with toxicity in humans at 10 mg/kg. Suggest q 24 h at 5 mg/kg	PK	Berg et al,[156] 2020
Cannabidiol	60,120	PO	Single dose	Hispaniolan Amazon parrots	Very high interindividual variability. Elimination half-life of 1.28 h at the higher dose evaluated	PK	Carpenter et al,[157] 2022
CBD CBDA, THC, tetrahydrocannabinolic acid, cannabigerol, cannabigerolic acid and cannabichromene	Dosing based on CBD/CBDA 30/32.5 mg/kg	PO	Single and multiple dose q 12 h for 7 d	Orange-winged Amazon parrots	In the multiple-dose study, elimination half-life of 8.6 and 6.3 h for CBD and CBDA respectively. Suggests q 12 h administration.	PK	Sosa-Higareda et al,[158] 2022

Abbreviations: CBD, cannabidiol; CBDA, cannabidiolic acid; PD, pharmacodynamic; PK, pharmacokinetic; PO, orally; THC, Δ -tetrahydrocannabinol 9.

2 mg/kg (2% preservative-free lidocaine, made up to 0.2 mL in saline). The onset of analgesia was 1.3 to 2 minutes, and the duration was 4.5 to 21.3 min.[162]

Bupivacaine

Bupivacaine is the most clinically useful perioperative local anesthetic in mammals because it is a long-acting local anesthetic. The commercial preparations of bupivacaine available are 0.25%, 0.5%, and 0.75% solutions (2.5, 5, 7.5 mg/mL, respectively), and the lower concentration may not need dilution for birds. Bupivacaine has been used conservatively in birds due to concerns that toxic effects may take longer to resolve due to this drug's longer duration of effect. The recommended maximum dose of bupivacaine for mammals is 2 mg/kg. Results from a study in which mallard ducks (*Anas platyrhynchos*) were administered bupivacaine 2 mg/kg SC suggested the drug is shorter acting than in mammals, and a potential for delayed toxicity based on increased plasma concentrations at 6 and 12 hours (see Table 4).[163] The cardiovascular tolerance of bupivacaine was evaluated in chickens anesthetized with isoflurane.[164] In this study 1.96 mg/kg IV bupivacaine was associated with a 50% probability of a clinically relevant change in mean arterial pressure and heart rate, whereas 1.33 mg/kg IV bupivacaine was associated with a 1% probability of causing the same effect. The analgesic effects have been seen in several studies. Intraarticular bupivacaine (3 mg in 0.3 mL saline) was effective for treating arthritic pain in chickens.[165] A 1:1 mixture of bupivacaine and dimethyl sulfoxide was applied to amputated chicken beaks immediately after amputation, and feed intake improved.[166] In 2-kg broiler chickens spinal anesthesia using 0.1, 0.25, and 0.5 mg/kg (0.5% bupivacaine hydrochloride, made up 0.2 mL in saline) was evaluated. The onset of analgesia was 3.3 to 9 minutes, and the duration was 11 to 54 min.[162]

Regional Techniques

Local line or splash blocks are the most common methods of regional infiltration used in birds. The SC space in most avian species is very thin, so a small-gauge needle is recommended to make several SC injections into the operative area. Brachial plexus blockade has been described in a variety of avian species, but neither bupivacaine (2 and 8 mg/kg) nor lidocaine (15 mg/kg) with epinephrine perineurally effectively blocked nerve transmission in the brachial plexus of mallard ducks.[160] Similar findings were reported in chickens with lidocaine (20 mg/kg) or bupivacaine (5 mg/kg) with epinephrine for brachial plexus blockade using a nerve locator.[167] In Hispaniolan Amazon parrots, neither palpation-guided nor ultrasound-guided brachial plexus blockade was found to result in an effective block using lidocaine at 2 mg/kg perineurally.[168] Ischiatic-femoral nerve block has also been described in peregrine falcons (*F peregrinus*), and was considered a feasible technique applying lidocaine at 2 mg/kg perineurally with the aid of a nerve locator.[169] In more recent studies in chickens, a technique for spinal anesthesia (also called subarachnoid or intrathecal block) was developed.[170] This technique was considered effective in these large birds, but further studies evaluating efficacy and safety in smaller birds and/or different species is warranted.

DIETARY SUPPLEMENTS

Omega-3 polyunsaturated fatty acids like eicosapentaenoic acid (EPA) and docosahexaenoic acid (DHA) have anti-inflammatory effects, which might reduce the pain associated with osteoarthritis. The total EPA and DHA doses are the primary factors to consider, and not so much the omega-3 to omega-6 fatty acid ratio. Other omega-3 fatty acids (eg, plant-based omega-3 fatty acids, alpha-linoleic acid) do not have similar effects.[171] There have been no studies in birds evaluating the effects and optimal dosage of EPA and DHA in osteoarthritic pain.

Glucosamine, chondroitin, methylsulfonylmethane, and undenatured form of type II collagen may have benefits in osteoarthritis through their anti-inflammatory affects, but there are no studies in birds evaluating dosages and adverse effects. Polysulfated glycosaminoglycans have also been used anecdotally in the management of degenerative joint disease in birds, but fatal coagulopathies following IM doses from 0.5 mg/kg to 100 mg/kg in different avian species (1 coraciiform, 2 raptors, and 1 psittacine) have been reported.[172] A recent in vitro study evaluating the hypocoagulability effects of the same specific formulation (100 mg/mL; Adequan) previously associated with adverse effects, paired with the anecdotal reports of one of the investigators of use in a wide range of species over 20 years, supports its safe and effective use in birds at 1 mg/kg SC once weekly for 4 doses, followed by once every other week for 2 doses, then once monthly until the problem is resolved, or chronically at this dose for long-term maintenance.[173]

PHYSICAL REHABILITATION

Treatment of pain in humans and companion mammal species may include physical modalities, manual therapy, and therapeutic exercise. The application of adjunctive therapy should be considered for acute and chronic pain in birds, although evidence-based information is not yet available for birds. Therapeutic exercises, such as static weight-bearing, can be generally used in the acute phase of injury with gradual progression of difficulty as healing occurs. Physical modalities such as thermotherapy and laser are used to diminish pain. Thermotherapy can have analgesic effects after the inflammatory effect has subsided. Low-level laser therapy (660 nm, 9 J/cm^2) has been shown to decrease indicators of neuropathic pain. Manual physical therapeutic techniques for joint mobilization can decrease pain but trigger point pressure techniques might induce central sensitization.[174] There are several anecdotal reports of the use of acupuncture in pain management protocols for birds; however, no objective studies have been published to date.

NURSING AND SUPPORTING CARE

The environment may affect pain; stress and anxiety can have a modulatory effect. The bird should be in an environment where it is emotionally and physically as comfortable as possible. Human presence or absence, decreasing light and noise, and separating other animals from the bird could reduce stress and anxiety. When handling and moving an animal, avoiding painful areas (surgical/trauma site, osteoarthritic joints, and so on), even when the animal is anesthetized or sedated, is important to prevent inflicting a painful stimulus, which can begin a new pain cascade.[174]

Cold compress during acute injury can reduce swelling and provide analgesia. Cold compress generally needs to be in place for 15 to 20 minutes to be effective. Warm compress is generally more comfortable after the acute phase has passed, but can aid tissue relaxation and as a precursor to massage or stretching. Warm compress generally needs to be in place for 10 to 15 minutes.[174]

DISCLOSURE

The authors have nothing to disclose.

REFERENCES

1. Mansour A, Khachaturian H, Lewis ME, et al. Anatomy of CNS opioid receptors. Trends Neurosci 1988;11:308–14.
2. Csillag A, Bourne RC, Stewart MG. Distribution of mu, delta, and kappa opioid receptor binding sites in the brain of the one-day-old domestic chick (Gallus domesticus): an in vitro quantitative autoradiographic study. J Comp Neurol 1990; 302:543–51.
3. Fousse SL, Golsen BM, Sanchez-Migallon Guzman D, et al. Varying expression of mu and kappa opioid receptors in cockatiels (Nymphicus hollandicus) and domestic pigeons (Columba livia domestica). Front Genet 2020;11:549558.
4. Duhamelle A, Raiwet DL, Langlois I, et al. Preliminary Findings of Structure and Expression of Opioid Receptor Genes in a Peregrine Falcon (Falco peregrinus), a Snowy Owl (Bubo scandiacus), and a Blue-fronted Amazon Parrot (Amazona aestiva). J Avian Med Surg 2018;32:173–84.
5. Paul-Murphy J, Brunson DB, Miletic V. Analgesic effects of butorphanol and buprenorphine in conscious African grey parrots (Psittacus erithacus erithacus and Psittacus erithacus timneh). Am J Vet Res 1999;60:1218–21.
6. Gaggermeier B, Henke J, Schatzmann U. Investigations on analgesia in domestic pigeons (C. livia, Gmel., 1789, var. dom.) using buprenorphine and butorphanol. Proc Eur Assoc Avian Vet 2001;70–3.
7. Riggs SM, Hawkins MG, Craigmill AL, et al. Pharmacokinetics of butorphanol tartrate in red-tailed hawks (Buteo jamaicensis) and great horned owls (Bubo virginianus). Am J Vet Res 2008;69:596–603.
8. Laniesse D, Sanchez-Migallon Guzman D, Smith DA, et al. Evaluation of the thermal antinociceptive effects of subcutaneous administration of butorphanol tartrate or butorphanol tartrate in a sustained-release poloxamer 407 gel formulation to orange-winged Amazon parrots (Amazona amazonica). Am J Vet Res 2020;81:543–50.
9. Laniesse D, Guzman DS, Knych HK, et al. Pharmacokinetics of butorphanol tartrate in a long-acting poloxamer 407 gel formulation administered to Hispaniolan Amazon parrots (Amazona ventralis). Am J Vet Res 2017;78:688–94.
10. Sanchez-Migallon Guzman D, Flammer K, Paul-Murphy JR, et al. Pharmacokinetics of butorphanol after intravenous, intramuscular, and oral administration in Hispaniolan Amazon parrots (Amazona ventralis). J Avian Med Surg 2011; 25:185–91.
11. Sladky K, Krugner-Higby L, Meek-Walker E, et al. Serum concentrations and analgesic effects of liposome-encapsulated and standard butorphanol tartrate in parrots. Am J Vet Res 2006;67:775–81.
12. Klaphake E, Schumacher J, Greenacre C, et al. Comparative anesthetic and cardiopulmonary effects of pre- versus postoperative butorphanol administration in Hispaniolan amazon parrots (Amazona ventralis) anesthetized with sevoflurane. J Avian Med Surg 2006;20:2–7.
13. Paul-Murphy JR, Krugner-Higby LA, Tourdot RL, et al. Evaluation of liposome-encapsulated butorphanol tartrate for alleviation of experimentally induced arthritic pain in green-cheeked conures (Pyrrhura molinae). Am J Vet Res 2009;70:1211–9.
14. Singh PM, Johnson CB, Gartrell B, et al. Analgesic effects of morphine and butorphanol in broiler chickens. Vet Anaesth Analg 2017;44:538–45.
15. Singh PM, Johnson C, Gartrell B, et al. Pharmacokinetics of butorphanol in broiler chickens. Vet Rec 2011;2011:588.

16. Clancy MM, KuKanich B, Sykes JMt. Pharmacokinetics of butorphanol delivered with an osmotic pump during a seven-day period in common peafowl (Pavo cristatus). Am J Vet Res 2015;76:1070–6.

17. Curro TG, Brunson DB, Paul-Murphy J. Determination of the ED50 of isoflurane and evaluation of the isoflurane-sparing effect of butorphanol in cockatoos (Cacatua spp.). Vet Surg 1994;23:429–33.

18. Curro TG. Evaluation of the isoflurane-sparing effects of butorphanol and flunixin in psittaciformes. Proc Assoc Avian Vet 1994;17–9.

19. Guzman DS, Drazenovich TL, KuKanich B, et al. Evaluation of thermal antinociceptive effects and pharmacokinetics after intramuscular administration of butorphanol tartrate to American kestrels (Falco sparverius). Am J Vet Res 2014; 75:11–8.

20. Mikoni N, Sanchez-Migallon Guzman D, Knych H, et al. Pharmacokinetics of butorphanol tartrate in a poloxamer P407 gel formulation administered to orange-winged Amazon parrots (Amazona amazonica). Am J Vet Res 2022;83. https://doi.org/10.2460/ajvr.22.01.0012.

21. Lichtenberger M, Lennox A, Chavez W, et al. The use of butorphanol constant rate infusion in psittacines. Proc Assoc Avian Veterinarians 2009;73.

22. Keller DL, Sanchez-Migallon Guzman D, Klauer JM, et al. Pharmacokinetics of nalbuphine hydrochloride after intravenous and intramuscular administration to Hispaniolan Amazon parrots (Amazona ventralis). Am J Vet Res 2011;72: 741–5.

23. Sanchez-Migallon Guzman D, KuKanich B, Keuler NS, et al. Antinociceptive effects of nalbuphine hydrochloride in Hispaniolan Amazon parrots (Amazona ventralis). Am J Vet Res 2011;72:736–40.

24. Sanchez-Migallon Guzman D, KuKanich B, Heath TD, et al. Pharmacokinetics of long-acting nalbuphine decanoate after intramuscular administration to Hispaniolan Amazon parrots (Amazona ventralis). Am J Vet Res 2013;74:191–5.

25. Sanchez-Migallon Guzman D, Braun JM, Steagall PV, et al. Antinociceptive effects of long-acting nalbuphine decanoate after intramuscular administration to Hispaniolan Amazon parrots (Amazona ventralis). Am J Vet Res 2013;74: 196–200.

26. Guzman DS, KuKanich B, Drazenovich TL, et al. Pharmacokinetics of hydromorphone hydrochloride after intravenous and intramuscular administration of a single dose to American kestrels (Falco sparverius). Am J Vet Res 2014;75:527–31.

27. Guzman DS, Drazenovich TL, Olsen GH, et al. Evaluation of thermal antinociceptive effects after intramuscular administration of hydromorphone hydrochloride to American kestrels (Falco sparverius). Am J Vet Res 2013;74:817–22.

28. Houck EL, Guzman DS, Beaufrere H, et al. Evaluation of the thermal antinociceptive effects and pharmacokinetics of hydromorphone hydrochloride after intramuscular administration to cockatiels (Nymphicus hollandicus). Am J Vet Res 2018;79:820–7.

29. Sanchez-Migallon Guzman D, Knych H, Douglas J, et al. Pharmacokinetics of hydromorphone hydrochloride after intramuscular and intravenous administration of a single dose to orange-winged Amazon parrots (Amazona amazonica). Am J Vet Res 2020;81:894–8.

30. Sanchez-Migallon Guzman D, Douglas JM, Beaufrere H, et al. Evaluation of the thermal antinociceptive effects of hydromorphone hydrochloride after intramuscular administration to orange-winged Amazon parrots (Amazona amazonica). Am J Vet Res 2020;81:775–82.

31. Singh PM, Johnson C, Gartrell B, et al. Pharmacokinetics of morphine after intravenous administration in broiler chickens. J Vet Pharmacol Ther 2010;33:515–8.
32. Schneider C. Effects of morphine-like drugs in chicks. Nature 1961;191:607–8.
33. Bardo MT, Hughes RA. Brief communication. Shock-elicited flight response in chickens as an index of morphine analgesia. Pharmacol Biochem Behav 1978;9:147–9.
34. Fan S, Shutt AJ, Vogt M. The importance of 5-hydroxytryptamine turnover for the analgesic effect of morphine in the chicken. Neuroscience 1981;6:2223–7.
35. Hughes RA. Strain-dependent morphine-induced analgesic and hyperalgesic effects on thermal nociception in domestic fowl (Gallus gallus). Behav Neurosci 1990;104:619–24.
36. Concannon KT, Dodam JR, Hellyer PW. Influence of a mu- and kappa-opioid agonist on isoflurane minimal anesthetic concentration in chickens. Am J Vet Res 1995;56:806–11.
37. Hoppes S, Flammer K, Hoersch K, et al. Disposition and analgesic effects of fentanyl in white cockatoos (Cacatua alba). J Avian Med Surg 2003;17:124–30.
38. Pascoe PJ, Pypendop BH, Pavez Phillips JC, et al. Pharmacokinetics of fentanyl after intravenous administration in isoflurane-anesthetized red-tailed hawks (Buteo jamaicensis) and Hispaniolan Amazon parrots (Amazona ventralis). Am J Vet Res 2018;79:606–13.
39. Pavez JC, Hawkins MG, Pascoe PJ, et al. Effect of fentanyl target-controlled infusions on isoflurane minimum anaesthetic concentration and cardiovascular function in red-tailed hawks (Buteo jamaicensis). Vet Anaesth Analgesia 2011; 38:344–51.
40. Waugh L, Knych H, Cole G, et al. Pharmacokinetic evaluation of a long-acting fentanyl solution after transdermal administration in helmeted guineafowl (Numida meleagris). J Zoo Wildl Med 2016;47:468–73.
41. Delaski KM, Gehring R, Heffron BT, et al. Plasma concentrations of fentanyl achieved with transdermal application in chickens. J Avian Med Surg 2017; 31:6–15.
42. da Rocha RW, Escobar A, Pypendop BH, et al. Effects of a single intravenous bolus of fentanyl on the minimum anesthetic concentration of isoflurane in chickens (Gallus gallus domesticus). Vet Anaesth Analg 2017;44:546–54.
43. Hawkins MG, Pascoe PJ, DiMaio Knych HK, et al. Effects of three fentanyl plasma concentrations on the minimum alveolar concentration of isoflurane in Hispaniolan Amazon parrots (Amazona ventralis). Am J Vet Res 2018;79:600–5.
44. Pavez JC, Pypendop BH, Pascoe PJ, et al. Pharmacokinetics of intravenous fentanyl in isoflurane-anesthetized red-tailed hawks (Buteo jamaicensis). Vet Anaesth Analg 2012;79(6):606–13.
45. Escobar A, Barletta M, Pypendop BH, et al. Pharmacokinetics and pharmacodynamics of methadone administered intravenously and intramuscularly to isoflurane-anesthetized chickens. Am J Vet Res 2021;82:181–8.
46. Escobar A, da Rocha RW, Pypendop BH, et al. Effects of Methadone on the Minimum Anesthetic Concentration of Isoflurane, and Its Effects on Heart Rate, Blood Pressure and Ventilation during Isoflurane Anesthesia in Hens (Gallus gallus domesticus). PLoS One 2016;11:e0152546.
47. Paul-Murphy J, Hess J, Fialkowski JP. Pharmokinetic properties of a single intramuscular dose of buprenorphine in African Grey Parrots (Psittacus erithacus erithacus). J Avian Med Surg 2004;18:224–8.
48. Guzman DS, Houck EL, Knych HKD, et al. Evaluation of the thermal antinociceptive effects and pharmacokinetics after intramuscular administration of

buprenorphine hydrochloride to cockatiels (Nymphicus hollandicus). Am J Vet Res 2018;79:1239–45.

49. Guzman DSM, Ceulemans SM, Beaufrere H, et al. Evaluation of the thermal antinociceptive effects of a sustained-release buprenorphine formulation after intramuscular administration to American kestrels (Falco sparverius). J Avian Med Surg 2018;32:1–7.

50. Sanchez-Migallon Guzman D, Knych, Olsen G, et al. Pharmacokinetics of a sustained release buprenorphine formulation after intramuscular and subcutaneous administration to American kestrels (Falco sparverius). J Avian Med Surg 2017; 31:102–7.

51. Guzman DS, Knych HK, Olsen GH, et al. Pharmacokinetics of a sustained release formulation of buprenorphine after intramuscular and subcutaneous administration to American kestrels (Falco sparverius). J Avian Med Surg 2017;31:102–7.

52. Gleeson MD, Guzman DS, Knych HK, et al. Pharmacokinetics of a concentrated buprenorphine formulation in red-tailed hawks (Buteo jamaicensis). Am J Vet Res 2018;79:13–20.

53. Gustavsen KA, Guzman DS, Knych HK, et al. Pharmacokinetics of buprenorphine hydrochloride following intramuscular and intravenous administration to American kestrels (Falco sparverius). Am J Vet Res 2014;75:711–5.

54. Ceulemans SM, Guzman DS, Olsen GH, et al. Evaluation of thermal antinociceptive effects after intramuscular administration of buprenorphine hydrochloride to American kestrels (Falco sparverius). Am J Vet Res 2014;75:705–10.

55. Souza MJ, Martin-Jimenez T, Jones MP, et al. Pharmacokinetics of intravenous and oral tramadol in the bald eagle (Haliaeetus leucocephalus). J Avian Med Surg 2009;23:247–52.

56. Black PA, Cox SK, Macek M, et al. Pharmacokinetics of tramadol hydrochloride and its metabolite O-desmethyltramadol in peafowl (Pavo cristatus). J Zoo Wildl Med 2010;41:671–6.

57. Souza MJ, Martin-Jimenez T, Jones MP, et al. Pharmacokinetics of oral tramadol in red-tailed hawks (Buteo jamaicensis). J Vet Pharmacol Ther 2011;34:86–8.

58. Souza MJ, Gerhardt L, Cox S. Pharmacokinetics of repeated oral administration of tramadol hydrochloride in Hispaniolan Amazon parrots (Amazona ventralis). Am J Vet Res 2013;74:957–62.

59. Geelen S, Sanchez-Migallon Guzman D, Souza MJ, et al. Antinociceptive effects of tramadol hydrochloride after intravenous administration to Hispaniolan Amazon parrots (Amazona ventralis). Am J Vet Res 2013;74:201–6.

60. Souza MJ, Sanchez-Migallon Guzman D, Paul-Murphy JR, et al. Pharmacokinetics after oral and intravenous administration of a single dose of tramadol hydrochloride to Hispaniolan Amazon parrots (Amazona ventralis). Am J Vet Res 2012;73:1142–7.

61. Sanchez-Migallon Guzman D, Souza MJ, Braun JM, et al. Antinociceptive effects after oral administration of tramadol hydrochloride in Hispaniolan Amazon parrots (Amazona ventralis). Am J Vet Res 2012;73:1148–52.

62. Guzman DS, Drazenovich TL, Olsen GH, et al. Evaluation of thermal antinociceptive effects after oral administration of tramadol hydrochloride to American kestrels (Falco sparverius). Am J Vet Res 2014;75:117–23.

63. Kilburn JJ, Cox SK, Kottyan J, et al. Pharmacokinetics of tramadol and its primary metabolite O-desmethyltramadol in African penguins (Spheniscus demersus). J Zoo Wildl Med 2014;45:93–9.

64. Bailey RS, Sheldon JD, Allender MC, et al. Analgesic Efficacy of Tramadol Compared With Meloxicam in Ducks (Cairina moschata domestica) Evaluated by Ground-Reactive Forces. J Avian Med Surg 2019;33:133–40.
65. Papich MG. An update on nonsteroidal anti-inflammatory drugs (NSAIDs) in small animals. Vet Clin North Am Small Anim Pract 2008;38:1243–66, vi.
66. Bergh MS, Budsberg SC. The coxib NSAIDs: potential clinical and pharmacologic importance in veterinary medicine. J Vet Intern Med 2005;19:633–43.
67. Mathonnet M, Lalloue F, Danty E, et al. Cyclo-oxygenase 2 tissue distribution and developmental pattern of expression in the chicken. Clin Exp Pharmacol Physiol 2001;28:425–32.
68. Dajani EZ, Islam K. Cardiovascular and gastrointestinal toxicity of selective cyclo-oxygenase-2 inhibitors in man. J Physiol Pharmacol 2008;59(Suppl 2): 117–33.
69. Gerstenfeld LC, Thiede M, Seibert K, et al. Differential inhibition of fracture healing by non-selective and cyclooxygenase-2 selective non-steroidal anti-inflammatory drugs. J Orthop Res 2003;21:670–5.
70. Pelligand L, King JN, Toutain PL, et al. Pharmacokinetic/pharmacodynamic modelling of robenacoxib in a feline tissue cage model of inflammation. J Vet Pharmacol Ther 2012;35:19–32.
71. Cramer K, Schmidt V, Richter A, et al. [Investigations on the acute, carrageenan-induced inflammatory reaction and pharmacology of orally administered sodium salicylate in turkeys]. Berl Munch Tierarztl Wochenschr 2015;128:240–51.
72. Baert K, De Backer P. Disposition of salicylate, flunixin, and meloxicam after intravenous administration in broiler chickens. J Vet Pharmacol Ther 2002;25: 449–53.
73. Baert K, De Backer P. Comparative pharmacokinetics of three non-steroidal anti-inflammatory drugs in five bird species. Comp Biochem Physiol C Toxicol Pharmacol 2003;134:25–33.
74. Castineiras D, Armitage L, Lamas LP, et al. Perioperative pharmacokinetics and pharmacodynamics of meloxicam in emus (Dromaius novaehollandiae) of different age groups using nonlinear mixed effect modelling. J Vet Pharmacol Ther 2021;44:603–18.
75. Souza MJ, Bailey J, White M, et al. Pharmacokinetics and Egg Residues of Meloxicam After Multiple Day Oral Dosing in Domestic Chickens. J Avian Med Surg 2018;32:8–12.
76. Souza MJ, Gerhardt LE, Shannon L, et al. Breed differences in the pharmacokinetics of orally administered meloxicam in domestic chickens (Gallus domesticus). J Am Vet Med Assoc 2021;259:84–7.
77. Baert K, De Backer P. Disposition of sodium salicylate, flunixin and meloxicam after intravenous administration in broiler chickens. J Vet Pharmacol Ther 2002;25:449–53.
78. Baert K, De Backer P. Disposition of sodium salicylate, flunixin, and meloxicam after intravenous administration in ostriches (Struthio camelus). J Avian Med Surg 2002;16:123–8.
79. Sartini I, Łebkowska-Wieruszewska B, Lisowski A, et al. Pharmacokinetic profiles of meloxicam after single IV and PO administration in Bilgorajska geese. J Vet Pharmacol Ther 2020;43:26–32.
80. Horgan MD, Knych HK, Siksay SE, et al. Pharmacokinetics of a Single Dose of Oral Meloxicam in Rehabilitated Wild Brown Pelicans (Pelecanus occidentalis). J Avian Med Surg 2020;34:329–37.

81. Turk E, Tekeli IO, Corum O, et al. Pharmacokinetics of meloxicam, carprofen, and tolfenamic acid after intramuscular and oral administration in Japanese quails (Coturnix coturnix japonica). J Vet Pharmacol Ther 2021;44:388–96.

82. Cetin G, Corum O, Corum D, et al. Pharmacokinetics of intravenous meloxicam, ketoprofen and tolfenamic acid in chukar partridge (Alectoris chukar). Br Poult Sci 2021;63(1):1–7.

83. Miller KA, Hill NJ, Carrasco SE, et al. Pharmacokinetics and Safety of Intramuscular Meloxicam in Zebra Finches (Taeniopygia guttata). J Am Assoc Lab Anim Sci 2019;58:589–93.

84. Wilson HG, Hernandez-Divers S, Budsberg SC. Pharmacokinetics and use of meloxican in psittacine birds. Proc Assoc Avian Veterinarians 2004;7–9.

85. Molter CM, Court MH, Cole GA, et al. Pharmacokinetics of meloxicam after intravenous, intramuscular, and oral administration of a single dose to Hispaniolan Amazon parrots (Amazona ventralis). Am J Vet Res 2013;74:375–80.

86. Montesinos A, Ardiaca M, Gilabert JA, et al. Pharmacokinetics of meloxicam after intravenous, intramuscular and oral administration of a single dose to African grey parrots (Psittacus erithacus). J Vet Pharmacol Ther 2017;40:279–84.

87. Dhondt L, Devreese M, Croubels S, et al. Comparative population pharmacokinetics and absolute oral bioavailability of COX-2 selective inhibitors celecoxib, mavacoxib and meloxicam in cockatiels (Nymphicus hollandicus). Sci Rep 2017;7:12043.

88. Zordan MA, Papich MG, Pich AA, et al. Population pharmacokinetics of a single dose of meloxicam after oral and intramuscular administration to captive lesser flamingos (Phoeniconaias minor). Am J Vet Res 2016;77:1311–7.

89. Lindemann DM, Carpenter JW, KuKanich B. Pharmacokinetics of a Single Dose of Oral and Subcutaneous Meloxicam in Caribbean Flamingos (Phoenicopterus ruber ruber). J Avian Med Surg 2016;30:14–22.

90. Boonstra JL, Cox SK, Martin-Jimenez T. Pharmacokinetics of meloxicam after intramuscular and oral administration of a single dose to American flamingos (Phoenicopertus ruber). Am J Vet Res 2017;78:267–73.

91. Morrison J, Greenacre CB, George R, et al. Pharmacokinetics of a Single Dose of Oral and Intramuscular Meloxicam in African Penguins (Spheniscus demersus). J Avian Med Surg 2018;32:102–8.

92. Lacasse C, Gamble KC, Boothe DM. Pharmacokinetics of a single dose of intravenous and oral meloxicam in red-tailed hawks (Buteo jamaicensis) and great horned owls (Bubo virginianus). J Avian Med Surg 2013;27:204–10.

93. Naidoo V, Wolter K, Cromarty AD, et al. The pharmacokinetics of meloxicam in vultures. J Vet Pharmacol Ther 2008;31:128–34.

94. Montesinos A, Encinas T, Ardiaca M, et al. Pharmacokinetics of meloxicam during multiple oral or intramuscular dose administration to African grey parrots (Psittacus erithacus). Am J Vet Res 2019;80:201–7.

95. Zorrilla I, Richards NL, Benítez JR, et al. Case study: detection of two nonsteroidal anti-inflammatory drugs (NSAIDs) in the eggs of captive-reared bearded vultures at a breeding center in southern Spain. J Wildl Rehabil 2018;38:15–7.

96. Guzman DS, Court MH, Zhu Z, et al. Pharmacokinetics of a Sustained-release Formulation of Meloxicam After Subcutaneous Administration to Hispaniolan Amazon Parrots (Amazona ventralis). J Avian Med Surg 2017;31:219–24.

97. Sim RR, Cox SK. Pharmacokinetics of a Sustained-Release Formulation of Meloxicam after Subcutaneous Administration to American Flamingos (Phoenicopterus Ruber). J Zoo Wildl Med 2018;49:839–43.

98. Hothersall B, Caplen G, Parker RM, et al. Thermal nociceptive threshold testing detects altered sensory processing in broiler chickens with spontaneous lameness. PLoS One 2014;9:e97883.
99. Nakhaee P, Mosleh N, Nazifi S, et al. Comparative effects of meloxicam and dexamethasone in chickens with experimental systemic inflammation: clinical outcome and cardiovascular parameters. Comp Clin Pathol 2021;30:681–91.
100. Pereira ME, Werther K. Evaluation of the renal effects of flunixin meglumine, ketoprofen and meloxicam in budgerigars (Melopsittacus undulatus). Vet Rec 2007;160:844–6.
101. Montesinos A, Ardiaca M, Juan-Sallés C, et al. Effects of Meloxicam on Hematologic and Plasma Biochemical Analyte Values and Results of Histologic Examination of Kidney Biopsy Specimens of African Grey Parrots (Psittacus erithacus). J Avian Med Surg 2015;29:1–8.
102. Desmarchelier M, Troncy E, Fitzgerald G, et al. Analgesic effects of meloxicam administration on postoperative orthopedic pain in domestic pigeons (Columba livia). Am J Vet Res 2012;73:361–7.
103. Sinclair KM, Church ME, Farver TB, et al. Effects of meloxicam on hematologic and plasma biochemical analysis variables and results of histologic examination of tissue specimens of Japanese quail (Coturnix japonica). Am J Vet Res 2012; 73:1720–7.
104. Summa NM, Guzman DS, Larrat S, et al. Evaluation of High Dosages of Oral Meloxicam in American Kestrels (Falco sparverius). J Avian Med Surg 2017;31: 108–16.
105. Dijkstra B, Guzman DS, Gustavsen K, et al. Renal, gastrointestinal, and hemostatic effects of oral administration of meloxicam to Hispaniolan Amazon parrots (Amazona ventralis). Am J Vet Res 2015;76:308–17.
106. Summa NM, Guzman DS-M, Larrat S, et al. Evaluation of high dosages of oral meloxicam in American Kestrels (Falco sparverius). J Avian Med Surg 2017; 31:108–16.
107. Oaks JL, Gilbert M, Virani MZ, et al. Diclofenac residues as the cause of vulture population decline in Pakistan. Nature 2004;427:630–3.
108. Naidoo V, Venter L, Wolter K, et al. The toxicokinetics of ketoprofen in Gyps coprotheres: toxicity due to zero-order metabolism. Arch Toxicol 2010;84:761–6.
109. Swarup D, Patra RC, Prakash V, et al. Safety of meloxicam to critically endangered Gyps vultures and other scavenging birds in India. Anim Conservation 2007;10:192–8.
110. Hoppes SM, Tizard I, Shivaprasad HL. Avian bornavirus and proventricular dilatation disease. Veterinary Clin North Am Exot Anim Pract 2013;13:339–55.
111. Escandon P, Heatley JJ, Tizard I, et al. Treatment With Nonsteroidal Anti-Inflammatory Drugs Fails To Ameliorate Pathology In Cockatiels Experimentally Infected With Parrot Bornavirus-2. Vet Med (Auckl) 2019;10:185–95.
112. Rossi G, Dahlhausen RD, Galosi L, et al. Avian Ganglioneuritis in Clinical Practice. Veterinary Clin North Am Exot Anim Pract 2018;21:33–67.
113. Lees P, Pelligand L, Elliott J, et al. Pharmacokinetics, pharmacodynamics, toxicology and therapeutics of mavacoxib in the dog: a review. J Vet Pharmacol Ther 2015;38:1–14.
114. Cox SR, Lesman SP, Boucher JF, et al. The pharmacokinetics of mavacoxib, a long-acting COX-2 inhibitor, in young adult laboratory dogs. J Vet Pharmacol Ther 2010;33:461–70.
115. Gasthuys E, Houben R, Haesendonck R, et al. Development of an in Vivo Lipopolysaccharide Inflammation Model to Study the Pharmacodynamics of COX-2

Inhibitors Celecoxib, Mavacoxib, and Meloxicam in Cockatiels (Nymphicus hol landicus). J Avian Med Surg 2019;33:349–60.

116. Cox SR, Liao S, Payne-Johnson M, et al. Population pharmacokinetics of mavacoxib in osteoarthritic dogs. J Vet Pharmacol Ther 2011;34:1–11.

117. Huckins GL, Carpenter JW, Dias S, et al. Pharmacokinetics of Oral Mavacoxib in Caribbean Flamingos (Phoenicopterus Ruber Ruber). J Zoo Wildl Med 2020; 51:53–8.

118. Lamb SK. Obstruction by fibrous foreign object ingestion in two green-cheeked conures (Pyrrhura molinae) and a jenday conure (Aratinga jandaya). J Exot Pet Med 2019;31:127–32.

119. McGeowen D, Danbury TC, Waterman-Pearson AE, et al. Effect of carprofen on lameness in broiler chickens. Vet Rec 1999;144:668–71.

120. Danbury TC, Weeks CA, Chambers JP, et al. Self-selection of the analgesic drug carprofen by lame broiler chickens. Vet Rec 2000;146:307–11.

121. Hadipour MM, Hadipourfard MR, Vakili MB, et al. Treatment of joint inflammatory diseases in the lame backyard chickens with NSAIDs. Int J Anim Vet Adv 2011; 3:73–6.

122. Paul-Murphy JR, Sladky KK, Krugner-Higby LA, et al. Analgesic effects of carprofen and liposome-encapsulated butorphanol tartrate in Hispaniolan parrots (Amazona ventralis) with experimentally induced arthritis. Am J Vet Res 2009; 70:1201–10.

123. Zollinger TJ, Hoover JP, Payton ME, et al. Clinicopathologic, gross necropsy, and histologic findings after intramuscular injection of carprofen in a pigeon (Columba livia) model. J Avian Med Surg 2011;25:173–84.

124. Naidoo V, Taggart MA, Duncan N, et al. The use of toxicokinetics and exposure studies to show that carprofen in cattle tissue could lead to secondary toxicity and death in wild vultures. Chemosphere 2018;190:80–9.

125. Graham JE, Kollias-Baker C, Craigmill AL, et al. Pharmacokinetics of ketoprofen in Japanese quail (Coturnix japonica). J Vet Pharmacol Ther 2005;28:399–402.

126. Machin KL, Tellier LA, Lair S, et al. Pharmacodynamics of flunixin and ketoprofen in mallard ducks (Anas platyrhynchos). J Zoo Wildl Med 2001;32:222–9.

127. Hajizadeh H, Abedi G, Asghari A, et al. Comparative evaluation of the biochemical effects of ketamine plus ketoprofen and midazolam in the premedication of pigeons. J Arch Razi Inst 2018;73:223–7.

128. Hajizadeh H, Abedi G, Asghari A, et al. Clinical and histopathological comparison of ketoprofen and midazolam as premedication in pigeon. J Vet Clin Pathol Q Scientific J 2018;12:273–80.

129. Awan AF, Ashraf M, Malik A, et al. Toxicity study of piroxicam in broilers. Lat Am J Pharm 2012;31:456–60.

130. Keiper NL, Cox SK, Doss GA, et al. Pharmacokinetics of piroxicam in cranes (Family Gruidae). J Zoo Wildl Med 2017;48:886–90.

131. Sharma AK, Saini M, Singh SD, et al. Diclofenac is toxic to the Steppe Eagle Aquila nipalensis: widening the diversity of raptors threatened by NSAID misuse in South Asia. Bird Conservation Int 2014;24:282–6.

132. Green RE, Donázar JA, Sánchez-Zapata JA, et al. Potential threat to Eurasian griffon vultures in Spain from veterinary use of the drug diclofenac. J Appl Ecol 2016;53:993–1003.

133. Swan GE, Cuthbert R, Quevedo M, et al. Toxicity of diclofenac to Gyps vultures. Biol Lett 2006;2:279–82.

134. Galligan TH, Mallord JW, Prakash VM, et al. Trends in the availability of the vulture-toxic drug, diclofenac, and other NSAIDs in South Asia, as revealed by covert pharmacy surveys. Bird Conservation Int 2021;31:337–53.

135. Chandramohan S, Mallord JW, Mathesh K, et al. Experimental safety testing shows that the NSAID tolfenamic acid is not toxic to Gyps vultures in India at concentrations likely to be encountered in cattle carcasses. Sci Total Environ 2022;809:152088.

136. Cuthbert RJ, Taggart MA, Mohini S, et al. Continuing mortality of vultures in India associated with illegal veterinary use of diclofenac and a potential threat from nimesulide. Oryx 2016;50:104–12.

137. Galligan TH, Green RE, Wolter K, et al. The non-steroidal anti-inflammatory drug nimesulide kills Gyps vultures at concentrations found in the muscle of treated cattle. Sci Total Environ 2022;807:150788.

138. Nambirajan K, Muralidharan S, Ashimkumar AR, et al. Nimesulide poisoning in white-rumped vulture Gyps bengalensis in Gujarat, India. Environ Sci Pollut Res 2021;28:1–7.

139. Stokstad E. Vultures face new toxic threat. Science 2021;373:1187.

140. Lascelles BD, Court MH, Hardie EM, et al. Nonsteroidal anti-inflammatory drugs in cats: a review. Vet Anaesth Analg 2007;34(4):228–50.

141. Corell T. Pharmacology of tolfenamic acid. Pharmacol Toxicol 1994;75(Suppl 2): 14–21.

142. Gómez-Ramírez P, Blanco G, García-Fernández AJ. Validation of Multi-Residue Method for Quantification of Antibiotics and NSAIDs in Avian Scavengers by Using Small Amounts of Plasma in HPLC-MS-TOF. Int J Environ Res Public Health 2020;17:4058.

143. Cetin G, Corum O, Corum DD, et al. Pharmacokinetics of intravenous meloxicam, ketoprofen and tolfenamic acid in chukar partridge (Alectoris chukar). Br Poult Sci 2022;63:14–20.

144. Turk E, Tekeli IO, Durna Corum D, et al. Pharmacokinetics of tolfenamic acid after different administration routes in geese (Anser cygnoides). J Vet Pharmacol Ther 2021;44:381–7.

145. Corum O, Atik O, Durna Corum D, et al. Pharmacokinetics of tolfenamic acid in red-eared slider turtles (Trachemys scripta elegans). Vet Anaesth Analgesia 2019;46:699–706.

146. Tekeli IO, Turk E, Durna Corum D, et al. Effect of dose on the intravenous pharmacokinetics of tolfenamic acid in goats. J Vet Pharmacol Ther 2020;43:435–9.

147. Rodriguez P, Paul-Murphy JR, Knych HK, et al. Pharmacokinetics of grapiprant administered to red-tailed hawks (Buteo jamaicensis) after food was withheld for 24 hours. Am J Vet Res 2021;82:912–9.

148. Rodriguez P, Paul-Murphy JR, Knych HK, et al. Absorption of grapiprant in red-tailed hawks (Buteo jamaicensis) is decreased when administered with food. Am J Vet Res 2022;83. https://doi.org/10.2460/ajvr.21.10.0170.

149. Baine K, Jones MP, Cox S, et al. Pharmacokinetics of Compounded Intravenous and Oral Gabapentin in Hispaniolan Amazon Parrots (Amazona ventralis). J Avian Med Surg 2015;29:165–73.

150. Yaw TJ, Zaffarano BA, Gall A, et al. Pharmacokinetic Properties of a Single Administration of Oral Gabapentin in the Great Horned Owl (Bubo Virginianus). J Zoo Wildl Med 2015;46:547–52.

151. Browning GR, Carpenter JW, Magnin GC, et al. Pharmacokinetics of Oral Gabapentin in Caribbean Flamingos (Phoenicopterus Ruber Ruber). J Zoo Wildl Med 2018;49:609–16.

152. KuKanich B. Outpatient oral analgesics in dogs and cats beyond nonsteroidal antiinflammatory drugs: an evidence-based approach. Vet Clin North Am Small Anim Pract 2013;43:1109–25.
153. Bujak-Gizycka B, Kacka K, Suski M, et al. Beneficial effect of amantadine on postoperative pain reduction and consumption of morphine in patients subjected to elective spine surgery. Pain Med 2012;13:459–65.
154. Elmawgood AA, Rashwan S, DJEJoA Rashwan. Tourniquet-induced cardiovascular responses in anterior cruciate ligament reconstruction surgery under general anesthesia: Effect of preoperative oral amantadine. Egypt J Anesth 2015; 31:29–33.
155. Lascelles BD, Gaynor JS, Smith ES, et al. Amantadine in a multimodal analgesic regimen for alleviation of refractory osteoarthritis pain in dogs. J Vet Intern Med 2008;22:53–9.
156. Berg KJ, Sanchez-Migallon Guzman D, Knych HK, et al. Pharmacokinetics of amantadine after oral administration of single and multiple doses to orange-winged Amazon parrots (Amazona amazonica). Am J Vet Res 2020;81:651–5.
157. Carpenter JW, Tully TN Jr, Rockwell K, et al. Pharmacokinetics of Cannabidiol in the Hispaniolan Amazon Parrot (Amazona ventralis). J Avian Med Surg 2022;36: 121–7.
158. Sosa-Higareda M, Guzman Sanchez-Migallon, Knych H, et al. Pharmacokinetics of cannabinoids and metabolites in orange-winged Amazon parrots (Amazona amazonica) following administration of a hemp extract. Proc Assoc Avian Veterinarians 2022;94.
159. Brandao J, da Cunha AF, Pypendop B, et al. Cardiovascular tolerance of intravenous lidocaine in broiler chickens (Gallus gallus domesticus) anesthetized with isoflurane. Vet Anaesth Analg 2015;42:442–8.
160. Brenner DJ, Larsen RS, Dickinson PJ, et al. Development of an avian brachial plexus nerve block technique for perioperative analgesia in mallard ducks (Anas platyrhynchos). J Avian Med Surg 2010;24:24–34.
161. Da Cunha AF, Messenger KM, Stout RW, et al. Pharmacokinetics of lidocaine and its active metabolite monoethylglycinexylidide after a single intravenous administration in chickens (Gallus domesticus) anesthetized with isoflurane. J Vet Pharmacol Ther 2012;35:604–7.
162. Khamisabadi A, Kazemi-Darabadi S, Akbari G. Comparison of Anesthetic Efficacy of Lidocaine and Bupivacaine in Spinal Anesthesia in Chickens. J Avian Med Surg 2021;35:60–7.
163. Machin KL, Livingstone AL. Plasma bupivicaine levels in mallard ducks (Anas platyrhynchos) following a single subcutaneous dose. Proc Am Assoc Zoo Vet 2001;159–63.
164. DiGeronimo PM, da Cunha AF, Pypendop B, et al. Cardiovascular tolerance of intravenous bupivacaine in broiler chickens (Gallus gallus domesticus) anesthetized with isoflurane. Vet Anaesth Analg 2017;44:287–94.
165. Hocking PM, Gentle MJ, Bernard R, et al. Evaluation of a protocol for determining the effectiveness of pretreatment with local analgesics for reducing experimentally induced articular pain in domestic fowl. Res Vet Sci 1997;63: 263–7.
166. Glatz PC, Murphy LB, Preston AP. Analgesic therapy of beak-trimmed chickens. Aust Vet J 1992;69:18.
167. Figueiredo JP, Cruz ML, Mendes GM, et al. Assessment of brachial plexus blockade in chickens by an axillary approach. Vet Anaesth Analgesia 2008; 35:511–8.

168. da Cunha AF, Strain GM, Rademacher N, et al. Palpation- and ultrasound-guided brachial plexus blockade in Hispaniolan Amazon parrots (Amazona ventralis). Vet Anaesth Analgesia 2013;40:1–7.
169. d'Ovidio D, Noviello E, Adami C. Nerve stimulator-guided sciatic-femoral nerve block in raptors undergoing surgical treatment of pododermatitis. Vet Anaesth Analg 2014;42:449–53.
170. Kazemi-Darabadi S, Akbari G, Shokrollahi S. Development and evaluation of a technique for spinal anaesthesia in broiler chickens. N Z Vet J 2019;67:241–8.
171. Heinze CR, Hawkins MG, Gillies LA, et al. Effect of dietary omega-3 fatty acids on red blood cell lipid composition and plasma metabolites in the cockatiel, Nymphicus hollandicus. J Anim Sci 2012;90:3068–79.
172. Anderson K, Garner MM, Reed HH, et al. Hemorrhagic diathesis in avian species following intramuscular administration of polysulfated glycosaminoglycan. J Zoo Wildl Med 2013;44:93–9.
173. Wonn AM, Brooks MB, Hu H, et al. Hypocoagulability effect of Adequan in domestic chickens (Gallus gallus) and chilean flamingos (Phoenicopterus chilensis). J Zoo Wildl Med 2022;53:126–32.
174. Mathews K, Kronen PW, Lascelles D, et al. Guidelines for recognition, assessment and treatment of pain: WSAVA Global Pain Council members and co-authors of this document. J small Anim Pract 2014;55:E10–68.
175. Hawkins MG, Paul-Murphy J, Guzman DS-M. Recognition, assessment, and management of pain in birds. Current therapy in Avian medicine and surgery. Elsevier; 2016. p. 616–30.
176. Escobar A, Valadao CA, Brosnan RJ, et al. Effects of butorphanol on the minimum anesthetic concentration for sevoflurane in guineafowl (Numida meleagris). Am J Vet Res 2012;73:183–8.
177. Bailey RS, Sheldon JD, Allender MC, et al. Pharmacokinetics of orally administered tramadol in Muscovy ducks (Cairina moschata domestica). J Vet Pharmacol Ther 2019;42:380–4.
178. Cole GA, Paul-Murphy J, Krugner-Higby L, et al. Analgesic effects of intramuscular administration of meloxicam in Hispaniolan parrots (Amazona ventralis) with experimentally induced arthritis. Am J Vet Res 2009;70:1471–6.
179. Hocking PM, Robertson GW, Gentle MJ. Effects of non-steroidal anti-inflammatory drugs on pain-related behaviour in a model of articular pain in the domestic fowl. Res Vet Sci 2005;78:69–75.
180. Mulcahy DM, Tuomi P, Larsen RS. Differential mortality of male spectacled eiders (Somateria fischeri) and king eiders (Somateria spectabilis) subsequent to anesthesia with propofol, bupivacaine, and ketoprofen. J Avian Med Surg 2003;17:117–23.
181. Musser JM, Heatley JJ, Phalen DN. Pharmacokinetics after intravenous administration of flunixin meglumine in budgerigars (Melopsittacus undulatus) and Patagonian conures (Cyanoliseus patagonus). J Am Vet Med Assoc 2013;242:205–8.
182. Hanley CS, Thomas NJ, Paul-Murphy J, et al. Exertional myopathy in whooping cranes (Grus americana) with prognostic guidelines. J Zoo Wildl Med 2005;36:489–97.

Pain Recognition in Rodents

Vanessa L. Oliver, DVM, MSc, DACLAM[a,b],
Daniel S.J. Pang, BVSc, PhD, DECVAA, DACVAA, FRCVS[c,d],*

KEYWORDS

- Rat • Mouse • Analgesia • Pain • Nociception

KEY POINTS

- Pain is a unique, individual experience that includes sensory and emotional components.
- Applying pain assessment methods facilitates individualized pain management.
- Available pain assessment methods vary in their level of validation, including sensitivity and specificity for identifying pain.

INTRODUCTION

In all animal species that have been studied, pain is underdiagnosed and under-treated, and pain is undertreated even when veterinarians identify that it is likely to be present.[1–3] In contrast with cats and dogs, data on analgesic use in companion rodents are very limited. The available evidence indicates that analgesic use in companion rodents is considerably lower than in cats and dogs.[3–7] Multiple factors contribute to this situation, including a limited availability of pain assessment tools.[1,2,8] The ability to recognize and assess pain is a fundamental requirement of good pain management. Reassuringly, there has been considerable and growing interest in developing pain assessment methods for rodents (primarily rats and mice), much of which has been driven by an increasing focus on the welfare of laboratory rodents and awareness of the role of pain in interfering with research outcomes.[9–11]

Why is pain assessment important? Our current assumption is that all mammals and birds are sentient, with the necessary neurobiology to experience pain.[12,13] If pain can be experienced, then an absence of appropriate treatment leads to suffering. This situation creates a professional obligation for veterinarians to minimize or prevent this experience through pain assessment and treatment. Although a less common

a Department of Comparative Biology and Experimental Medicine, Faculty of Veterinary Medicine, University of Calgary, Calgary, Alberta, Canada; b Animal Health Unit, VP Research, University of Calgary, 3280 Hospital Dr NW, Calgary, Alberta, T2N 4Z6, Canada; c Department of Veterinary Clinical and Diagnostic Sciences, Faculty of Veterinary Medicine, University of Calgary, 3280 Hospital Dr NW, Calgary, Alberta, T2N 4Z6, Canada; d Department of Clinical Sciences, Faculty of Veterinary Medicine, Université de Montréal, Québec, Canada
* Corresponding author.
E-mail address: dsjpang@ucalgary.ca

Vet Clin Exot Anim 26 (2023) 121–149
https://doi.org/10.1016/j.cvex.2022.07.010
1094-9194/23/© 2022 Elsevier Inc. All rights reserved.

situation, pain assessment also helps to prevent analgesic overmedication, with the risk of increasing adverse effects.

As presented in the Definition of Pain section, pain is a unique, individual experience. As a result, there are clear limitations to applying a one-size-fits-all approach to analgesia; for a given procedure, the individual pain experience (and response to analgesics) varies. This point is the basis for routinely assessing pain in our patients and using these assessments to guide analgesia provision. Unfortunately, there are inherent hurdles to pain assessment in many veterinary species, but especially small mammals and exotic species. These include a lack of familiarity with a given species, an inherent subjectivity in pain assessment in nonverbal species, an absence of validated pain assessment methods, and incomplete information regarding analgesic drug options and dosing. In this article, we present an overview of pain assessment scale validation methods, available pain assessment methods, and a rational approach to pain assessment and decision-making. This discussion is primarily within the context of acute pain.

Definition of Pain

For consistency, when discussing pain in this article, we use the widely accepted definition of the International Association for the Study of Pain. This defines pain as "An unpleasant sensory and emotional experience associated with, or resembling that associated with, actual or potential tissue damage."[14] This definition is accompanied by several guidance notes, of which the most relevant to veterinary medicine are presented in **Table 1**.

Table 1
Guidance notes accompanying the International Association for the Study of Pain definition of pain[14]

Guidance Note	Elaboration
"Pain is always a personal experience that is influenced to varying degrees by biological, psychological, and social factors."	This reflects the individual experience of pain
"Pain and nociception are different phenomena. Pain cannot be inferred solely from activity in sensory neurons."	For example, while under general anesthesia, animals cannot experience pain but may respond to a nociception[a] (such as with an increase in heart rate in response to a surgical incision).
"Although pain usually serves as an adaptive role, it may have adverse effects on function and social and psychological well-being."	This underlines the negative emotional (affective) component of pain.
"Verbal description is only one of several behaviors to express pain; inability to communicate does not negate the possibility that a human or a nonhuman animal experiences pain."	The inability to verbalize pain does not mean it is not present.

[a] Nociception is "The neural process of encoding noxious stimuli."[14] The consequences of encoding may include activation of the autonomic nervous system (as commonly seen during surgery) or a behavioral response (eg, withdrawal reflex to a toe pinch); however, the sensation (experience) of pain is not necessarily present.

Table 2	
Key validation concepts with pain assessment scale examples	
Concept	**Pain Assessment Scale Examples**
Face validity	Discussion among experts to evaluate items that may be incorporated into a pain scale. Items might include, for example, attention to a surgical site, facial expression, response to interaction[15,23–25] Alternatively, scale items can be derived from behavioral observations.[26–31]
Criterion validity	Comparison between existing and novel pain scales, such as the RGS and a composite measure scale[32–34]
Construct validity	Testing hypotheses, for example, a pain scale, should be able to identify animals that have received analgesia after surgery versus those that have not.[15,21,27,29,31,35,36]
Reliability	Reproducibility of pain assessment results under different conditions, such as different raters.[15,21,23,35]

Critically, the definition of pain includes the emotional experience, so that pain can be described in terms of a negative emotional experience (a negative affective state) and there is experimental evidence that of the pain assessment methods described below, at least the grimace scales reflect the negative emotional state of pain.[15,16]

Traditionally, pain is often classified as acute or chronic. Acute pain is considered adaptive, serving to protect the animal from further injury. By contrast, chronic pain is considered maladaptive, with pain present beyond recovery from the initial injury. Although chronic pain is also defined based on its duration, there is no consensus as to the number of days or weeks needed to pass before pain can be described as chronic. This article focuses on acute pain; however, acute pain can transition to chronic pain if undertreated.[17]

Validation of Pain Assessment Methods

The term validated is widely misunderstood and tends to be applied loosely when discussing health assessment scales, such as pain scales. It is often used with the assumption that scale validation is a discrete, one-time process, when it is really an ongoing continual process. The aim of this section is to give a brief, simplified overview of key concepts of scale validation to assist readers in evaluating new and existing health assessment scales. The example of pain is used here (**Table 2**), but the concepts described apply to all health assessment scales. For an in-depth discussion of scale development and validation testing, interested readers are referred to Streiner and colleagues[18] and Streiner.[19] Validation can be considered to comprise several concepts. These concepts are validity, reliability, generalizability and, practicality.

Validity asks, "Does a scale measure what it claims to measure?"; that is, does a proposed pain assessment scale measure pain?[20,21] Aspects of this question can be examined explicitly by considering whether the items contained within a scale (such as ear position, in many grimace scales) are necessary and important (content validity), how a scale performs when compared directly against the current best measurement method, should one exist (criterion validity), and if a scale identifies important changes in the attribute being measured, for example, pain (construct validity). In veterinary medicine, because we work with nonverbal species, content validity is usually determined by face validity; identifying and initially selecting scale items based on the views of a group of experts. An alternative approach, as applied for some composite measure pain scales (discussed elsewhere in this article), is to generate an ethogram to identify behaviors that change in painful or nonpainful states. In humans, criterion validity is usually tested against a patient's verbal self-report. In animal species, a comparison is made against an existing scale, assuming one is available and believed to measure the attribute of interest. This task may be difficult to do owing to the limited number of well-developed scales and interpreting results may be challenging. Consequently, it is much more common in veterinary medicine to use construct validity instead of criterion validity. Construct validation is testing a hypothesis based on what is known (or assumed) about the construct of interest (eg, pain). This process commonly undertaken during pain scale development and frequently tested hypotheses are (1) a surgical procedure results in pain and (2) providing a known analgesic results in a decrease in pain after surgery. Importantly, as discussed further elsewhere in this article, construct validation should be viewed as an ongoing process: scale performance within the testing context (population, procedure, and environment) should not be assumed to extend to all possible contexts.

Reliability reflects the reproducibility of the results of a scale under different conditions. It is the measurement error associated with a scale. If measurement error is large, important or relevant changes in pain will not be detected. Measurement error is most commonly assessed for differences that result from scale use by different assessors (inter-rater reliability). Inter-rater reliability is important when an animal is assessed by different members of the veterinary team, as often happens over the course of hospitalization in larger clinics. Good inter-rater reliability means that the scores obtained by different assessors are believable. This factor facilitates good pain management; trends in pain levels can be identified and response to analgesics assessed. From this, it should be apparent that reliability may change when a scale is used by different assessors and may be affected by training and experience, although few scale developers draw attention to this important consideration.

As more studies are published assessing scale validity and reliability under different conditions (animal populations, painful diseases, pain types, assessors, and environment), this process contributes toward generalizability, which reflects how a scale performs in a wide range of settings. Ideally, a scale should work well regardless of setting; however, this assumption is risky without support from continued validation and reliability testing. Sadly, testing of existing scales is not frequently performed. Because of their role in biomedical research, the Mouse Grimace Scale (MGS) and the Rat Grimace Scale (RGS) remain the most completely developed and evaluated of existing rodent pain assessment methods.[20]

A frequently overlooked consideration with pain assessment scales, probably because most formally developed scales are created for use in research, is whether scales are practical to apply. In a research setting, in contrast with clinical applications, it is often feasible for a single assessor to perform all observations, have ample time to do so, and without time pressure to produce results within a short timeframe (minutes). Realistically, for a scale to be widely adopted in clinical practice, it needs to be quick to apply (<1–2 minutes), produce interpretable results immediately, and produce reliable results when used by multiple assessors with varying levels of experience and training. As discussed elsewhere in this article for the MGS and RGS, both scales currently have some practical limitations. Additionally, for a pain scale to be of practical clinical value, it must provide users with guidance regarding decisions on analgesic use. To achieve this goal, identifying an intervention threshold (a scale score above which the probability of pain being present is increased) is a valuable aspect of scale development. Unfortunately, this goal has not been a priority for most scales developed for research use, where identifying pain is based on statistical analyses of groups of animals, with the advantage of having baseline values for comparison. An intervention threshold has been derived for the RGS, but not the MGS.[21]

Table 3
Summary of rodent pain assessment methods

Test	Construct Validity Demonstrated	Reliability Assessed	Potential Confounding Factors	Assessor Training Recommended
Physiologic variables	Mice Rats	Not applicable (objective measure)	Stress Restraint Disease states	Not applicable (objective measure)
Nesting	Mice	Mice	Cold stress Group housing Genetics Type of nesting material provided Analgesics Disease states	Yes
Burrowing	Mice Rats Hamsters Gerbils	Not applicable (objective measure)	Disease Cage flooring Surroundings Diet Estrous cycle	Not applicable (objective measure)
Ethograms and composite measure pain scales	Mice Rats Guinea pigs	Rats	Analgesia Anesthesia Observer presence	Yes
Grimace scales	Mice Rats	Mice Rats	Anesthesia Hypothermia Sex Strain Observer presence Restraint	Rats, not investigated for mice

When adopting pain assessment scales in clinics, there is often a temptation to adapt scales to suit local conditions. This modification could be in the form of assessing some, but not all, of the scale items; applying the scale to a different species; or adjusting the scores assigned to individual items. From the preceding discussion, it should be clear that adapting scales risks compromising validity and reliability, and the impact of adaptations should be assessed. To facilitate use, some pain assessment scales have been assessed for performance with items removed, but research in this area is limited in rodents.[15,21–24]

Potential Pain Assessment Methods

The methods described in this section are presented in order of level of supporting evidence for their use, from least to most. It is important to consider that other negative affective states (such as illness and distress) will influence some of these methods. A summary of their current validity, reliability, known confounding factors and training requirements is presented in **Table 3**.

Physiological markers
Hormones and physiological variables. Pain can act as a stressor, affecting the secretion of hormones, neurotransmitters, and enzymes within the body. Of particular

importance is the effect of pain on the hypothalamic–pituitary–adrenal and sympathetic axes, leading to the release of corticosteroids from the adrenal cortex, as well as epinephrine and norepinephrine from the adrenal medulla.[37] In rodents, the principal corticosteroid is corticosterone.[38] These hormones, among others, increase physiological variables such as heart rate, respiratory rate, blood pressure, and body temperature, which have been widely used in veterinary medicine to identify and monitor pain.[39,40] In addition, tissue injury releases inflammatory mediators that may also act as biomarkers of pain, as well as activate the hypothalamic–pituitary–adrenal axis, further contributing to alterations in these parameters.

Changes in the concentrations of these hormones or altered physiologic variables may be used as indirect indicators for acute pain. The response of physiologic variables to pain can be altered with the administration of analgesics.[30,41] It is important to note that these variables are not specific to pain and can be altered by other processes, such as stress[42–44] and disease.[45,46] Corticosterone, one of the more common hormones measured to infer stress levels associated with pain in rodents, has also been reported to be altered with handling,[42,47–53] cage changing,[49,54–57(p2002),58,59] removal of social housing,[60] circadian rhythm,[41] clinical procedures,[41,59,61,62] and surgery.[30,31,42] Some studies have also found significant variation in hormone responses across individuals and strains.[30,31] Traditionally, these variables require invasive techniques such as serial blood collection and surgical implantation of telemetry devices; however, noninvasive approaches such as fecal corticosterone sampling,[63] infrared thermography,[64,65] visual imaging,[66,67] or capacitive sensing[68] have been described or are under development in the research and laboratory animal medicine fields.

Although clinical incorporation of measuring hormonal parameters is likely impractical owing to the accessibility and time delay of laboratory analysis for these hormones, the measurement of vitals such as heart rate, respiratory rate, body temperature (with or without blood pressure) can be accessible in a clinical setting. The drawbacks of depending on these vital signs for the assessment of pain is that the changes may not be sensitive or specific measures of pain, collection may require sedation or restraint (which may affect the measured values), and values may vary according to circadian rhythm.[69(p199),70] Ultimately, these variables should not be used as the sole method for pain evaluation.

Mice Changes in physiologic variables after surgical and soft tissue sampling procedures have been described in the literature. Studies investigating pain or analgesic efficacy following surgery note short-term changes in heart rate, heart rate variability, blood pressure, and body temperature that can be detected for several hours to days. Alteration in physiologic variables has been noted to last up to 5 to 7 days after surgery in some cases.[71] After telemetry implantation surgery without analgesia, mice commonly display an increased heart rate, decreased heart rate variability, elevated mean arterial pressure, and increases in body temperature.[71,72] One study noted no significant changes in heart rate and blood pressure after a mock ova implantation surgery that compared the analgesics buprenorphine and flunixin with a saline control.[73] For less invasive procedures like tissue biopsy sampling, significant increases in heart rate and core body temperature, which were more pronounced than changes seen with restraint alone, can be seen within the first few hours after the procedure.[41,62,74–78] Although physiologic changes have been noted for painful procedures, these studies recommend that physiologic outcomes be evaluated in combination with other pain assessment methods as they are exclusive measures of pain and can be influenced by other factors.

Rats Similar changes to those reported in mice are seen in rats with respect to heart rate, heart rate variability, and mean arterial pressure after noxious visceral stimuli and surgery.[75,79–81] A study evaluating pain following surgical implantation of a telemetry device found elevated heart rate and heart rate variability that followed increases in mechanical allodynia and decreases in mobility tests.[81] These changes were reversed after local anesthetic was administered, indicating pain played a role in the changes observed but could not always be distinguished from other stressors.

Guinea pigs Although telemetry studies in guinea pigs measuring physiological parameters during experimental manipulations are described in the literature, there is limited evidence on associations with pain. One study comparing preoperative and postoperative values, found heart rate and temperature to increase and respiratory rate and body weight to decrease after orchiectomy surgery.[70] However, no changes between treatment groups were identified (meloxicam vs saline postoperatively). This could reflect a limited analgesic effect of postoperative meloxicam, a lack of discriminative ability of the physiologic variables to distinguish between analgesic treatments or relatively small differences in pain levels between treatment groups (all animals also received perioperative analgesia: butorphanol, intratesticular lidocaine, meloxicam).[70] Further work is needed in this species.

Chinchillas Studies evaluating changes in physiological parameters associated with pain have yet to be described in the literature. Further work is required in this area.

Other rodents Telemetry studies evaluating the relationship of blood pressure, heart rate, and body temperature during torpor in hamsters have been reported in the literature[164,165], but currently lack investigation into changes associated with pain.

Weight loss. Weight loss (and slow growth) is commonly used in pain assessment. Although a decrease in body mass can reflect pain causing reduced food consumption (or drinking), it is neither specific nor sensitive for pain, because these factors may also be affected by a variety of factors (nonpainful illness, environmental and social stress, handling, and drugs). A study of a mouse cancer model that used a conditioned place preference design showed that animals displayed analgesia-seeking behavior up to 10 days before the common experimental end point of a 15% weight loss occurred.[82] This finding suggests that, when weight loss is considered as an indicator of illness (including, but not exclusive to pain), smaller changes (in the region of ≤5%) than historically applied should be used.[82] Similar weight losses of approximately 5% have been noted in mice after a laparotomy surgery and correlated with decreases in nesting, grooming, and mechanical threshold testing over a 48-hour postoperative period.[76] In mice, handling can serve as a stressor, affecting weight loss after surgery.[83] In rats, weight loss did not distinguish between animals that received analgesia (carprofen or buprenorphine) versus a saline control group, despite changes in behavior.[29] Weight loss and food consumption are associated with postoperative buprenorphine treatment in rats (0.03 mg/kg, twice daily for 3 days) and may extend several days beyond the end of treatment.[84] In guinea pigs, weight loss remained below a 10% threshold for providing analgesia, despite changes in heart and respiratory rates, food consumption, and mechanical hypersensitivity.[70]

Food consumption. Although a decrease in food consumption is a widely accepted indicator of compromised well-being, and frequently advocated as an outcome measure by veterinarians, there is little evidence that it is either a sensitive or specific indicator of pain, although it may serve as an item within a composite measure pain scale.[70] Additionally, because the majority of food intake by rodents takes place at night, observable changes may be delayed, and assessing food consumption can be very difficult with ad libitum feeding from a relatively large volume of food or in group housing. Weighing food can help to address the former situation. Species that cache food may give the impression of food consumption as food is removed from the bowl but not eaten.

Perhaps unexpectedly, food consumption may be decreased as an adverse effect of some analgesics. The best known example of this is the effect of buprenorphine in Sprague-Dawley rats, where its administration is associated with decreased food consumption and pica when repeated doses are given or with a single dose of a sustained release formulation.[84–86] Pica behavior has also been reported in Wistar rats given buprenorphine 3 times daily (every 8 hours, 0.05 mg/kg subcutaneously)[87] and hydromorphone (0.5, 1 and 2 mg/kg subcutaneously) has been associated with decreased food intake in chinchillas.[88] In guinea pigs, opioid agonists (mu and kappa) decrease gastrointestinal motility, although the importance of this effect postoperatively is unclear; both pain and stress also decrease gastrointestinal motility.[70,89]

Response to touch. Gentle stroking or palpation around an injury or incision site is a potentially useful indicator of pain and is included in several well-developed composite measure pain scales in larger companion species (eg, dogs and cats).[23–25] Response to touch reflects mechanical hypersensitivity (allodynia), as may occur after surgery. When incorporated as part of a composite scale or alongside other indicators of pain, the response to touch constitutes a valuable part of pain assessment. When used alone, responses to touch should be interpreted cautiously. Differentiating between a nociceptive response (eg, reflex limb withdrawal) versus pain (eg, vocalizing or turning toward the injured site) is not always straightforward and nociceptive responses are considered less significant.[15,90,91] In biomedical research, the response to touch is a well-established form of evoked response testing used in laboratory rodents, usually tested with von Frey filaments. An increase in sensitivity has been reported in guinea pigs following surgery, though current reliance on comparing preoperative and postoperative may limit its application to elective procedures when preoperative responses can be recorded.[70] It is also possible that evoked responses may be altered when performed by an unfamiliar individual, and a more useful response may be elicited when performed by an owner.

Nesting. Nesting is an innate, highly motivated behavior that many wild and domesticated rodents perform, including outside of maternal, brood-rearing purposes. In many rodent species, both sexes can be highly driven to participate in nest building,[77] to boost overall survivability through provision of thermoregulation, as well as creating shelter from the elements and protection from predators. The drive to perform this behavior can be used as a measurement of well-being, where part or all the behavior may be decreased by clinical conditions, including pain. Owing to these qualities, it has been suggested that nest building can be a useful tool in evaluating the impact of pain on an individual's overall quality of life.[76,78]

In laboratory rodents, several nest building assessments have been developed to assess pain. Materials such as compressed cotton, shredded paper, facial tissue, paper towel, hay, wood shavings, and/or twine are provided for the animal to forage, shred, and arrange into a nest.[77,92–96] Assessments include measuring the quality or complexity of the nest,[76,92,94,97] latency to begin to build a nest,[97] time to build a nest,[76,98–100] consolidation of nesting material (**Fig. 1**),[76,101] or incorporation of new material into the nest (**Fig. 2**).[102,103] Nest building has been seen to be decreased after surgical procedures,[72,76,97,100,102] as well as during clinical disease associated with pain.[99,103]

The benefits of these assessments are that they follow robust, innate behaviors that require basic, readily available materials and, in some instances, such as the time-to-integrate-to-nest test, may be tracked on an ongoing, on-demand basis. Nesting scores follow expected pain trajectories, where impaired nesting is associated with painful stimuli and improves after the administration of analgesics (construct validity).[76,97,104] Disadvantages of these assessments are that they can be relatively subjective with poor inter-rater reliability.[105,106] Many of the assessments focus on parameters that are binary and may not be able to track changes in pain after a nest has been built. Assessment also becomes difficult when animals are housed in groups as other cage mates can compensate in nest building activities for any affected individuals, thus skewing the nesting score. Other factors, such as cold ambient temperatures, can increase nesting behavior,[107] genetics can alter the motivation and quality of nest building behavior,[102,108] type of nest material provided can impact the quality of nest built,[92] analgesics or other drugs that cause behavioral changes, such as sedation, can impair nest building,[76,100] and some neurological diseases can decrease nesting.[99,109] Many of these factors can be managed easily when taken into consideration before the test is performed and when interpreting results. It is recommended to use detailed scoring systems, train observers, and use mean values of scores provided by a group of raters to increase the robustness of findings.[76,105,106]

Burrowing. Burrowing is a spontaneous, highly motivated, innate behavior seen in many rodent species. Burrows can serve as shelters away from the elements, defense against predators, food stores, and safe places to rear young.[110] Owing to the nature of this behavior, burrowing can also be used as an indicator of overall well-being and quality of life.[106] It has been reported to decrease during pain states such as postoperative pain and peripheral nerve injury, as well as inflammatory conditions, and can be reversed with the administration of analgesics.[111–118] The behavior of burrowing

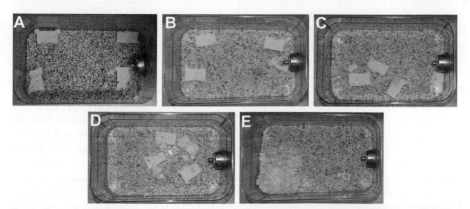

Fig. 1. The nest consolidation test measures a mouse's ability to retrieve 4 pieces of nesting material, consolidate the pieces to within a specific distance of one another, and then shred the material to build a nest. The nest can be built anywhere in the cage. (*A*) Start of test, no nesting squares grouped together. (*B*) Nesting squares paired together in 1 or 2 pairs. (*C*) Three nesting squares grouped together. (*D*) All 4 nesting squares grouped together. (*E*) Four nesting squares grouped together and completely shredded. (From Turner et al. 2019; with permission.)[158]

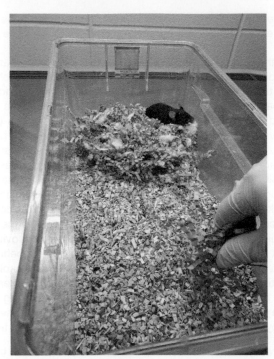

Fig. 2. After a nest has been built, nest building behavior as a potential reflection of pain can continue to be assessed by providing small amounts of nesting material in the cage and monitoring if it becomes incorporated into the existing nest within 10 minutes. In the picture, 4 strands of new nesting material (shredded paper) is being added to the cage.

involves the animal using its front and hind feet to push material just outside of the burrow and can be distinguished from similar behaviors such as hoarding, where edible material is carried from the burrow by mouth to be stored away from the burrow, as well as digging, which is performed with bedding in the greater cage area instead of the burrowing container.[110] Animals primarily burrow during the dark phase when they are most active; however, they have also been noted perform this behavior during the light cycle.[114]

A detailed protocol for performing burrowing assessments in various rodent species is provided by Deacon.[110,119] To perform this test, the animal is given a long tube that is sealed at one end (eg, water bottle) and filled with a preweighed amount of substrate (see species section elsewhere in this article for suitable substrate options) (**Fig. 3**). The amount of substrate remaining in the tube is measured after 2 hours. A limitation to evaluating burrowing is that the behavior varies between individuals and increases with practice.[110,120] Knowledge of whether an individual burrows when healthy is needed to interpret burrowing behavior postoperatively or when sick. Soliciting information from clients about their pet's burrowing behavior at home could help to identify if burrowing could be useful to assess during a hospital stay. A potential approach for motivated clients could involve having them take home a burrowing testing kit consisting of a plastic tube or water bottle, instructions and monitoring sheet ahead of their scheduled procedure. The clients can make notes on the burrowing behavior (eg, substrate used, time to clear the burrow, or amount of substrate remaining after 2 hours) in the days leading up to the procedure that can be used as baseline information to be compared with testing performed after the procedure.

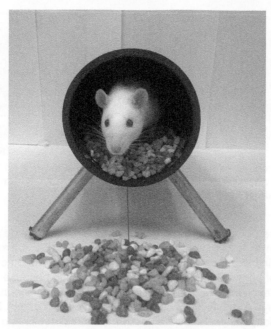

Fig. 3. Burrowing is a highly motivated, innate behavior in many rodents species that can be used as a potential indicator of pain using supplies that are readily available.

The implementation of this test is relatively easy because the supplies used (eg, plastic tube or water bottle, food, bedding) are readily available. In addition, if the test can be performed within the animal's home cage, confounding factors such as stress associated with handling or novel environments can be minimized. In addition to individual variability, various other conditions beyond pain can influence burrowing. These factors include cognitive dysfunction, neurodegenerative diseases, anxiety, infection, and inflammation.[32,109,110,121–128] Alterations in the cage flooring,[129] surroundings,[97] diet,[130] and estrous cycle[131] have also been noted to alter burrowing.

Ethograms
Ethograms for pain evaluation have been described in many rodents and involve observing the animal for a catalog of species-specific normal and abnormal behaviors. In pain assessments, ethograms rely on detecting a decrease or absence of normal behaviors (eg, rearing, grooming, coprophagy) and an increase in pain-specific behaviors (eg, writhing, back arch, squinting, weight shifting) (**Fig. 4**). Changes that may be associated with pain include changes in vocalizations (eg, number, duration, intensity), posture (eg, abnormal standing, sitting, lying), activity (eg, decreases in rearing, increases or decreases in locomotion, decreases in responses to external stimuli, and changes to grooming such as increased licking, biting, or scratching) and daily routines (eg, social isolation, loss of appetite, sleep disturbance, and increases in attention to a painful area).[9] Descriptions of general ethograms in rodents are available through the National Center for the Replacement Refinement and Reduction of Animals in Research and can be a useful starting point in identifying potentially relevant behaviors.[132] Because many of the parameters assessed in ethograms involve spontaneous, routine activities or behaviors, these assessments also provide the benefit of serving as an indicator of overall well-being and quality of life. It should also be noted

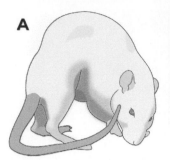
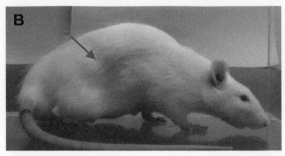

Fig. 4. Pain-associated behaviors demonstrated after laparotomy in a rat. (*A*) Back arch, (*B*) Writhe (created by contraction of the abdominal muscles, *arrow*). (Illustration by Dr Vivian SY Leung.) (From Turner et al. 2019; with permission.)[158]

that many of these behaviors are not specific to pain and may be altered owing to other factors such as anesthetic and analgesic drugs.[133] For example, guinea pigs given buprenorphine experience sedation, resulting in lower locomotive scores.[133]

The detection of behavioral changes can be challenging because rodents are prey species and have evolved to hide or mask these conditions to increase their likelihood of survival. Displays of these behaviors can be difficult to detect by the untrained observer. In addition, many rodents are nocturnal or crepuscular and have their active periods during the dark phase of the light cycle. Monitoring behaviors outside of their normal active period can decrease the likelihood of detecting these changes. Rodents are also known to depress their behaviors in the presence of other animals, such as a human observer.[133,134] The results of ethograms may be incorporated into composite measure pain scales (see the Composite Measure Pain Scales section).

Under controlled conditions (ie, in research settings), the animal is observed in its home cage using remote video monitoring. Environmental items such as huts or nesting material, as well as other animals, may be removed or reduced from the cage environment to observe the animal more clearly. Observers are trained on the behaviors in advance to improve interrater reliability and minimize subjectivity in scoring. Some of these strategies may not be possible in a clinical setting and could limit the observer's ability to detect these behaviors. When using behavioral observations, it is recommended to evaluate multiple items (see the Composite Measure Pain Scales section) to improve the sensitivity and specificity for pain detection.[133] A number of automated monitoring devices are under development in the laboratory animal medicine field and may serve as more practical tools for the implementation of these assessments in the future. More detailed descriptions of these tools are discussed elsewhere in this article.

Composite measure pain scales

Composite measure pain scales combine evaluation of several behaviors to assess pain.[25] Such behaviors might include posture/body position, demeanor, response to interaction and mobility.[25–31] These scales contrast with historic, unidimensional scales that focus on a single measure, typically pain intensity (eg, 0 = no pain, 1 = mild pain, 2 = moderate pain, and 3 = severe pain). Such scales are generally unvalidated and perform poorly in a clinical setting.[69] Although the intuitive use of a composite of behaviors to assess pain is commonplace, and many clinicians combine evaluation of several behaviors when performing an informal (gut feeling) assessment of pain (such as activity, interaction, and general demeanor), this approach can be highly subjective and at risk of confirmation bias. Ideally, composite measure pain scales should go through validation testing as described elsewhere in this article.

Rats and mice. Partially validated composite measure pain scales exist for rats[26-29] and mice.[30,31] These scales were developed using a rigorous ethogram approach to identify behavioral changes after surgery (content validity). The result was to identity the following key behaviors associated with pain following laparotomy (rat) and vasectomy (mouse) surgeries: rearing, attention to surgical incision, posture, writhing, back arch, and gait.[28,31] For both scales, construct validation testing has been performed: identifying the presence of pain after surgery and responses to opioid and nonsteroidal anti-inflammatory drug analgesia. However, it is unclear to what extent these scales are being used, and a short period of training may be required for reliable use.[135] Practically, the rat scale has been shown to be fairly quick to apply, and an assessment can be performed within approximately 5 minutes.[28] Unfortunately, analgesia intervention thresholds have not been defined for either scale. Because these scales were developed using surgical models, it is unclear to what extent they apply to other sources of pain. Some overlap in behaviors (hump-backed [hunched] position, licking of the lower abdomen or flank, repeated waves of flank muscle contractions, stretching of the body, and pressing of the abdomen against the floor) has been identified occurring in rats with urethral stones.[136] It is possible that alternative or additional behaviors are required to effectively evaluate pain, and response to analgesics.[29] A number of general behavior descriptions in Norway rats are available online and may serve as a useful starting point for scale development.[137] For mice, a free resource providing descriptions and videos of common behaviors in mice is available through the Garner Laboratory at Stanford School of Medicine.[138] Although little is known about factors that may confound composite measure pain scales in rats and mice, buprenorphine alters activity and has the potential to interfere with these scales.[26,31] Evidence from canine and feline composite measure scales suggests that other confounds are likely and could include anesthesia, sedation, and demeanor.[24,139,140]

Interestingly, it may be the case that some existing scales used for well-being assessment in research partially reflect pain. For example, a comparison of the RGS, burrowing behavior, a composite measure pain scale, and the Disease Activity Index (a composite scale containing items for weight loss, stool consistency and blood in stools) found both the Disease Activity Index and RGS scores to increase with acute and chronic colitis, indicating that the Disease Activity Index reflect pain associated with colitis.[32] By contrast, the composite measure pain scale and burrowing showed limited sensitivity to the presence of pain. In mice undergoing experimental thoracotomy and myocardial infarct creation, the MGS was found to be more sensitive in identifying pain than a generic well-being assessment scale (items included body position, activity, response to handling, and respiratory rate).[34]

Guinea pigs. Postsurgical ethograms and composite measure scales have been described for male and female guinea pigs.[70,133,141,142] One validated scale focused on the detection of passive and active behaviors that increase and decrease in frequency during pain, respectively.[133] Passive behaviors include eyes closed or squinting, piloerection, weight shifting, subtle body movements, and incomplete movements. Active behaviors include forward or backward movement, body turn, head or neck movement, rearing, and coprophagy.

Chinchillas. There is currently no literature on the use of ethograms or composite measure pain scales for pain assessment. Pain is a commonly considered differential when fur chewing is observed in chinchillas. Fur chewing is often a manifestation of stress rather than a pain-specific behavior, but sources of pain should be ruled out.[143] Further work is required in this species.

Other rodents. A general rodent ethogram is freely available for golden hamsters and gerbils through the National Center for the Replacement, Refinement, and Reduction of Animals in Research.[132] A postoperative ethogram in golden hamsters has been developed; however, further work is required for its use as a reliable postoperative pain assessment.[144]

Grimace Scales

Grimace scales are an example of facial expression scales that were developed to identify pain. After the publication of the initial scales, for use in mice (MGS)[15] and rats (RGS),[35] grimace scales were rapidly developed for a wide range of species (**Fig. 5**) (see Mogil and colleagues 2020[20] for a comprehensive review of grimace scales). The most compelling aspect of these scales is that they reflect the pain experience, that is, the emotional experience of pain.[52,91] The MGS and RGS have undergone considerable validation and reliability testing, greater than for other grimace scales. They exhibit construct validity for acute pain and very good reliability for trained, experienced assessors.[20] An attractive feature of grimace scales is that they do not require interaction, minimizing potentially stressful handling. However, they are not without limitations. These limitations include practicality and a potential requirement for observer training.

The concept of grimace scales is similar across species: individual facial action units (AUs) are assessed and assigned a numerical score. The MGS and RGS differ in which AUs apply in each species. For the MGS, there are 5 AUs: eyes, ears, nose, cheek, and whiskers. For the RGS, there are 4: eyes, ears, nose/cheek, and whiskers. Additionally, the assessment of the nose/cheek area differs: in mice, the nose and cheek areas bulge when pain is present, whereas in rats these areas flatten.[15,35] In assessing each AU, the assessor is determining how far the appearance of the AU deviates from normal (**Fig. 6**). A score of 0 is assigned when the assessor has high confidence that the AU is absent, a score of 2 for high confidence that the AU is present, and a score of 1 when either there is high confidence that the AU is moderately present or equivocation over its presence or absence.[15] The scores for the AUs are then summed and averaged.

Posters illustrating the key features of the MGS and RGS are available freely through the National Center for the Replacement Refinement and Reduction of Animals in Research[145] and an RGS training manual is freely available online.[146]

Of the AUs, eyes tend to be the easiest to score and whiskers the most difficult. It is unclear if whisker scoring is inherently difficult or whether problems obtaining high-quality images is a major factor. Usefully, both the MGS and RGS continue to perform well if whiskers are not scored.[15,21]

For the RGS, an analgesic intervention threshold has been developed. At scores of more than 0.67, the probability of pain being present increases (sensitivity of 84.6%; specificity of 88.6%).[21] This threshold serves to aid users in guiding decisions around providing analgesia. The analgesic intervention threshold can be increased or decreased to increase specificity or sensitivity, respectively, and Oliver and colleagues[21] provided the information required to support setting a different intervention threshold. The threshold developed from this work was shown to be applicable in spinal cord injury, an example of generalizability.[147]

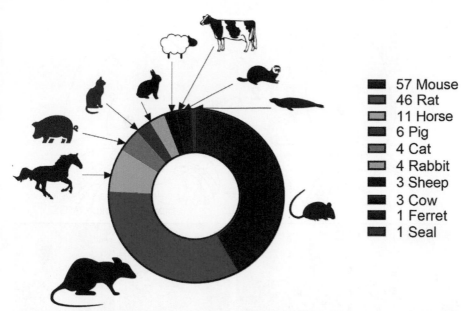

Fig. 5. Number of published journal articles (2010–2019 inclusive) featuring the grimace scales, separated by species. (From Mogil et al. 2020; with permission.)[20]

In terms of practicality, the original grimace scale descriptions relied on a fairly labor intensive video- and image-based data collection method, reflecting their application in biomedical research. This approach is impractical for clinical use owing to the time and labor required and delay in identifying pain. Since the initial publications, real-time scoring has been found to be successful with the RGS, with some indication of success for the MGS.[134,148] Leung and colleagues[148] found that scores collected in real time (2 minutes of continuous observation) were comparable with the standard method. It should be noted that, in this study, animals were placed in an observation cage to facilitate scoring, they were familiar with the observer and the observer was trained in use of the scale.

One aspect of pain scales that is seldom discussed is the potential requirement for observer training. It is often assumed that scales can be applied with little to no training, but this factor is rarely investigated. The very limited evidence on training suggests that it may be needed for some, but not all, grimace scales. For the RGS, training improved scoring, so that scores were comparable with those of an expert rater.[36] The training process was straightforward, requiring scoring of randomized, blinded images, including a brief discussion to clarify how to apply the RGS. The requirement or benefit of training in the MGS is largely unknown, although differences in scores assigned by different assessors has been reported.[34] In contrast with research use, in clinics the decision to withhold or provide analgesia may be based on the scores of a single assessor so that confirming assessor performance would be prudent.

There is some potential for MGS and RGS scores to be influenced by confounding factors. To date, there has been limited research identifying confounding factors, but factors shown to potentially interfere with scores include general anesthesia, hypothermia, sex and strain, observer effects, and restraint. General anesthesia with isoflurane inflates MGS and RGS scores, although the effect is short lasting (<3 hours) and can be minimized by supporting normothermia.[33,149–151] Concerningly, scores

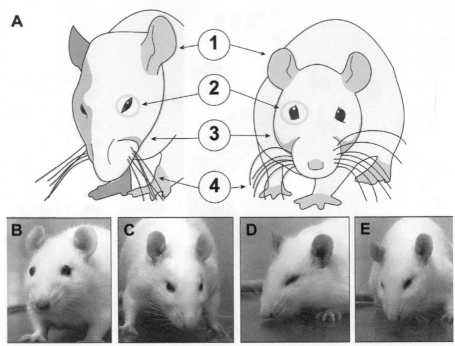

Fig. 6. The RGS. (*A*) Rat depicted with "pain" (*left*) and with "no pain" (*right*). The pain rat has (1) folded ears that are angled away from the front of the face, (2) partial eye closure, (3) a flattened and elongated nose, and (4) whiskers that are bunched together and directed away from the face. The no pain rat has (1) rounded ears that face forward, (2) no eye closure, (3) a rounded nose and ,cheeks and (4) whiskers that are fanned and droopy at the ends. (*B*) The face of a normal male Wistar rat with no pain. Its eyes are round and open. Its ears are rounded, facing forward and roughly perpendicular to the top of its head. Its nose and cheeks are rounded with an evident bulge and crease between the nose and cheeks. Lasy, the whiskers are spread apart and droop downward at the ends. (AU scores—eyes, 0; ears, 0; nose/cheek, 0; whiskers, 0). (*C*) An adult male Wistar rat grimacing with orbital tightening, nose/cheek flattening with only a slight crease between the nose and cheeks and straightened whiskers that are pulled toward the cheeks. Its ears are curled and slightly rotated outwards. (AU scores—eyes, 1; ears, 1; nose/cheek, 1; whiskers, 1; overall score of 1 [from average of 4 AUs]). (*D*) An adult male Wistar rat grimacing with an overall score of 2. It has a tightly closed eyelid. Its nose and cheeks are flattened with the nose appearing elongated. The nose and cheek flatten with no crease evident between them. The whiskers are straightened, bunched together, and horizontal to the cheeks. Its ears are rotated outwards and curled inwards (AU scores—eyes, 2; ears, 2; nose/cheek, 2; whiskers, 2). (*E*) An adult male Wistar rat grimacing with an overall score of 1.75. Its eyelids are tightly closed. The ears are curled and rotated away from the front of the rat's face. Its nose and cheeks are flattened with no crease evident between them. The whiskers are straight and pulled toward the cheeks (AU scores—eyes, 2; ears, 2; nose/cheek, 2; whiskers, 1). (Illustration by Dr Vivian SY Leung.) ([B-E] From Turner et al. 2019; with permission.)[158]

increased by anesthesia and hypothermia can be high enough to exceed the RGS analgesia intervention threshold, risking misidentifying pain as being present.[33] In mice, the MGS is inflated with ketamine–xylazine anesthesia, although the duration of the effect is unclear.[152] The possibility of sex and strain differences in MGS scores have been identified, although the size of observed differences was small and the study was performed in healthy, nonpainful animals so the impact of pain could not be determined.[134] There is some concern that expressed behaviors, perhaps including facial expressions, may be suppressed in the presence of male observers or potential predators.[153,154] Stressful restraint, such as prolonged immobilization, increases the MGS, whereas gentle restraint does not.[20] In contrast with many of the proposed pain assessment methods described elsewhere in this article, the MGS and RGS do not seem to be affected by opioid administration.[35,155]

Additionally, because facial expressions reflect affective states, it is unsurprising that there is the potential for overlap between AUs indicative of pain and facial expressions associated with other negative affective states (eg, fear,[156] nonpainful illness[15]) or behaviors involving the face (eg, sleep, grooming[15]). The degree of overlap in AUs between painful and nonpainful disease states requires further research. Knowledge of these confounding factors are important in avoiding mistakes in identifying the presence or absence of pain.[139,140]

The MGS and RGS were originally thought to be limited to acute pain over the time course encountered with surgery. However, there is increasing evidence that at least some forms of chronic pain lasting several weeks (such as nerve injury) can also be identified with these scales.[20]

Practical Guidelines for Pain Assessment

Which pain assessment method(s)?

From the preceding discussion, it is clear that although we know much more about assessing pain now than just a few years ago, there is a strong need for further work to evaluate the performance limits of existing pain assessment methods and identify methods suitable for other rodent species. For species in which validated scales do not currently exist or in situations when existing scales may not apply, a "triangulation method" has been proposed.[157,158] This reflects what many veterinarians already do, that is, using a variety of measures and behaviors to reach a decision regarding the presence of pain.[70] Although this approach offers a means of performing pain assessment, it comes with a risk of (1) inconsistency owing to variability in the methods used, (2) cognitive biases (particularly confirmation bias), (3) interindividual and intraindividual variability (low reliability), and (4) poor validity (outcomes assessed may not reflect pain at all, or be influenced by other factors, as discussed elsewhere in this article). For instance, evaluating postoperative pain with a visual analogue scale (a method of subjective pain assessment based on unstructured user evaluation) revealed highly variable results between assessors, highlighting a lack of reliability and validity with subjective (gut feeling) assessments.[135] To have any success with applying a triangulation method requires meticulous record keeping and review of notes to attempt to establish what methods seem to be useful. This type of an approach should be considered secondary to validated methods as they become available.

Timing of pain assessment

There are currently no guidelines regarding the frequency of pain assessment in animals, with current practice reflecting a balance of performing assessments frequently enough so that animals are not suffering for long periods should pain be present versus disturbing the animal in a period when rest is an important part of recovery (and demands on staff time and labor).

The time course of acute postoperative pain is difficult to predict because it will vary according to procedure, surgical trauma, use and type of analgesia, and presence of

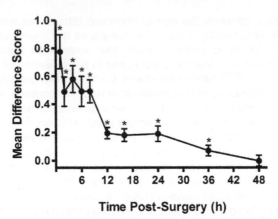

Fig. 7. Time course of postoperative pain after surgery in mice as revealed by facial grimacing. Bars represent mean ± standard error of the mean difference scores. *$P < 0.05$ compared with 0 (no change from baseline) according to a 1-sample t test. (From Matsumiya and colleagues 2012[155]; with permission.)

preexisting pain. In mice and rats undergoing laparotomy surgery without analgesia provided, the duration of pain varies from a few hours to close to 2 days (**Fig. 7**).[29,33,35,155] Pain involving orthopedic procedures may last considerably longer (1 week or more).[159] This is the period during which efforts should be focused on pain assessment. A pragmatic approach would be to coincide pain assessments with (1) the early postoperative period, once the animal is fully recovered from anesthesia and normothermic (in many cases approximately 1–3 hours after the end of surgery), (2) the predicted duration of activity of analgesics (see "Treatment of pain in rodents" in this issue), and (3) the time at which pain would be expected to no longer be present (to confirm the animal is pain free, accounting for individual variability in the pain experience). As discussed in the Grimace Scale section, assessing pain in the immediate postoperative period is difficult owing to the presence of potential confounds.

When to treat?
Ideally, each pain assessment method should include an analgesic intervention threshold that can be used to guide pain management. However, the RGS is currently the only scale for which an intervention threshold has been defined. One of the key challenges of pain assessment in veterinary species, but particularly those with which we are less familiar or in which signs of pain may be subtle (at least without specific training) or for which no validated pain assessment scales exist, is achieving a reasonable degree of confidence in identifying pain. This uncertainty creates the possibility of failing to treat pain when it is present. In such cases, an anthropomorphic approach known as critical anthropomorphism is justified.[160] This method takes the view that procedures or diseases that cause pain in humans may cause pain in animals. This approach is further supported by widespread recognition that all mammals are sentient (have the capacity to feel or experience subjectively).[12,13] The following options exist to help guide the decision to administer analgesics when there is the possibility that pain is present:

1. Provide analgesia and reassess the patient at a predetermined time. The timing of assessment should be matched to the predicted time to onset of the analgesic.

2. Withhold analgesia and plan to reassess the patient to establish if a change in behavior has occurred. This approach is only appropriate if difficulty in identifying pain is presumed to reflect a potentially low level of pain and the time to reassessment is short (within 30–90 minutes). If a pain scale is used, comparing sequential scores is invaluable in identifying trends (eg, a gradual increase or decrease in scores over time). The first of these options is generally preferred because it decreases the risk of suffering and promotes a proactive approach to pain management (vs a reactive approach, whereby animals are allowed to become painful before analgesia is provided).

Future of Pain Assessment

Advances in pain assessment methods driven by biomedical research will soon extend to include automated scoring systems. Proofs of concept have already been established for both partial and full automation of the MGS and RGS, with ongoing work to refine the accuracy and ease of use.[35,161,162] Full automation uses machine learning (artificial intelligence) to select and score facial images. The process is initially intensive, requiring a large library of video/images but has the appeal of potentially identifying novel AUs and being able to distinguish between negative affective states (eg, pain, fear, anxiety). Automated systems for general activity recording have been available for a number of years and are attractive in providing continuous observations of a wide variety of in-cage behaviors, but have had mixed success in identifying pain.[163]

SUMMARY

Considerable progress has been made in pain assessment of rodents over the last 10 to 15 years. These advances are largely limited to mice and rats, reflecting their role in biomedical research. Of the available methods, those that show the greatest promise as specific measures of pain and have undergone the most development and validation are the RGS and RGS. However, more work is needed to establish their value in clinical settings, including confirming performance for cage-side assessments and more fully describing potential confounding factors. Composite measure scales are highly effective in larger companion species but their development in rodents is currently limited. Further research is needed to develop these scales for clinical use. When well-validated and established pain assessment methods are unavailable or cannot be applied, combining assessments of multiple variables (physiologic and behavioral) can be useful provided they are performed consistently, and detailed records maintained. Methods that assess well-being (such as nest building and burrowing) can be usefully applied to gain an overview of a patient's condition (including the presence or absence of pain and response to analgesia).

CLINICS CARE POINTS

- Whenever possible, pain assessment methods that have undergone some degree of validation should be used in preference over subjective assessments.

- Composite measure pain scales and grimace scales currently have the greatest evidence supporting their use.

- It is likely that no single pain assessment method is perfect. Clinicians should become familiar with their preferred methods, including appreciating confounding factors that interfere with their use.

- When pain assessment methods that have undergone validation cannot be applied, the use of multiple assessment methods, applied consistently, can help create a picture of pain behavior that can be used to identify changes over time or in response to analgesia.

- If it is unclear if pain is present, and the procedure is known to cause pain in other species, analgesia should be provided unless the adverse effects of analgesics outweigh their likely benefit.

- Performing repeated assessments before (when possible) and after pain is anticipated (eg, postoperatively) will establish a baseline for an individual animal, facilitating observing postoperative changes.

- Recording observations from pain assessment is helpful in identifying early trends and facilitates proactive pain management.

DISCLOSURE

The authors have no commercial or financial conflicts of interest to declare.

Dr D. S. Pang receives funding from the Natural Sciences and Engineering Research Council of Canada (Discovery Grant) and Zoetis.

ACKNOWLEDGMENTS

The authors thank Dr Samantha Swisher (The Ohio State University) and Dr Juliette Raulic (Université de Montreal) for their insightful comments on an earlier version of this article.

REFERENCES

1. Dohoo SE, Dohoo IR. Postoperative use of analgesics in dogs and cats by Canadian veterinarians. Can Vet J 1996;37(9):546–51.
2. Hunt JR, Knowles TG, Lascelles BDX, et al. Prescription of perioperative analgesics by UK small animal veterinary surgeons in 2013. Vet Rec 2015;176(19):493.
3. Capner CA, Lascelles BD, Waterman-Pearson AE. Current British veterinary attitudes to perioperative analgesia for dogs. Vet Rec 1999;145(4):95–9.
4. Stokes EL, Flecknell PA, Richardson CA. Reported analgesic and anaesthetic administration to rodents undergoing experimental surgical procedures. Lab Anim 2009;43(2):149–54.
5. Uhlig C, Krause H, Koch T, et al. Anesthesia and monitoring in small laboratory mammals used in anesthesiology, respiratory and critical care research: a systematic review on the current reporting in top-10 impact factor ranked journals. PLoS One 2015;10(8):e0134205.
6. Carbone L, Austin J. Pain and laboratory animals: publication practices for better data reproducibility and better animal welfare. PLoS One 2016;11(5): e0155001.
7. Keown AJ, Farnworth MJ, Adams NJ. Attitudes towards perception and management of pain in rabbits and guinea pigs by a sample of veterinarians in New Zealand. N Z Vet J 2011;59(6):305–10.
8. Hugonnard M, Leblond A, Keroack S, et al. Attitudes and concerns of French veterinarians towards pain and analgesia in dogs and cats. Vet Anaesth Analg 2004;31(3):154–63.
9. Mogil JS, Crager SE. What should we be measuring in behavioral studies of chronic pain in animals? PAIN 2004;112(1):12–5.

10. Huss MK, Felt SA, Pacharinsak C. Influence of pain and analgesia on orthopedic and wound-healing models in rats and mice. Comp Med 2019;69(6):535–45.
11. Taylor DK. Influence of pain and analgesia on cancer research studies. Comp Med 2019;69(6):501–9.
12. Mellor DJ. Welfare-aligned sentience: enhanced capacities to experience, interact, anticipate, choose and survive. Animals (Basel) 2019;9(7):E440.
13. The Cambridge Declaration on Consciousness. Animal Cognition. 2015. Available at: http://www.animalcognition.org/2015/03/25/the-declaration-of-nonhuman-animal-conciousness/. Accessed January 11, 2022.
14. Terminology | International Association for the Study of Pain. International Association for the Study of Pain (IASP). Available at: https://www.iasp-pain.org/resources/terminology/. Accessed January 11, 2022.
15. Langford DJ, Bailey AL, Chanda ML, et al. Coding of facial expressions of pain in the laboratory mouse. Nat Methods 2010;7(6):447–9.
16. Mendl M, Burman OHP, Paul ES. An integrative and functional framework for the study of animal emotion and mood. Proc Biol Sci 2010;277(1696):2895–904.
17. Clark L. Chronic (or persistent) postsurgical pain: a veterinary problem? Vet Anaesth Analg 2021;48(1):4–6.
18. Streiner DL, Norman GR, Cairney J. Health measurement scales: a practical guide to their development and use. Oxford University Press. 2014. https://oxfordmedicine.com/view/10.1093/med/9780199685219.001.0001/med-9780199685219.
19. Streiner DL. A checklist for evaluating the usefulness of rating scales. Can J Psychiatry 1993;38(2):140–8.
20. Mogil JS, Pang DSJ, Silva Dutra GG, et al. The development and use of facial grimace scales for pain measurement in animals. Neurosci Biobehav Rev 2020;116:480–93.
21. Oliver V, De Rantere D, Ritchie R, et al. Psychometric assessment of the Rat Grimace Scale and development of an analgesic intervention score. PLoS One 2014;9(5):e97882.
22. Evangelista-Vaz R, Bergadano A, Arras M, et al. Analgesic efficacy of subcutaneous-oral dosage of tramadol after surgery in C57BL/6J Mice. J Am Assoc Lab Anim Sci 2018;57(4):368–75.
23. Brondani JT, Mama KR, Luna SPL, et al. Validation of the English version of the UNESP-Botucatu multidimensional composite pain scale for assessing postoperative pain in cats. BMC Vet Res 2013;9:143.
24. Reid J, Nolan A, Hughes J, et al. Development of the short-form Glasgow Composite Measure Pain Scale (CMPS-SF) and derivation of an analgesic intervention score. Anim Welfare 2007;16(2):97–104.
25. Holton L, Reid J, Scott EM, et al. Development of a behaviour-based scale to measure acute pain in dogs. Vet Rec 2001;148(17):525–31.
26. Roughan JV, Flecknell PA. Effects of surgery and analgesic administration on spontaneous behaviour in singly housed rats. Res Vet Sci 2000;69(3):283–8.
27. Roughan JV, Flecknell PA. Behavioural effects of laparotomy and analgesic effects of ketoprofen and carprofen in rats. Pain 2001;90(1–2):65–74.
28. Roughan JV, Flecknell PA. Evaluation of a short duration behaviour-based postoperative pain scoring system in rats. Eur J Pain 2003;7(5):397–406.
29. Roughan JV, Flecknell PA, Davies BR. Behavioural assessment of the effects of tumour growth in rats and the influence of the analgesics carprofen and meloxicam. Lab Anim 2004;38(3):286–96.

30. Wright-Williams SL, Courade JP, Richardson CA, et al. Effects of vasectomy surgery and meloxicam treatment on faecal corticosterone levels and behaviour in two strains of laboratory mouse. Pain 2007;130(1–2):108–18.

31. Wright-Williams S, Flecknell PA, Roughan JV. Comparative effects of vasectomy surgery and buprenorphine treatment on faecal corticosterone concentrations and behaviour assessed by manual and automated analysis methods in C57 and C3H mice. PLoS One 2013;8(9):e75948.

32. Leung VSY, Benoit-Biancamano MO, Pang DSJ. Performance of behavioral assays: the Rat Grimace Scale, burrowing activity and a composite behavior score to identify visceral pain in an acute and chronic colitis model. Pain Rep 2019; 4(2):e718.

33. Klune CB, Larkin AE, Leung VSY, et al. Comparing the Rat Grimace Scale and a composite behaviour score in rats. PLoS One 2019;14(5):e0209467.

34. Faller KME, McAndrew DJ, Schneider JE, et al. Refinement of analgesia following thoracotomy and experimental myocardial infarction using the Mouse Grimace Scale. Exp Physiol 2015;100(2):164–72. https://doi.org/10.1113/expphysiol.2014.083139.

35. Sotocinal SG, Sorge RE, Zaloum A, et al. The Rat Grimace Scale: a partially automated method for quantifying pain in the laboratory rat via facial expressions. Mol Pain 2011;7:55.

36. Zhang EQ, Leung VS, Pang DS. Influence of rater training on inter- and intrarater reliability when using the rat grimace scale. J Am Assoc Lab Anim Sci 2019; 58(2):178–83.

37. National Research Council (US) Committee on Recognition and Alleviation of Pain in Laboratory Animals. Recognition and alleviation of pain in laboratory animals. National Academies Press (US); 2009. Available at: http://www.ncbi.nlm.nih.gov/books/NBK32658/. Accessed December 19, 2021.

38. Woodman DD. Laboratory animal endocrinology: hormonal action, control mechanisms and interactions with drugs. Wiley; 1997. Available at: https://www.wiley.com/en-gb/Laboratory+Animal+Endocrinology%3A+Hormonal+Action%2C+Control+Mechanisms+and+Interactions+with+Drugs-p-9780471972624. Accessed December 20, 2021.

39. Hernandez-Avalos I, Mota-Rojas D, Mora-Medina P, et al. Review of different methods used for clinical recognition and assessment of pain in dogs and cats. Int J Vet Sci Med 2019;7(1):43–54.

40. Prunier A, Mounier L, Le Neindre P, et al. Identifying and monitoring pain in farm animals: a review. Animal 2013;7(6):998–1010.

41. Arras M, Rettich A, Seifert B, et al. Should laboratory mice be anaesthetized for tail biopsy? Lab Anim 2007;41(1):30–45.

42. Benedetti M, Merino R, Kusuda R, et al. Plasma corticosterone levels in mouse models of pain. Eur J Pain 2012;16(6):803–15.

43. Vachon P, Moreau JP. Serum corticosterone and blood glucose in rats after two jugular vein blood sampling methods: comparison of the stress response. Contemp Top Lab Anim Sci 2001;40(5):22–4.

44. Gärtner K, Büttner D, Döhler K, et al. Stress response of rats to handling and experimental procedures. Lab Anim 1980;14(3):267–74.

45. Abe R, Shimosegawa T, Kimura K, et al. The role of endogenous glucocorticoids in rat experimental models of acute pancreatitis. Gastroenterology 1995;109(3): 933–43.

46. Kojima K, Naruse Y, Iijima N, et al. HPA-axis responses during experimental colitis in the rat. Am J Physiol Regul Integr Comp Physiol 2002;282(5):R1348–55.
47. Ghosal S, Nunley A, Mahbod P, et al. Mouse handling limits the impact of stress on metabolic endpoints. Physiol Behav 2015;150:31–7.
48. Goldkuhl R, Jacobsen KR, Kalliokoski O, et al. Plasma concentrations of corticosterone and buprenorphine in rats subjected to jugular vein catheterization. Lab Anim 2010;44(4):337–43.
49. Sharp J, Zammit T, Azar T, et al. Stress-like responses to common procedures in individually and group-housed female rats. Contemp Top Lab Anim Sci 2003; 42(1):9–18.
50. Gallaher EJ, Egner DA, Swen JW. Automated remote temperature measurement in small animals using a telemetry/microcomputer interface. Comput Biol Med 1985;15(2):103–10.
51. Armario A, Montero JL, Balasch J. Sensitivity of corticosterone and some metabolic variables to graded levels of low intensity stresses in adult male rats. Physiol Behav 1986;37(4):559–61. https://doi.org/10.1016/0031-9384(86)90285-4.
52. De Boer SF, Koopmans SJ, Slangen JL, et al. Plasma catecholamine, corticosterone and glucose responses to repeated stress in rats: effect of interstressor interval length. Physiol Behav 1990;47(6):1117–24.
53. Barrett AM, Stockham MA. The effect of housing conditions and simple experimental procedures upon the corticosterone level in the plasma of rats. J Endocrinol 1963;26:97–105.
54. Balcombe JP, Barnard ND, Sandusky C. Laboratory routines cause animal stress. Contemp Top Lab Anim Sci 2004;43(6):42–51.
55. Rasmussen S, Miller MM, Filipski SB, et al. Cage change influences serum corticosterone and anxiety-like behaviors in the mouse. J Am Assoc Lab Anim Sci 2011;50(4):479–83.
56. Sharp JL, Zammit TG, Azar TA, et al. Stress-like responses to common procedures in male rats housed alone or with other rats. Contemp Top Lab Anim Sci 2002;41(4):8–14.
57. Sharp JL, Zammit TG, Lawson DM. Stress-like responses to common procedures in rats: effect of the estrous cycle. Contemp Top Lab Anim Sci 2002; 41(4):15–22.
58. Duke JL, Zammit TG, Lawson DM. The effects of routine cage-changing on cardiovascular and behavioral parameters in male Sprague-Dawley rats. Contemp Top Lab Anim Sci 2001;40(1):17–20.
59. Conn CA, Borer KT, Kluger MJ. Body temperature rhythm and response to pyrogen in exercising and sedentary hamsters. Med Sci Sports Exerc 1990;22(5): 636–42.
60. Ferland CL, Schrader LA. Cage mate separation in pair-housed male rats evokes an acute stress corticosterone response. Neurosci Lett 2011;489(3): 154–8.
61. Raşid O, Chirita D, Iancu AD, et al. Assessment of routine procedure effect on breathing parameters in mice by using whole-body plethysmography. J Am Assoc Lab Anim Sci 2012;51(4):469–74.
62. Cinelli P, Rettich A, Seifert B, et al. Comparative analysis and physiological impact of different tissue biopsy methodologies used for the genotyping of laboratory mice. Lab Anim 2007;41(2):174–84.
63. Siswanto H, Hau J, Carlsson HE, et al. Corticosterone concentrations in blood and excretion in faeces after ACTH administration in male Sprague-Dawley rats. Vivo 2008;22(4):435–40.

64. Pereira CB, Kunczik J, Zieglowski L, et al. Remote welfare monitoring of rodents using thermal imaging. Sensors (Basel) 2018;18(11):E3653.

65. Vainer BG. A novel high-resolution method for the respiration rate and breathing waveforms remote monitoring. Ann Biomed Eng 2018;46(7):960–71.

66. Zhao F, Li M, Qian Y, et al. Remote measurements of heart and respiration rates for telemedicine. PLoS One 2013;8(10):e71384.

67. Kunczik J, Barbosa Pereira C, Zieglowski L, et al. Remote vitals monitoring in rodents using video recordings. Biomed Opt Express 2019;10(9):4422–36.

68. González-Sánchez C, Fraile JC, Pérez-Turiel J, et al. Capacitive sensing for non-invasive breathing and heart monitoring in non-restrained, non-sedated laboratory mice. Sensors (Basel) 2016;16(7):E1052.

69. Holton LL, Scott EM, Nolan AM, et al. Relationship between physiological factors and clinical pain in dogs scored using a numerical rating scale. J Small Anim Pract 1998;39(10):469–74.

70. Gleeson M, Hawkins M, Howerton CL, et al. Evaluating postoperative parameters in guinea pigs (cavia porcellus) following routine orchiectomy. J Exot Pet Med 2016;25(3):242–52.

71. Butz GM, Davisson RL. Long-term telemetric measurement of cardiovascular parameters in awake mice: a physiological genomics tool. Physiol Genomics 2001;5(2):89–97.

72. Arras M, Rettich A, Cinelli P, et al. Assessment of post-laparotomy pain in laboratory mice by telemetric recording of heart rate and heart rate variability. BMC Vet Res 2007;3:16.

73. Goecke JC, Awad H, Lawson JC, et al. Evaluating postoperative analgesics in mice using telemetry. Comp Med 2005;55(1):37–44.

74. Taitt KT, Kendall LV. Physiologic stress of ear punch identification compared with restraint only in mice. J Am Assoc Lab Anim Sci 2019;58(4):438–42.

75. Greene AN, Clapp SL, Alper RH. Timecourse of recovery after surgical intraperitoneal implantation of radiotelemetry transmitters in rats. J Pharmacol Toxicol Methods 2007;56(2):218–22.

76. Oliver VL, Thurston SE, Lofgren JL. Using cageside measures to evaluate analgesic efficacy in mice (mus musculus) after surgery. J Am Assoc Lab Anim Sci 2018;57(2):186–201.

77. Sherwin CM. Observations on the prevalence of nest-building in non-breeding TO strain mice and their use of two nesting materials. Lab Anim 1997;31(2):125–32.

78. Deacon R. Assessing burrowing, nest construction, and hoarding in mice. J Vis Exp 2012;59:e2607.

79. Nijsen MJMA, Ongenae NGH, Coulie B, et al. Telemetric animal model to evaluate visceral pain in the freely moving rat. Pain 2003;105(1–2):115–23.

80. Wassermann L, Helgers SOA, Riedesel AK, et al. Monitoring of heart rate and activity using telemetry allows grading of experimental procedures used in neuroscientific rat models. Front Neurosci 2020;14:587760.

81. Charlet A, Rodeau JL, Poisbeau P. Radiotelemetric and symptomatic evaluation of pain in the rat after laparotomy: long-term benefits of perioperative ropivacaine care. J Pain 2011;12(2):246–56.

82. Roughan JV, Coulter CA, Flecknell PA, et al. The conditioned place preference test for assessing welfare consequences and potential refinements in a mouse bladder cancer model. PLoS One 2014;9(8):e103362.

83. Roughan JV, Bertrand HGMJ, Isles HM. Meloxicam prevents COX-2-mediated post-surgical inflammation but not pain following laparotomy in mice. Eur J Pain 2016;20(2):231–40.
84. Bourque SL, Adams MA, Nakatsu K, et al. Comparison of buprenorphine and meloxicam for postsurgical analgesia in rats: effects on body weight, locomotor activity, and hemodynamic parameters. J Am Assoc Lab Anim Sci 2010;49(5): 617–22.
85. Clark JA, Myers PH, Goelz MF, et al. Pica behavior associated with buprenorphine administration in the rat. Lab Anim Sci 1997;47(3):300–3.
86. Allen M, Johnson RA. Evaluation of self-injurious behavior, thermal sensitivity, food intake, fecal output, and pica after injection of three buprenorphine formulations in rats (Rattus norvegicus). Am J Vet Res 2018;79(7):697–703.
87. Schaap MWH, Uilenreef JJ, Mitsogiannis MD, et al. Optimizing the dosing interval of buprenorphine in a multimodal postoperative analgesic strategy in the rat: minimizing side-effects without affecting weight gain and food intake. Lab Anim 2012;46(4):287–92.
88. Evenson EA, Mans C. Analgesic Efficacy and Safety of Hydromorphone in Chinchillas (Chinchilla lanigera). J Am Assoc Lab Anim Sci 2018;57(3):282–5.
89. Culpepper-Morgan J, Kreek MJ, Holt PR, et al. Orally administered kappa as well as mu opiate agonists delay gastrointestinal transit time in the guinea pig. Life Sci 1988;42(21):2073–7.
90. Gould HJ. Complete Freund's adjuvant-induced hyperalgesia: a human perception. Pain 2000;85(1–2):301–3.
91. De Rantere D, Schuster CJ, Reimer JN, et al. The relationship between the Rat Grimace Scale and mechanical hypersensitivity testing in three experimental pain models. Eur J Pain 2016;20(3):417–26.
92. Hess SE, Rohr S, Dufour BD, et al. Home improvement: C57BL/6J mice given more naturalistic nesting materials build better nests. J Am Assoc Lab Anim Sci 2008;47(6):25–31.
93. Van de Weerd HA, Van Loo PL, Van Zutphen LF, et al. Preferences for nesting material as environmental enrichment for laboratory mice. Lab Anim 1997; 31(2):133–43.
94. Deacon RMJ. Assessing nest building in mice. Nat Protoc 2006;1(3):1117–9.
95. Van Loo PLP, Baumans V. The importance of learning young: the use of nesting material in laboratory rats. Lab Anim 2004;38(1):17–24.
96. Manser CE, Broom DM, Overend P, et al. Operant studies to determine the strength of preference in laboratory rats for nest-boxes and nesting materials. Lab Anim 1998;32(1):36–41.
97. Jirkof P, Fleischmann T, Cesarovic N, et al. Assessment of postsurgical distress and pain in laboratory mice by nest complexity scoring. Lab Anim 2013;47(3): 153–61.
98. Lijam N, Paylor R, McDonald MP, et al. Social interaction and sensorimotor gating abnormalities in mice lacking Dvl1. Cell 1997;90(5):895–905.
99. Torres-Lista V, Giménez-Llort L. Impairment of nesting behaviour in 3xTg-AD mice. Behav Brain Res 2013;247:153–7.
100. Gallo MS, Karas AZ, Pritchett-Corning K, et al. Tell-tale TINT: does the time to incorporate into nest test evaluate postsurgical pain or welfare in mice? J Am Assoc Lab Anim Sci 2020;59(1):37–45.
101. Negus SS, Neddenriep B, Altarifi AA, et al. Effects of ketoprofen, morphine, and kappa opioids on pain-related depression of nesting in mice. Pain 2015;156(6): 1153–60.

102. Rock ML, Karas AZ, Rodriguez KBG, et al. The time-to-integrate-to-nest test as an indicator of wellbeing in laboratory mice. J Am Assoc Lab Anim Sci 2014; 53(1):24–8.

103. Häger C, Keubler LM, Biernot S, et al. Time to Integrate to Nest Test Evaluation in a Mouse DSS-Colitis Model. PLoS One 2015;10(12):e0143824.

104. Garner JB, Marshall LS, Boyer NM, et al. Effects of ketoprofen and morphine on pain-related depression of nestlet shredding in male and female mice. Front Pain Res (Lausanne) 2021;2:673940.

105. Schwabe K, Boldt L, Bleich A, et al. Nest-building performance in rats: impact of vendor, experience, and sex. Lab Anim 2020;54(1):17–25.

106. Jirkof P. Burrowing and nest building behavior as indicators of well-being in mice. J Neurosci Methods 2014;234:139–46.

107. Gaskill BN, Gordon CJ, Pajor EA, et al. Heat or insulation: behavioral titration of mouse preference for warmth or access to a nest. PLoS One 2012;7(3):e32799.

108. Lee CT. Genetic analyses of nest-building behavior in laboratory mice (Mus musculus). Behav Genet 1973;3(3):247–56.

109. Deacon RMJ, Croucher A, Rawlins JNP. Hippocampal cytotoxic lesion effects on species-typical behaviours in mice. Behav Brain Res 2002;132(2):203–13.

110. Deacon RMJ. Burrowing in rodents: a sensitive method for detecting behavioral dysfunction. Nat Protoc 2006;1(1):118–21.

111. Andrews N, Legg E, Lisak D, et al. Spontaneous burrowing behaviour in the rat is reduced by peripheral nerve injury or inflammation associated pain. Eur J Pain 2012;16(4):485–95.

112. Jirkof P, Leucht K, Cesarovic N, et al. Burrowing is a sensitive behavioural assay for monitoring general wellbeing during dextran sulfate sodium colitis in laboratory mice. Lab Anim 2013;47(4):274–83.

113. Bryden LA, Nicholson JR, Doods H, et al. Deficits in spontaneous burrowing behavior in the rat bilateral monosodium iodoacetate model of osteoarthritis: an objective measure of pain-related behavior and analgesic efficacy. Osteoarthritis Cartilage 2015;23(9):1605–12.

114. Jirkof P, Cesarovic N, Rettich A, et al. Burrowing behavior as an indicator of post-laparotomy pain in mice. Front Behav Neurosci 2010;4:165.

115. Gould SA, Doods H, Lamla T, et al. Pharmacological characterization of intraplantar Complete Freund's Adjuvant-induced burrowing deficits. Behav Brain Res 2016;301:142–51.

116. Rutten K, Gould SA, Bryden L, et al. Standard analgesics reverse burrowing deficits in a rat CCI model of neuropathic pain, but not in models of type 1 and type 2 diabetes-induced neuropathic pain. Behav Brain Res 2018;350: 129–38.

117. Rutten K, Robens A, Read SJ, et al. Pharmacological validation of a refined burrowing paradigm for prediction of analgesic efficacy in a rat model of subchronic knee joint inflammation. Eur J Pain 2014;18(2):213–22.

118. Rutten K, Schiene K, Robens A, et al. Burrowing as a non-reflex behavioural readout for analgesic action in a rat model of sub-chronic knee joint inflammation. Eur J Pain 2014;18(2):204–12.

119. Deacon RMJ. Burrowing: a sensitive behavioural assay, tested in five species of laboratory rodents. Behav Brain Res 2009;200(1):128–33.

120. McLinden KA, Kranjac D, Deodati LE, et al. Age exacerbates sickness behavior following exposure to a viral mimetic. Physiol Behav 2012;105(5):1219–25.

121. de Sousa AA, Reis R, Bento-Torres J, et al. Influence of enriched environment on viral encephalitis outcomes: behavioral and neuropathological changes in albino Swiss mice. PLoS One 2011;6(1):e15597.

122. Deacon RM, Raley JM, Perry VH, et al. Burrowing into prion disease. Neuroreport 2001;12(9):2053–7.

123. Deacon RMJ, Rawlins JNP. Hippocampal lesions, species-typical behaviours and anxiety in mice. Behav Brain Res 2005;156(2):241–9.

124. Whittaker AL, Lymn KA, Nicholson A, et al. The assessment of general well-being using spontaneous burrowing behaviour in a short-term model of chemotherapy-induced mucositis in the rat. Lab Anim 2015;49(1):30–9.

125. Teeling JL, Felton LM, Deacon RMJ, et al. Sub-pyrogenic systemic inflammation impacts on brain and behavior, independent of cytokines. Brain Behav Immun 2007;21(6):836–50.

126. Teeling JL, Cunningham C, Newman TA, et al. The effect of non-steroidal anti-inflammatory agents on behavioural changes and cytokine production following systemic inflammation: implications for a role of COX-1. Brain Behav Immun 2010;24(3):409–19.

127. Püntener U, Booth SG, Perry VH, et al. Long-term impact of systemic bacterial infection on the cerebral vasculature and microglia. J Neuroinflammation 2012; 9:146.

128. Muralidharan A, Kuo A, Jacob M, et al. Comparison of Burrowing and Stimuli-Evoked Pain Behaviors as End-Points in Rat Models of Inflammatory Pain and Peripheral Neuropathic Pain. Front Behav Neurosci 2016;10:88.

129. Bangsgaard Bendtsen KM, Krych L, Sørensen DB, et al. Gut microbiota composition is correlated to grid floor induced stress and behavior in the BALB/c mouse. PLoS One 2012;7(10):e46231.

130. Lavin DN, Joesting JJ, Chiu GS, et al. Fasting induces an anti-inflammatory effect on the neuroimmune system which a high-fat diet prevents. Obesity (Silver Spring) 2011;19(8):1586–94.

131. Christensen SLT, Petersen S, Sørensen DB, et al. Infusion of low dose glyceryl trinitrate has no consistent effect on burrowing behavior, running wheel activity and light sensitivity in female rats. J Pharmacol Toxicol Methods 2016;80:43–50.

132. Approach 1: monitoring behaviour using an ethogram | NC3Rs. Available at: https://nc3rs.org.uk/approach-1-monitoring-behaviour-using-ethogram. Accessed December 23, 2021.

133. Oliver VL, Athavale S, Simon KE, et al. Evaluation of pain assessment techniques and analgesia efficacy in a female guinea pig (cavia porcellus) model of surgical pain. J Am Assoc Lab Anim Sci 2017;56(4):425–35.

134. Miller AL, Leach MC. The mouse grimace scale: a clinically useful tool? PLoS One 2015;10(9):e0136000.

135. Roughan JV, Flecknell PA. Training in behaviour-based post-operative pain scoring in rats—An evaluation based on improved recognition of analgesic requirements. Appl Anim Behav Sci 2006;96(3):327–42.

136. Affaitati G, Giamberardino MA, Lerza R, et al. Effects of tramadol on behavioural indicators of colic pain in a rat model of ureteral calculosis. Fundam Clin Pharmacol 2002;16(1):23–30.

137. Norway Rat Behavior Repertoire. Available at: http://www.ratbehavior.org/norway_rat_ethogram.htm. Accessed December 23, 2021.

138. Garner Laboratory, Stanford School of Medicine. Mouse Ethograms. Available at: https://mousebehavior.org/ethogram. Accessed December 23, 2021.

139. Buisman M, Hasiuk MMM, Gunn M, et al. The influence of demeanor on scores from two validated feline pain assessment scales during the perioperative period. Vet Anaesth Analg 2017;44(3):646–55.

140. Buisman M, Wagner MC, Hasiuk MM, et al. Effects of ketamine and alfaxalone on application of a feline pain assessment scale. J Feline Med Surg 2016; 18(8):643–51.

141. Dunbar ML, David EM, Aline MR, et al. Validation of a behavioral ethogram for assessing postoperative pain in guinea pigs (Cavia porcellus). J Am Assoc Lab Anim Sci 2016;55(1):29–34.

142. Ellen Y, Flecknell P, Leach M. Evaluation of using behavioural changes to assess post-operative pain in the guinea pig (cavia porcellus). PLoS One 2016;11(9): e0161941.

143. Ponzio MF, Monfort SL, Busso JM, et al. Adrenal activity and anxiety-like behavior in fur-chewing chinchillas (Chinchilla lanigera). Horm Behav 2012; 61(5):758–62.

144. Edmunson AM, Boynton FDD, Rendahl AK, et al. Indicators of postoperative pain in Syrian hamsters (mesocricetus auratus). Comp Med 2021;71(1):76–85.

145. National centre for the replacement refinement and reduction of animals in research. grimace scales. grimace scales. Available at: https://nc3rs.org.uk/grimacescales. Accessed January 9, 2022.

146. Pang, Daniel. RGS Training Manual. 2022. Available at: https://doi.org/10.7910/DVN/57K7PE/3DOR8F. Accessed January 11, 2022.

147. Schneider LE, Henley KY, Turner OA, et al. Application of the rat grimace scale as a marker of supraspinal pain sensation after cervical spinal cord injury. J Neurotrauma 2017;34(21):2982–93.

148. Leung V, Zhang E, Pang DS. Real-time application of the Rat Grimace Scale as a welfare refinement in laboratory rats. Sci Rep 2016;6:31667.

149. Hohlbaum K, Bert B, Dietze S, et al. Severity classification of repeated isoflurane anesthesia in C57BL/6JRj mice—Assessing the degree of distress. PLoS One 2017;12(6):e0179588.

150. Miller A, Kitson G, Skalkoyannis B, et al. The effect of isoflurane anaesthesia and buprenorphine on the mouse grimace scale and behaviour in CBA and DBA/2 mice. Appl Anim Behav Sci 2015;172:58–62.

151. Miller AL, Golledge HDR, Leach MC. The Influence of Isoflurane Anaesthesia on the Rat Grimace Scale. PLoS One 2016;11(11):e0166652.

152. Hohlbaum K, Bert B, Dietze S, et al. Impact of repeated anesthesia with ketamine and xylazine on the well-being of C57BL/6JRj mice. PLoS One 2018; 13(9):e0203559.

153. Lester LS, Fanselow MS. Exposure to a cat produces opioid analgesia in rats. Behav Neurosci 1985;99(4):756–9.

154. Sorge RE, Martin LJ, Isbester KA, et al. Olfactory exposure to males, including men, causes stress and related analgesia in rodents. Nat Methods 2014;11(6): 629–32.

155. Matsumiya LC, Sorge RE, Sotocinal SG, et al. Using the Mouse Grimace Scale to reevaluate the efficacy of postoperative analgesics in laboratory mice. J Am Assoc Lab Anim Sci 2012;51(1):42–9.

156. Defensor EB, Corley MJ, Blanchard RJ, et al. Facial expressions of mice in aggressive and fearful contexts. Physiol Behav 2012;107(5):680–5.

157. Bateson P. Assessment of pain in animals. Anim Behav 1991;42(5):827–39.

158. Turner PV, Pang DS, Lofgren JL. A review of pain assessment methods in laboratory rodents. Comp Med 2019;69(6):451–67.

159. Sperry MM, Yu YH, Welch RL, et al. Grading facial expression is a sensitive means to detect grimace differences in orofacial pain in a rat model. Sci Rep 2018;8(1):13894.
160. Karlsson F. Critical Anthropomorphism and Animal Ethics. J Agric Environ Ethics 2012;25(5):707–20.
161. Tuttle AH, Molinaro MJ, Jethwa JF, et al. A deep neural network to assess spontaneous pain from mouse facial expressions. Mol Pain 2018;14. 1744806918763658.
162. Andresen N, Wöllhaf M, Hohlbaum K, et al. Towards a fully automated surveillance of well-being status in laboratory mice using deep learning: starting with facial expression analysis. PLoS One 2020;15(4):e0228059.
163. Zhang H, Lecker I, Collymore C, et al. Cage-lid hanging behavior as a translationally relevant measure of pain in mice. Pain 2021;162(5):1416–25.
164. Batavia M, Nguyen G, Harman K, et al. Hibernation patterns of Turkish hamsters: influence of sex and ambient temperature. J Comp Physiol B 2013; 183(2):269–77.
165. Horwitz BA, Chau SM, Hamilton JS, et al. Temporal relationships of blood pressure, heart rate, baroreflex function, and body temperature change over a hibernation bout in Syrian hamsters. Am J Physiol Regul Integr Comp Physiol 2013;7: R759–68.

Treatment of Pain in Rats, Mice, and Prairie Dogs

Rhonda Oates, DVM, MPVM, DACLAM[a],*, Danielle K. Tarbert, DVM[b]

KEYWORDS

- Rodent • Myomorph • Sciuromorph • Analgesia • Nociception • Opioid
- Nonsteroidal anti-inflammatory drug

KEY POINTS

- Although caution is necessary when extrapolating laboratory rodent analgesia studies to clinical patients, the extensive available laboratory research provides an excellent foundation for analgesia decisions.
- Rodents often require higher and more frequent analgesic dosing compared with other species.
- A multimodal analgesic approach aids in increased efficacy and reduced doses.
- Analgesic options include local anesthetics, nonsteroidal anti-inflammatory drugs, opioids, and adjuvants such as serotonin-norepinephrine reuptake inhibitors and anticonvulsants.

INTRODUCTION

Myomorph rodents, including rats, mice, gerbils, and hamsters, are common companion species.[1] Sciuromorph rodents such as prairie dogs and squirrels are also encountered as companion animals or in zoologic collections. Rodents, especially mice and rats, are commonly used in laboratory animal research, necessitating appropriate analgesia protocols to ensure animal welfare and produce valid scientific outcomes.[2] As a result, much investigation has been dedicated to the recognition and alleviation of pain in laboratory rodents.[3] Despite this growing body of information, recent literature reviews reveal inconsistent adequate pain relief in rodents, which may stem from socio-zoologic bias, with underuse of perioperative analgesics in mice and rats compared with larger animals.[4–7] It is essential to remember that all mammals have nearly identical nociceptive pathways and pain signaling mechanisms and that rodents are not "less sentient" species compared with others such as primates and

[a] Research and Teaching Animal Care Program, University of California – Davis, One Shields Avenue, Davis, CA 95616, USA; [b] Companion Exotic Animal Medicine and Surgery Service, Veterinary Medical Teaching Hospital, School of Veterinary Medicine, University of California – Davis, One Shields Avenue, Davis, CA 95616, USA
* Corresponding author.
E-mail address: rsoates@ucdavis.edu

Vet Clin Exot Anim 26 (2023) 151–174
https://doi.org/10.1016/j.cvex.2022.07.005
1094-9194/23/Published by Elsevier Inc.

dogs.[7] In fact, rodent dose requirements are often higher than other species, due to high metabolic rate.[8]

Some fundamentals of laboratory animal studies should be considered when extrapolating information to clinical patients.[3] Pharmacokinetic studies often target "therapeutic levels" extrapolated from other species, which may not always translate to rodents.[7] When pharmacodynamic studies are performed, analgesiometric tests such as thermal stimuli may not perfectly represent clinical pain.[3] Additionally, laboratory studies are generally performed in young, healthy animals, and dose adjustment may be needed for geriatric or diseased companion animals.[3] Some clinicians advocate starting with half of the low end of the dose range when first using a laboratory animal protocol.[8] Conversely, studies targeting the "effective dose 50" (ED50) measure the dose with a desired effect in 50% of the test subjects, meaning that the dose will be too low for many individuals.[9] Finally, although a few drugs are indexed for use in rodents under the Minor Use and Minor Species Animal Health Act of 2004, most are not approved through the United States Food and Drug Administration (FDA) and client education regarding off-label use, even if well studied in research animals, is essential.[3,10]

Despite limitations, laboratory rodent analgesia research provides an excellent foundation for companion animals. Pharmacologic agents with varied mechanisms of action are available for pain alleviation in rodents. A multimodal analgesic approach aids in overcoming research study limitations while also allowing for increased efficacy and reduced doses.[7] In the absence of studies in rodents such as gerbils and hamsters, the available literature can be used as a starting point for extrapolation.

The first step of the traditional World Health Organization (WHO) analgesic ladder recommends treatment of mild pain with nonopioid analgesics such as nonsteroidal anti-inflammatory drugs (NSAIDs) or acetaminophen, with or without adjuvants or coanalgesics.[11] Adjuvants include tricyclic antidepressants, serotonin-norepinephrine reuptake inhibitors, anticonvulsants, topical anesthetics, corticosteroids, bisphosphonates, and cannabinoids.[11] Pain persisting or increasing despite first-step interventions is considered moderate and treatment should be moved to the second step, with weak opioids such as hydrocodone, codeine, and tramadol used, with or without nonopioid analgesics and adjuvants.[7,11] The third step represents severe and persistent pain, with the use of potent opioids such as morphine, methadone, fentanyl, buprenorphine, and hydromorphone, again with or without nonopioid analgesics and adjuvants.[11] For acute pain, the strongest analgesic needed for the pain intensity should be administered, then stepped down as pain decreases.[11] For chronic pain, a stepwise approach from bottom to top should be considered.[11] However, in some cases an approach focused on the specific pain type is beneficial.[11] For example, in some types of neuropathic pain, adjuvant drugs may be the most appropriate first-line drug.[11] A newer WHO model incorporates a fourth step encompassing interventional and minimally invasive procedures such as nerve blocks and epidurals.[11] More recently, models such as the "multimodal trolley approach" have been developed, which consider the physical, psychological, and emotional causes of pain, and incorporates nonpharmacologic strategies such as acupuncture and physical therapy (covered in other articles of this text).[12] Evaluation of pain intensity, pathophysiology, complexity, comorbidities, and social context, as well as response to analgesic therapy, should guide patient assessment and treatment decisions.[11,12]

Local Anesthetics

Local anesthetics are used either individually or more commonly as part of a multimodal strategy to manage pain in surgical and nonsurgical procedures. Local anesthetics include aminoamides (lidocaine, prilocaine, and bupivacaine) and amino-esters (benzocaine), which inhibit voltage-gated sodium channels resulting in the blockade of sensory nerve fibers.[13] Administration routes include topical, as a splash, infiltration into a tissue, intravenous regional, and nerve block techniques. In smaller animals such as rodents, the topical, splash, and tissue infiltration routes are more easily used. There are also extended release local anesthetics available. The historical agents include lidocaine and bupivacaine, and more recently the literature includes liposomal bupivacaine. If lidocaine or bupivacaine are being administered to an un-anesthetized animal consider buffering.[14] In general, local anesthetics are relatively safe when used appropriately (**Table 1**).[13]

Lidocaine-prilocaine cream can be applied topically before minor procedures. Per the manufacturer, onset of analgesia in humans occurs at 1 hour after application to the skin, reaches maximum effect at 2 to 3 hours and persists for 1 to 2 hours after removal.[15] The application of lidocaine-prilocaine with an occlusive bandage was shown to provide effective analgesia for ear tattooing in rabbits after 20 minutes.[16] Rodent studies are few and have not shown efficacy. The use of lidocaine-prilocaine was found to be ineffective for preventing tail vein injection pain in mice after 30 to 45 minutes of application.[17] The use of lidocaine-prilocaine was also shown to be ineffective for 7 to 15 day old mice that received tail tip biopsies at 5 and 60 minutes after application.[18] The ineffectiveness may have been due to removal by environmental contact or the animals.[18] Perhaps, the addition of an occlusive bandage would increase effectiveness; alternatively, the scales on rodent tails may be resistant to absorption of local anesthetics.[17]

Lidocaine is a fast-acting local anesthetic with a relatively short duration of action. The onset of action is less than 5 minutes with up to 2 hours duration.[19] Compared with lidocaine, bupivacaine has a slower onset of action with a much longer duration. The onset of action is approximately 10 to 15 minutes with up to 8 hours duration.[19] The use of topical bupivacaine applied after tail biopsies in mice 7 to 15 days old was shown to decrease parameters indicative of pain and likely provide effective analgesia; however, the use of ice-cold 70% ethanol was considered superior because it also prevented a reaction to the biopsy.[18]

Liposomal bupivacaine has been approved for human use, and a 1 mg/kg dose administered subcutaneously provided effective analgesia for 4 days after use in a plantar incisional model in rats.[20] Increased dosing up to 6 mg/kg may be effective if not administered to a limited space such as the paw.[20]

Epidurals

Epidural analgesia studies in rodents are limited. One report successfully used lidocaine in a tail flick model.[21] Another report used bupivacaine, buprenorphine, or a combination in tail flick and colorectal distension models; the combination of bupivacaine and buprenorphine resulted in adequate analgesia comparable to morphine.[22]

Nonsteroidal Anti-Inflammatory Drugs

NSAIDs have become increasingly popular analgesics and are easier to obtain and manage than many other drug classes because they are not controlled. NSAIDs inhibit both the cyclooxygenase (COX)-1 and COX-2 pathways, or preferentially inhibit the COX-2 pathway greater than the COX-1 pathway. NSAIDs are associated with adverse effects on platelet function, gastrointestinal tract ulceration, and nephrotoxicity.[23] They have also been shown to inhibit bone healing in a research setting.[24] Historical doses were based primarily on clinical experience. More recent doses (**Tables 2–4**) are generally higher than the historical doses. It is critical that animals be regularly

Table 1
Selected local anesthetic drugs used in rodents

Drug	Route	Dose	Study Type	Comments
Bupivicaine	SC/infiltrated	≤4 mg/kg total dose	EU[14]	
Bupivicaine	SC/infiltrated	≤8 mg/kg total dose	EU[113]	Dilute to 0.25%
Bupivacaine, liposomal	SC/infiltrated	1 mg/kg	PD[20]	Attenuated mechanical and thermal hypersensitivity (incisional pain model) for 4 d
Butorphanol	Infiltrated	1 mg/kg	PD[62]	Thermal paw withdrawal latency; provides 15 min of analgesia
Lidocaine	SC/infiltrated	≤7 mg/kg total dose	EU[113]	Dilute to 0.5%
Lidocaine	SC/infiltrated	≤10 mg/kg total dose	EU[14]	
Lidocaine and bupivicaine	SC/infiltrated	10 mg/kg (L) and 3 mg/kg (B)	PD[42]	Laparotomy model
Lidocaine-prilocaine cream	Topical		PD[16]	Ear tattooing; apply 20–60 min before procedure; may be ineffective on rodent tails[17,18]

Abbreviations: EU, empirical use; PD, pharmacodynamic study; SC, subcutaneously.

assessed to ensure that dose and dosing frequency are appropriate for the animal's clinical condition and surgical procedure. Dosing of NSAIDs is most commonly via oral, intramuscular, and subcutaneous routes. Bioavailability and appropriate dosing must be considered when using oral routes. The small muscle mass of rodents makes intramuscular dosing challenging to accomplish and volumes must be carefully considered.

Ketoprofen
Ketoprofen is a nonselective inhibitor of the COX-1 and COX-2 pathways. Historically, ketoprofen was dosed in mice and rats at 2 to 5 mg/kg subcutaneously.[25–28] More recent sources recommend ketoprofen at 20 mg/kg for mice based on pain relief observed at 1 hour after surgery in a laparotomy surgical study.[7,29,30] Please note that this higher dose may exceed the threshold for gastrointestinal ulcerogenesis.[29,30] In 2015, a study showed that the only dose of ketoprofen that was effective for a surgical study in rats was 25 mg/kg; however, this dose results in toxicity.[31] The administration of ketoprofen at 5 to 10 mg/kg in rats has been shown to result in gastrointestinal damage after a single dose.[32–34] The authors recommend careful consideration regarding the use of ketoprofen in rats.

Carprofen
Carprofen inhibits the COX-2 pathway and was the first COX-2 selective NSAID approved for use in dogs.[23] Historically, carprofen was dosed in mice and rats at 2

Table 2
Selected nonsteroidal anti-inflammatory drugs used in mice

Drug	Route	Dose (mg/kg)	Frequency	Reference	Comments
Carprofen	PO, SC	2–5	q12–24 h	EU[114]	
	SC	5	q12 h	EU,[26,28] PD[7]	Vasectomy model115; dose may be inadequate[29]
	PO	10		PK[116]	Dose may be inadequate[29]
	SC	20	q24 h	PD[7,29,30]	Laparotomy model[29]; dose is near or at ulcerogenic dose[30]
Ibuprofen	PO	30		EU[28]	
Ketoprofen	IM, SC	2–5	q12–24 h	EU[28,114]	Doses may be inadequate[29]
	SC	20	q24 h	PD[7,29,30]	Laparotomy model[29]; dose is near or at ulcerogenic dose[30]
Meloxicam	PO, SC	1–2	q12 h?	EU[26]	
	IP, PO, SC	1–5	q24 h	EU, PD[114]	Laparotomy model
	PO, SC	5		EU[28]	
	SC	5–10	q8–12h	PD[7]	Vasectomy model
	SC	5–20		PD[30]	Vasectomy model; dose is near or at ulcerogenic dose[30]
	SC	20	q24 h	PD[38,117]	Vasectomy model; dose near or at ulcerogenic dose in one study[30]; no gastrointestinal, liver, or kidney damage after 6 d of administration in another study[38]

Abbreviations: EU, empirical use; IM, intramuscularly; IP, intraperitoneally; PO, orally; PD, pharmacodynamic study; PK, pharmacokinetic study; SC, subcutaneously.

to 5 mg/kg subcutaneously and up to 10 mg/kg in a few references.[25–28,35,36] More recent sources recommend carprofen at 20 mg/kg for mice.[7,29,30] Please note that this higher dose may exceed the threshold for gastrointestinal ulcerogenesis.[29,30] In 2015, a study showed that carprofen doses of 5 to 25 mg/kg administered subcutaneously for laparotomy in rats were ineffective based on assessments performed 45 minutes after surgery.[31] Carprofen gel with an estimated oral dose of 5 mg/kg administered daily was found to be ineffective in a rat paw incision model using mechanical and thermal sensitivity testing.[37]

Meloxicam
Meloxicam preferentially inhibits the COX-2 pathway.[23] The dose of 20 mg/kg subcutaneously once daily was shown to be safe when administered at a concentration of 1 mg/mL for up to 6 days in mice.[38]

The administration of SR meloxicam may result in injection site reactions in mice and rats.[39,40] Additionally, meloxicam-SR administered once at 4 mg/kg subcutaneously was found to be ineffective in a rat paw incision model.[37]

Acetaminophen
Acetaminophen is an analgesic and antipyretic, and its exact mechanism of action is not fully understood. When administered at doses ranging from 65.8 to 450 mg/kg subcutaneously in mice, it was ineffective at providing postoperative analgesia for laparotomies and vasectomies, with the 450 mg/kg dose approaching toxicity.[29,41]

Table 3
Selected nonsteroidal anti-inflammatory drugs used in rats

Drug	Route	Dose (mg/kg)	Frequency	Reference	Comments
Carprofen	PO, SC	2–5	q12–24 h	PD[114]	Laparotomy model; doses <5 mg/kg may be inadequate
	SC	5	q6–24 h	EU,[26,28] PD[7,25,30,115]	Vasectomy model; laparotomy model
	SC	5–10		PD[35]	Laparotomy model
Carprofen and buprenorphine	SC	5 (C) and 0.05 (B)		PD[35]	Laparotomy model
Ibuprofen	SC	5, 15, 30		PD[31]	Laparotomy model
	PO	15		EU[28]	
Ketoprofen	IM, SC	2–5	q12–24 h	PD[114]	Laparotomy model; doses <5 mg/kg may be inadequate
	IM, PO, SC	5	q24 h	EU,[26] PD[25,28,30]	Laparotomy model; vasectomy model
Meloxicam	PO, SC	0.5–2	q24 h	EU,[26] PD[36,118]	Laparotomy model; doses <1 mg/kg may be inadequate
	PO, SC	1	q12–24 h	PD[7,28,30,]	Vasectomy model; laparotomy model
Meloxicam-SR	SC	4	q72 h	PK, PD[37,119]	Manufacturer dosage recommendation[119], attenuated mechanical hypersensitivity for 48 h but not thermal hypersensitivity[37]

Abbreviations: EU, empirical use; IM, intramuscularly; PO, orally; PD, pharmacodynamic study; PK, pharmacokinetic study; SC, subcutaneously; SR, sustained-release.

Table 4
Selected nonsteroidal anti-inflammatory drugs used in prairie dogs

Drug	Route	Dose (mg/ kg)	Frequency	Reference	Comments
Carprofen	PO	1	q12–24 h	EU[120]	
	PO, SC	1–4	q24 h	EU[120]	
Ketoprofen	IM, SC	1–5	q12–24 h	EU[120]	
Meloxicam	PO, SC	0.1–0.2	q24 h	EU[120]	Dosing may be inadequate[81]

Abbreviations: EU, empirical use; IM, intramuscularly; PO, orally; SC, subcutaneously.

Another study reported that acetaminophen administration in the drinking water before laparotomy provided adequate analgesia in mice for 24 hours after surgery (**Table 5**); however, the mouse grimace pain scale was highest in animals treated with systemic acetaminophen alone compared with acetaminophen and local anesthetics or local anesthetics alone.[42] The authors do not recommend the use of acetaminophen alone for major surgery.

Opioid Drugs

Opioids provide analgesia by mimicking endogenous opioid peptide action on cell membrane opioid receptors, ultimately inhibiting transmission of nociceptive input.[8,43] Opioid receptors include mu opioid receptor (MOR), kappa opioid receptor (KOR), delta opioid receptors (DOR), and nociception or opioid receptor-like 1 (ORL-1) receptors, with activation of each receptor type having specific effects.[44–46] Opioid analgesics include full agonists, partial agonists, and agonist-antagonists. Opioids may also be classified as weak or potent.[11] Some opioids have additional analgesic mechanisms, such as serotonin and norepinephrine reuptake inhibition (methadone, tramadol) or N-methyl-D-aspartate (NMDA) receptor antagonism (methadone).[47,48] Opioids are generally metabolized in the liver, with metabolites excreted via glomerular filtration.[8] Sex-associated and strain-associated differences in analgesic effect can be seen.[49] Dosing appropriate for species and condition (**Tables 6–8**) is important for immediate safety and efficacy, as well as for long-term effects. Opioid-induced hyperalgesia, defined as increased sensitivity to painful stimuli as a result of opioid use, may occur following high intraoperative doses or chronic use.[50–53] Hyperalgesia was also seen immediately with ultra-low buprenorphine doses in a rat model.[54] Tolerance, defined as an increased opioid dose requirement to achieve the same analgesic effect, may be accelerated by high doses.[50,53–55] Tolerance developed within hours in a rat morphine model; importantly, tolerance to the analgesic effects may occur without tolerance to adverse effects, making opioid-tolerant patients higher risk.[53] General opioid adverse effects include central nervous system depression or stimulation, ataxia, hypothermia or hyperthermia, respiratory depression or apnea, nausea, initial increased intestinal peristalsis followed by ileus or constipation, urine retention, oliguria (MOR-agonists), increased diuresis (KOR-agonists), and histamine release (intravenous morphine).[8,43,56,57] Although rodents do not vomit, nausea may manifest through weight loss or pica.[7,58] Opioids are commonly reversed with naloxone or naltrexone.[8,43] Administration of peripheral opioid antagonists such as methylnaltrexone may be beneficial in reducing morphine-induced nausea and ileus in rats.[59,60] In contrast to naloxone and naltrexone, methylnaltrexone does not cross the blood–brain

Table 5
Selected adjuvant and miscellaneous analgesics used in rodents

Drug	Species	Route	Dose	Frequency	Study Type	Comments
Acetaminophen	Mouse	PO	200 mg/kg		EU[3]	Dose may be ineffective[29]
		PO	4 mg/mL in drinking water	Ad lib	PD[42]	Laparotomy model; assumes water intake of 3 mL/24 h
	Rat	PO	200 mg/kg		EU[3]	
Amitriptyline	Mouse	IP	30 mg/kg		PD[104]	Cisplatin-induced neuropathy
Dexmedetomidine	Mouse	SC	0.004–0.03 mg/kg		PD[9]	ED50, hot plate and tail immersion (higher doses required for tail immersion); peak effect at 0.5 h; motor impairment at 0.009 mg/kg (ED50)
	Rat	IV	0.004–0.02 mg/kg/h	CRI	PD[121]	Somatosensory-evoked and auditory-evoked potentials, which relate to analgesia and sedation, respectively; analgesia could not be produced without sedation
		IV	0.01 mg/kg		PD[107]	Hot plate and tail-flick tests
		IP	0.03–0.18 mg/kg		PD[105]	Dose-dependent increase in tail-flick latency; deep sedation with motor impairment
Dexmedetomidine and butorphanol	Mouse	SC	0.0029–0.0067 mg/kg (D) and 0.29–0.67 mg/kg (B)		PD[9]	Fixed-dose ratio (1 D: 3 B); hot-plate and tail immersion tests (acute nociceptive pain, ED50); synergism; peak effect at 0.5 h; motor impairment at 0.0052 mg/kg (D) and 4.81 mg/kg (B) (ED50)
Dexmedetomidine and maropitant	Rat	IV	0.005 mg/kg (D) and 10 mg/kg (Ma)		PD[107]	Hot plate and tail-flick tests; caution with IV maropitant
Dexmedetomidine and midazolam	Rat	IP	0.09–0.12 mg/kg (D) and 15–20 mg/kg (Mi)		PD[105]	Tail-flick test; no change with Mi alone but significantly enhanced with D + Mi compared with D alone; onset of

Drug	Species	Route	Dose	Duration/Frequency	Reference	Effect
						sedation 1–3 min; profound analgesia within 5–10 min; sedation/analgesia >60 min
Duloxetine	Mouse	IP	10, 30 mg/kg		PD[100]	Spinally integrated reflex (tail flick), no effect; supraspinal reflex (hot plate), modest effect (ED50 16.4 mg/kg); persistent inflammatory pain, dose-related inhibition (ED50 4.6–10.7 mg/kg)
	Rat	PO	11.8 mg/kg	8–18 h duration	PD[100]	Visceral inflammatory pain, ED50
		PO	30 mg/kg		PD[100]	Capsaicin-induced mechanical allodynia (ED50 9.2 mg/kg)
Gabapentin	Mouse	PO	3–100 mg/kg		PD[100]	No motor impairment; thermal hyperalgesia, ED50 4.4 mg/kg; mechanical allodynia, ED50 29.3 mg/kg
	Prairie dog	PO, SC	30, 80 mg/kg		PK[95]	Oral bioavailability poor but sustains concentrations longer
	Rat	PO	101–133 mg/kg	Once daily	PD[99]	Attenuated postoperative mechanical hypersensitivity, less consistent for thermal hypersensitivity (incisional pain models)
Gabapentin and carprofen	Rat	PO	86–137 mg/kg (G) and 1.9–3 mg/kg (C)	Once daily	PD[99]	Attenuated postoperative mechanical hypersensitivity, no reduction in thermal hypersensitivity (incisional pain models)
Gabapentin and tramadol	Rats		80 mg/kg SC q24 h (G) and 10 mg/kg IP q12 h (T)		PD[94]	Incisional pain model
Pregabalin	Mice		200–400 mg/kg IP		PD[101]	Tail flick test; peak effect between 1 and 1.25 h (ED50 246 mg/kg)
Pregabalin and tramadol	Mice		10 mg/kg IP (P) and 30 mg/kg IP (T)		PD[101]	Tail flick test

Abbreviations: CRI, constant rate infusion; ED50, effective dose 50; EU, empirical use; IM, intramuscularly; IP, intraperitoneally; IV, intravenously; PO, orally; PD, pharmacodynamic study; PK, pharmacokinetic study; SC, subcutaneously.

Table 6
Selected opioids used in mice

Drug	Route	Dose (mg/kg)	Frequency	Study Type	Comments
Buprenorphine, HCl (standard)	SC	0.1	q4–8 h	PD, PK[65,77,122]	Thermal sensitivity and laparotomy models; peak at 2 h; 8 h interval too long; insufficient for abdominal procedures
	SC	1		PD, PK[71]	Less than therapeutic threshold by 12 h; decreased body weight at 1.5 mg/kg (not recommended)[123]
	PO	1		PD[72]	Hot plate test; in Nutella; 1 h for effect
Buprenorphine, high concentration	SC	0.9	q6–12 h	PD, PK[124]	Shorter analgesia duration in female CD1 strain compared with male B6 strain; females evaluated with ovariectomy model
	SC	1		PD, PK[71]	Less than therapeutic threshold by 16 h
Buprenorphine, SR	SC	0.6	q24–48 h	PD[65,122]	Peak at 4 h; laparotomy model
	SC	1		PD, PK[71]	24 h duration
	SC	1.5		PD[123]	Significant nociception (tail flick and hot plate tests) for 48 h without substantial adverse effects; lower respiratory rate; no significant decrease in body weight unlike mice receiving BH
	SC	2.2		PD, PK[77]	Thermal sensitivity and laparotomy models; 24–48 h duration; no significant decrease in body weight unlike mice receiving BH
Butorphanol	SC	1–2	q4 h	EU[26]	Hot plate, ED50; peak effect at 0.5 h
	SC	2		PD[9]	Hot plate and tail flick tests; injection may be painful
	SC	5	q1–2 h	PD[64]	
	SC	7.3		PD[9]	Tail immersion, ED50; peak effect at 0.5 h; motor impairment at 9.6 mg/kg
Butorphanol, SR	SC	18		PK[65]	Less than suspected therapeutic levels at 8 h
Fentanyl, SR	SC	3.5		PK[65]	Maintained levels >12 h; decreased activity first 12 h, may approach anesthetic dose
Morphine	SC	1, 3, 10, 30		PD[100]	Dose-related nociception (tail flick, ED50 3.2 mg/kg; hot plate, ED 0.58 mg/kg; visceral inflammation, ED 0.31 mg/kg); motor impairment; apnea and hypotension with IV administration (not recommended)
Nalbuphine	SC	10		PK[86]	
Tramadol		25 mg/kg SC + 25 mg/kg PO		PD[92]	Laparotomy model; insufficient

Abbreviations: ED50, effective dose 50; EU, empirical use; IP, intraperitoneally; IV, intravenously; PO, orally; PD, pharmacodynamic study; PK, pharmacokinetic study; SC, subcutaneously; SR, sustained-release

Table 7
Selected opioid drugs used in rats

Drug	Route	Dose (mg/kg)	Frequency	Study Type	Comments
Buprenorphine, HCl (standard)	SC	0.03		PD[49]	Thermal pain (capsaicin); pica, self-mutilation possible with all buprenorphine formulations
	SC	0.05	q8–12 h	PD[37,58,82,94,118,125]	Reduced mechanical and thermal hypersensitivity (incisional pain models)[125], ovariohysterectomy model[118]
	SC	0.1	Twice daily	PD[118]	Ovariohysterectomy model; no clear advantage over 0.05 mg/kg
	PO	0.3		PD[73]	Flank laparotomy model
	PO	0.5–0.6		PD[49]	Thermal pain (capsaicin); analgesic efficacy only in males
Buprenorphine, SR	SC	0.3		PD[125]	Reduced mechanical but not thermal hypersensitivity (incisional pain models) for 48 h
	SC	0.65		PD, PK[82,126]	Hypoxemia[82]
	SC	1.2		PD[37,58,82,118,125]	Reduced mechanical and thermal hypersensitivity (incisional pain model) for 72 h[125], hypoxemia,[82] mild-moderate sedation[125], marked sedation and weight loss at 4.5 mg/kg (not recommended)[125], ovariohysterectomy model[118]
	SC	1.3		PK[126]	
Buprenorphine, high concentration	SC	0.075, 0.15		PD[74]	Not recommended; adverse effects (decreased food intake and fecal output, self-injurious behavior) without significant change in thermal withdrawal latency
	SC	0.3		PD[58,74]	Increase in thermal withdrawal latency at 1 h only; adverse effects (decreased food intake and fecal output, self-injurious behavior) limit clinical utility
	SC	0.5		PD, PK[127]	Laparotomy model; 12–24 h duration
Butorphanol	SC	2	q1–2 h	PD[64]	Hot plate and tail flick tests; injection may be painful

(continued on next page)

Table 7
(continued)

Drug	Route	Dose (mg/kg)	Frequency	Study Type	Comments
Codeine	SC	5–30		PD[57]	Spinal cord injury models; peak at 0.5 h; effect up to 3 h; no motor impairment at doses up to 960 mg/kg
Methadone	SC	0.5–3		PD[57]	Peripheral neuropathic pain and spinal cord injury models; dose-dependent antinociception; peak between 0.5 and 1.5 h; dose-dependent motor impairment at ≥1 mg/kg
Morphine	IV	3		PD[107]	Hot plate and tail-flick tests; respiratory depression not evaluated, use with caution
	SC	1–6		PD[57]	Peripheral neuropathic pain and spinal cord injury models; dose-dependent antinociception; peak at 0.5 h; effects up to 2 h; motor impairment at ≥ 6 mg/kg
	SC	3, 10		PD[100]	Capsaicin-induced mechanical allodynia ED50 1.9 mg/kg
Morphine and dexmedetomidine	IV	1.5 (Mo) and 0.005 (D)		PD[107]	Hot plate and tail-flick tests
Morphine and maropitant	IV	1.5 (Mo) and 10 (Ma)		PD[107]	Hot plate and tail-flick tests; supraadditive effect with Mo and Ma in tail-flick test; caution with IV maropitant
Morphine and dexmedetomidine and maropitant	IV	1 (Mo) and 0.0035 (D) and 6.5 (Ma)		PD[107]	Hot plate and tail-flick tests; caution with IV maropitant
Nalbuphine	2 mg/kg SC + 1 mg/kg/h IV (CRI)			PD, PK[85]	Intraperitoneal sepsis model
Tramadol	PO	20–40		PD[49]	Thermal pain (capsaicin); analgesia at all doses for females, only at 40 mg/kg for males
	IP	10	q12 h	PD[94]	Incisional pain model, insufficient

Abbreviations: CRI, constant rate infusion; ED50, effective dose 50; IP, intraperitoneally; IV, intravenously; PO, orally; PD, pharmacodynamic study; PK, pharmacokinetic study; SC, subcutaneously; SR, sustained-release.

Table 8
Selected opioid drugs used in prairie dogs

Drug	Route	Dose (mg/ kg)	Frequency	Study Type	Comments
Butorphanol	IM, SC	0.1–0.5	q6–8 h	EU[128]	
Buprenorphine HCl (standard)	SC	0.1	q12 h	EU[129]	
Buprenorphine, SR	SC	0.9, 1.2		PK[81]	Mild erythematous reactions

Abbreviations: BH; Buprenorphine HCl standard; EU, empirical use; IM, intramuscularly; PK, pharmacokinetic study; SC, subcutaneously; SR, sustained-release.

barrier, sparing central nervous system effects such as analgesia antagonism while blocking unwanted peripheral effects.[59]

Butorphanol

Butorphanol is a KOR agonist with mild antagonistic properties at the MOR, although some research suggests partial MOR agonist activity in mice.[9,61] It suppresses sodium and calcium channels resulting in suppression of the ascending pain pathways.[62] Intraplantar injection of butorphanol was shown to be safe and effective at providing 15 minutes of local analgesia based on thermal nociceptive paw withdrawal testing and may indicate the ability to achieve local analgesia for use in minor procedures in rats.[62]

Parenteral butorphanol is generally used for the treatment of mild pain of short duration.[63,64] As with many drugs, higher doses are required for mice compared with rats.[64] For some types of pain maximum analgesia effects cannot be reached without approaching a lethal dose.[61] Subcutaneous injection of butorphanol in mice and rats may be painful.[64] A sustained-release (SR) formulation was evaluated at a dose of 18 mg/kg in mice; although therapeutic levels of butorphanol are unknown in mice, plasma levels dropped less than those known to be therapeutic in other species between 4 and 8 hours.[65] Further investigation of SR options is warranted.

Buprenorphine

Buprenorphine is a MOR partial agonist, a DOR and KOR antagonist, and an ORL-1 receptor agonist.[44,45] Binding affinity is very high for the MOR, high for the DOR and KOR, and low for the ORL-1 receptor.[44,45] Dissociation from the MOR is slow compared with other opioids, contributing to prolonged analgesia.[45] Despite classification as a partial MOR agonist, buprenorphine has shown analgesic efficacy similar to full MOR agonists; partial agonism does not infer partial analgesic efficacy.[45] In contrast to full MOR agonists, a ceiling effect for respiratory depression is seen; however, as documented in humans, it seems no ceiling effect for analgesia occurs.[45,66,67] Due to these unique characteristics, some advocate for its classification as a full MOR agonist.[43,67]

Available parenteral formulations include standard buprenorphine hydrochloride (BH), SR buprenorphine (SRB), high-concentration buprenorphine (HCB), and transdermal buprenorphine patches.[43] Dilution of BH may be required for accurate dosing of small rodents; aseptically diluted BH can be stored refrigerated or at room temperature in glass vials protected from light for 180 days.[68]

SR refers to formulations providing a controlled rate of drug release via a vehicle or membrane, theoretically with constant amount per unit time metabolized (zero-order kinetic profile).[43] Two compounded SRB formulations are currently indexed through the FDA for control of postprocedural pain in rats and mice (BUPRELAB-RAT,

1 mg/mL, Wildlife Pharmaceuticals Inc., Windsor, CO, US, rats only; ETHIQA XR, 1.3 mg/mL, Fidelis Pharmaceuticals, North Brunswick, NJ, USA, rats and mice).[10] Alternatively, due to the long half-life of buprenorphine and respiratory depression ceiling, high doses of buprenorphine can be used to provide prolonged antinociception without an SR mechanism.[43] An HCB formulation FDA-approved for subcutaneous use in cats (SIMBADOL, Zoetis, Florham Park, NJ, US) allows a high dose to be administered while maintaining a small injection volume.[69] Injection volume can potentially affect pharmacokinetics, such as in mice where caudal thigh intramuscular injection volumes of 100 μL and above resulted in leakage into the extramuscular tissues.[70] Similar to BH formulations, metabolism of HCB formulations is expected at a constant fraction per unit time (first-order kinetics).[43,69] In mice, HCB did not offer an advantage over BH at a dose of 1 mg/kg, due to decrease in concentration by 16 hours and clinical signs of discomfort such as increased activity.[71]

Orally administered buprenorphine results in antinociception in rats; however, compared with subcutaneous administration, the effect is not as marked, has a later onset, and requires a 10-fold dose increase in part due to significant first-pass liver metabolism.[72,73] In the authors' experience, this dosing can be cost-prohibitive.

Administration of any buprenorphine formulation may result in pica, especially in rats, leading to poor weight gain, gastrointestinal obstruction, or self-injurious behavior.[7,58,74,75] This can be partially managed by removing indigestible bedding; however, in some cases, pica is replaced by excessive grooming or self-mutilation.[76] As this behavior can be directed at incisions, the authors recommend cautious postoperative use, with consideration of alternative analgesics and treatment of nausea. Behavioral changes such as circling and increased activity are reported with BH formulations.[77] SRB formulation administration may result in inflammatory and necrotic skin lesions lasting up to 3 weeks, presumably caused when the drug seeps out of injection site during injection.[78–81] Technique modifications such as slowly withdrawing the needle and pinching the injection site for 15 seconds resolved this reaction in rats but may be challenging in smaller species, especially when conscious.[78,79] Despite the respiratory ceiling effect, SRB products are not recommended in rats with respiratory compromise, and hypoxemia has been documented in healthy animals.[10,82] Naloxone reverses some effects but may need to be redosed as the duration of action is generally 3 hours or less.[10] Additionally, due to enterohepatic circulation of the drug, treated rodents and cagemates may have exposure through coprophagy.[10] SR formulations may not be absorbed in athymic nude rats, potentially due to lack of immune response needed to dissolve the vehicle.[83]

Similar to many opioids, SRB and HCB formulations contain human risk warnings, including abuse potential and life-threatening respiratory depression with accidental exposure.[10] Naloxone may not be effective in reversing human respiratory depression.[10]

Nalbuphine
Use of nalbuphine, a KOR agonist and MOR antagonist, is uncommon but preferred in some situations because it is not a controlled substance.[84] A ceiling effect is seen for both analgesia and respiratory depression, and it is a good choice for dystocia because it does not antagonize prostaglandins.[84–86] Administration improved Rat Grimace Scale scores in a rat sepsis model.[85]

Full mu Opioid receptor agonists
Oral and parenteral forms of MOR agonists are available. MOR agonist potencies in rodents are similar to humans, with fentanyl > buprenorphine > morphine > oxycodone > codeine for intramuscular administration, and

oxycodone > hydrocodone > morphine > codeine for oral administration.[56] In some cases, a lower potency may be acceptable, especially when combined with another analgesic.[56] In a neuropathic pain model, the weak opioid codeine had a superior therapeutic window (antinociception without ataxia) to morphine and methadone.[57] Short-acting MOR agonists such as fentanyl can be administered as constant rate infusions (CRI), through osmotic pumps, or transdermally.[43]

Intravenous morphine administration resulted in apnea at all doses tested in mice; alternative routes and lower doses should be used if animals are not intubated.[87] SR fentanyl has been studied but an apparent initial burst effect resulted in profound sedation, with labored breathing at higher doses.[65] Transdermal fentanyl patches have been investigated in rodents experimentally but should be used with extreme caution due to risk of fatal overdose via ingestion.[88–90] Subcutaneously implanted osmotic pumps may be a viable patch alternative.[91]

Tramadol
The synthetic opioid tramadol is a weak MOR agonist, as well as a serotonin and norepinephrine reuptake inhibitor.[47,63] Analgesia is provided primarily via the metabolite O-desmethyl-tramadol. Similar to findings in other taxa, analgesic studies thus far show mixed results (see **Tables 5–7**), with an incisional pain model in rats showing insufficient analgesia at 10 mg/kg intraperitoneally as a sole agent.[49,92–94] Although oral doses of 20 to 40 mg/kg provided analgesia in female Sprague-Dawley rats, 40 mg/kg was required for males.[49]

Adjuvants/Coanalgesics

Anticonvulsants
The anticonvulsants gabapentin and pregabalin can be used for analgesia, especially for neuropathic and chronic pain. These drugs provide analgesia by binding to alpha-2-delta ligands of calcium-voltage–gated subunit receptors, reducing excitatory neurotransmitter secretions, and have neuroprotective and anti-inflammatory properties.[95,96] Gabapentin benefits include a wide safety margin and lack of classification as a controlled substance in most states; pregabalin is currently a Schedule V drug.[95,97]

Oral and subcutaneous administration of gabapentin has been evaluated in mice, rats, and prairie dogs, and intraperitoneally administered pregabalin has been studied in mice (see **Table 5**).[95,98–101] Analgesia has been demonstrated in mice and rats, with some oral doses exceeding 100 mg/kg.[99,100] In prairie dogs, orally administered gabapentin had poor bioavailability but sustained presumed half maximal effective concentrations (concentration expected to induce a response halfway between baseline and maximum; extrapolated from rats in this case) longer than subcutaneous administration.[95] In mice, tail-flick test antinociception was demonstrated with intraperitoneal doses of 200 to 400 mg/kg pregabalin.[101] Adverse effects reported across species including humans include ataxia, sedation, dizziness, tremors, myoclonus, and peripheral edema; however, these were not noted in mice and prairie dogs at doses up to 100 and 80 mg/kg, respectively.[95,99,102] Both gabapentin and pregabalin are renally excreted, necessitating dose adjustments if renal dysfunction is present.[102] Synergism occurs between gabapentinoids and opioids, resulting in lower effective concentrations.[7,95] In a rat incisional pain model, gabapentin (80 mg/kg subcutaneously every 24 hours) plus tramadol (10 mg/kg intraperitoneally every 12 hours) provided analgesia, whereas tramadol alone did not.[94] Pregabalin and tramadol also showed synergism in an acute pain mouse model when used intraperitoneally at sufficient doses and ratios (10 and 30 mg/kg, respectively).[101]

Cannabinoids

Preliminary studies using injection of cannabinoids into the periaqueductal region of the rat brain show potential antinociceptive effects on neuropathic, osteoarthritic, incisional, and inflammatory pain.[103] Synergistic effects may be seen with opioids such as morphine.[103] Adverse effects include ataxia, sedation, nausea, and diarrhea.[103] Legal status of this drug is complex but further investigation is warranted.

Antidepressants

Duloxetine, a serotonergic and noradrenergic reuptake inhibitor, showed analgesic efficacy without significant motor impairment in rodent models of persistent and inflammatory pain.[100] These doses (see **Table 5**) had minimal effect on acute nociception.[100] Tricyclic antidepressants such as amitriptyline have shown analgesic efficacy for neuropathic pain in mice (see **Table 5**).[104]

Other Analgesic Classes

N-methyl-ᴅ-aspartate receptor antagonists

Low doses of noncompetitive NMDA receptor antagonists such as ketamine may be used as part of a multimodal analgesic approach, including in CRIs. In a mouse orthopedic surgery model, preemptive ketamine use not only improved morphine efficacy but also diminished short-term and long-term hyperalgesia.[52] Ketamine depresses the thalamoneocortical system, activates the limbic system, inhibits binding of gamma-aminobutyric acid, prevents central sensitization, and may block serotonin, norepinephrine, and dopamine in the central nervous system.[8] Metabolism is through hepatic biotransformation followed by renal excretion; renal impairment can prolong recovery.[8] Side effects include increased heart rate and myocardial contractility, increased myocardial oxygen demand, increased peripheral vascular resistance, increased salivation, depressed or apneustic ventilation, and increased intracranial pressure.[8] Muscle rigidity also occurs, making this drug less commonly used as a single agent.[8] The acidic pH may cause pain, irritation, or necrosis at injection sites.[8]

Alpha-2 adrenergic receptor antagonists

Alpha-2-adrenergic receptor agonists, including dexmedetomidine, medetomidine, and xylazine, may produce sedation, analgesia, muscle relaxation, anxiolysis, and dose-sparing anesthetic effects through arteriolar alpha-2 receptor stimulation.[8,105] Dexmedetomidine, the active isomer of medetomidine, has high receptor specificity and can be readily reversed with atipamezole.[105] Antinociception is dose-dependent.[9] Side effects of dexmedetomidine include bradycardia, peripheral and cardiac vasoconstriction, decreased respiratory rate, hypothermia, increased urine production, and transient hyperglycemia.[8,105] Metabolism is primarily hepatic; nonactive metabolites are excreted via urine and feces.[8] Although the sedating effects of alpha-2-adrenergic receptor agonists may limit their analgesic use, as with ketamine, a multimodal approach can permit lower doses (see **Table 5**).[106,107] The alpha-2-adrenergic receptor agonist clonidine showed analgesic synergism with morphine in a low back pain rodent model, without synergistic sedation or motor incoordination.[106]

Potential drug interactions must be considered with alpha-2 agonists and their reversals. Although the benzodiazepine midazolam exhibited no analgesic effect on its own, midazolam coadministration enhanced the analgesic effect of dexmedetomidine as measured by the tail-flick test.[105] Similarly, synergistic nociception was seen with coadministration of dexmedetomidine and butorphanol in mice.[9] Conversely, administration of atipamezole attenuates analgesic effects of butorphanol in rats, potentially because of colocation of KOR and alpha-2 receptors on descending serotonergic pathways.[108,109] Although this finding was not repeatable in mice,[110] use of additional or alternative analgesics might be considered with use of alpha-2 antagonists.[109]

Maropitant

In addition to its antiemetic properties, the neurokinin-1 receptor antagonist maropitant may also block substance-P mediated transmission of noxious stimuli.[107] Further investigation is needed but preliminary studies suggest this drug could be useful for visceral and inflammatory pain.[107,111] A synergistic effect with morphine was demonstrated in a rat tail-flick model.[107] Adverse effects include pain and irritation from subcutaneous injections, which can be reduced by maintaining at refrigerated temperature.[112] Due to noncardiogenic edema and death in one animal following intravenous administration in a recent study, the authors recommend further toxicity evaluation before intravenous use in rodents.[107]

SUMMARY

Although careful interpretation of laboratory animal rodent studies is necessary when extrapolating to clinical patients, a wealth of information is available in the literature. Pharmacokinetic and pharmacodynamic studies often demonstrate that rodent analgesic dosing requirements are higher and more frequent than historic recommendations. Analgesic classes including local anesthetics, anticonvulsants, antidepressants, and NMDA antagonists should be considered in addition to nonsteroidal anti-inflammatories and opioids. Continued efforts toward evidence-based, multimodal, and individualized approaches to rodent analgesia will improve patient welfare and clinical outcomes.

DISCLOSURE

The authors do not have any commercial or financial conflicts of interest or funding sources to disclose.

REFERENCES

1. Market Research Statistics. U.S. Pet Ownership 2012. American Veterinary Medical Association. Available at: https://www.avma.org/resources/reports-statistics/market-research-statistics-us-pet-ownership-2012.   Accessed December 27, 2021.
2. Turner P, Kirchain S, DiVincenti L, et al. ACLAM position statement on pain and distress in research animals. J Am Assoc Lab Anim Sci 2016;55(6):821.
3. Miller AL, Richardson CA. Rodent analgesia. Vet Clin North Am Exot Anim Pract 2011;14(1):81–92.
4. Coulter CA, Flecknell PA, Richardson CA. Reported analgesic administration to rabbits, pigs, sheep, dogs and non-human primates undergoing experimental surgical procedures. Lab Anim 2009;43(3):232–8.
5. Richardson CA, Flecknell PA. Anaesthesia and post-operative analgesia following experimental surgery in laboratory rodents: Are we making progress? Altern Lab Anim 2005;33(2):119–27.
6. Stokes EL, Flecknell PA, Richardson CA. Reported analgesic and anaesthetic administration to rodents undergoing experimental surgical procedures. Lab Anim 2009;43(2):149–54.
7. Foley PL, Kendall LV, Turner PV. Clinical management of pain in rodents. Comp Med 2019;69(6):468–89.

8. Bennett K, Lewis K. Sedation and anesthesia in rodents. Vet Clin North Am Exot Anim Pract 2022;25(1):211–55.

9. Ahsan MZ, Khan FU, Zhao MJ, et al. Synergistic interaction between butorphanol and dexmedetomidine in antinociception. Eur J Pharm Sci 2020;149:105322.

10. FDA. The Index of Legally Marketed Unapproved New Animal Drugs for Minor Species. 2009. 2022. Available at: https://www.fda.gov/animal-veterinary/minor-useminor-species/index-legally-marketed-unapproved-new-animal-drugs-minor-species. Accessed December 21, 2021.

11. Yang J, Bauer BA, Wahner-Roedler DL, et al. The modified WHO analgesic ladder: Is it appropriate for chronic non-cancer pain? J Pain Res 2020;13:411–7.

12. Cuomo A, Bimonte S, Forte CA, et al. Multimodal approaches and tailored therapies for pain management: the trolley analgesic model. J Pain Res 2019;12:711.

13. Lemke KA, Dawson SD. Local and regional anesthesia. Vet Clin Small Anim Pract 2000;30(4):839–57.

14. Flecknell P. Basic principles of anaesthesia. In: Flecknell P, editor. Laboratory animal anaesthesia. 4th edition. San Francisco, CA: Academic Press; 2016. p. 1–75.

15. FDA. EMLA CREAM (lidocaine 2.5% and Prilocaine 2.5%). Updated November 2018. Available at: https://www.accessdata.fda.gov/drugsatfda_docs/label/2018/019941s021lbl.pdf. Accessed March 2, 2022.

16. Keating SCJ, Thomas AA, Flecknell PA, et al. Evaluation of EMLA cream for preventing pain during tattooing of rabbits: Changes in physiological, behavioural and facial expression responses. PLoS One 2012;7(9).

17. David JM, Duarte Vogel S, Longo K, et al. The use of eutectic mixture of lidocaine and prilocaine in mice (*Mus musculus*) for tail vein injections. Vet Anaesth Analg 2014;41(6):654–9.

18. Dudley ES, Johnson RA, French DC, et al. Effects of topical anesthetics on behavior, plasma corticosterone, and blood glucose levels after tail biopsy of C57BL/6NHSD mice (*Mus musculus*). J Am Assoc Lab Anim Sci 2016;55(4):443–50.

19. Lascelles BDX, Kirkby Shaw K. An extended release local anaesthetic: Potential for future use in veterinary surgical patients? Vet Med Sci 2016;2(4):229–38.

20. Kang SC, Jampachaisri K, Seymour TL, et al. Use of liposomal bupivacaine for postoperative analgesia in an incisional pain model in rats (*Rattus norvegicus*). J Am Assoc Lab Anim Sci 2017;56(1):63–8.

21. Ouchi K, Sekine J, Koga Y, et al. Establishment of an animal model of epidural anesthesia and sedative tail-flick test for evaluating local anesthetic effects in rats. Exp Anim 2013;62(2):137–44.

22. Morimoto K, Nishimura R, Matsunaga S, et al. Epidural analgesia with a combination of bupivacaine and buprenorphine in rats. J Vet Med A Physiol Pathol Clin Med 2001;48(5):303–12.

23. Clark TP. The clinical pharmacology of cyclooxygenase-2–selective and dual inhibitors. Vet Clin North Am Small Anim Pract 2006;36(5):1061–85.

24. Harder AT, An YH. The mechanisms of the inhibitory effects of nonsteroidal anti-inflammatory drugs on bone healing: A concise review. J Clin Pharmacol 2003;43(8):807–15.

25. Flecknell PA, Orr HE, Roughan JV, et al. Comparison of the effects of oral or subcutaneous carprofen or ketoprofen in rats undergoing laparotomy. Vet Rec 1999;144(3):65–7.

26. Flecknell PA. Analgesia of Small Mammals. Vet Clin North Am Exot Anim Pract 2001;4(1):47–56.
27. Hawkins MG, Pascoe PJ. Anesthesia, analgesia, and sedation of small mammals. In: Quesenberry KE, Orcutt CJ, Mans C, et al, editors. Ferrets, rabbit, and rodents. 4th edition. St. Louis, MO: WB Saunders; 2021. p. 536–58.
28. Flecknell P. Analgesia and post-operative care. In: Flecknell P, editor. Laboratory animal anaesthesia. 4th edition. San Francisco, CA: Academic Press; 2016. p. 141–92.
29. Matsumiya LC, Sorge RE, Sotocinal SG, et al. Using the mouse grimace scale to reevaluate the efficacy of postoperative analgesics in laboratory mice. J Am Assoc Lab Anim Sci 2012;51(1):42–9.
30. Flecknell P. Rodent analgesia: Assessment and therapeutics. Vet J 2018; 232:70–7.
31. Waite ME, Tomkovich A, Quinn TL, et al. Efficacy of common analgesics for postsurgical pain in rats. J Am Assoc Lab Anim Sci 2015;54(4):420–5.
32. Takagi-Matsumoto H, Ng B, Tsukimi Y, et al. Effects of NSAIDs on bladder function in normal and cystitis rats: A comparison study of aspirin, indomethacin, and ketoprofen. J Pharmacol Sci 2004;95(4):458–65.
33. Lamon TK, Browder EJ, Sohrabji F, et al. Adverse effects of incorporating ketoprofen into established rodent studies. J Am Assoc Lab Anim Sci 2008; 47(4):20–4.
34. Shientag LJ, Wheeler SM, Garlick DS, et al. A therapeutic dose of ketoprofen causes acute gastrointestinal bleeding, erosions, and ulcers in rats. J Am Assoc Lab Anim Sci 2012;51(6):832–41.
35. Liles JH, Flecknell PA. A comparison of the effects of buprenorphine, carprofen and flunixin following laparotomy in rats. J Vet Pharmacol Ther 1994;17(4): 284–90.
36. Roughan JV, Flecknell PA. Evaluation of a short duration behaviour-based postoperative pain scoring system in rats. Eur J Pain 2003;7(5):397–406.
37. Seymour TL, Adams SC, Felt SA, et al. Postoperative analgesia due to sustained- release buprenorphine, sustained-release meloxicam, and carprofen gel in a model of incisional pain in rats (*Rattus norvegicus*). J Am Assoc Lab Anim Sci 2016;55(3):300–5.
38. Sarfaty AE, Zeiss CJ, Willis AD, et al. Concentration-dependent toxicity after subcutaneous administration of meloxicam to C57BL/6N mice (*Mus musculus*). J Am Assoc Lab Anim Sci 2018;58(6):802–9.
39. Stewart LA, Imai DM, Beckett L, et al. Injection-site reactions to sustained-release meloxicam in sprague dawley rats. J Am Assoc Lab Anim Sci 2020; 59(6):726–31.
40. Fuetsch SR, Stewart LA, Imai DM, et al. Injection reactions after administration of sustained-release meloxicam to BALB/cJ, C57BL/6J, and Crl:CD1(ICR) mice. J Am Assoc Lab Anim Sci 2021;60(2):176–83.
41. Dickinson AL, Leach MC, Flecknell PA. The analgesic effects of oral paracetamol in two strains of mice undergoing vasectomy. Animals 2009;43:357–61.
42. Durst MS, Arras M, Palme R, et al. Lidocaine and bupivacaine as part of multimodal pain management in a C57BL/6J laparotomy mouse model. Sci Rep 2021;11(1):1–17.
43. Emerson JA, Guzman DSM. Sustained-release and long-acting opioid formulations of interest in zoological medicine. In: Miller RE, Lamberski N, Calle PP, editors. Fowler's Zoo Wild Anim Curr Ther, vol. 9. St. Louis, MO: WB Saunders; 2019. p. 151–63.

44. Warner NS, Warner MA, Cunningham JL, et al. A practical approach for the management of the mixed opioid agonist-antagonist buprenorphine during acute pain and surgery. Mayo Clin Proc 2020;95(6):1253–67.

45. Gudin J, Fudin J. A narrative pharmacological review of buprenorphine: A unique opioid for the treatment of chronic pain. Pain Ther 2020;9(1):41–54.

46. Gopalakrishnan L, Chatterjee O, Ravishankar N, et al. Opioid receptors signaling network. J Cell Commun Signal 2021;1–9. https://doi.org/10.1007/s12079-021-00653-z. Epub ahead of print.

47. Codd EE, Shank RP, Schupsky JJ, et al. Serotonin and norepinephrine uptake inhibiting activity of centrally acting analgesics: structural determinants and role in antinociception. J Pharmacol Exp Ther 1995;274(3):1263–70.

48. Ebert B, Thorkildsen C, Andersen S, et al. Opioid analgesics as noncompetitive N-methyl-D-aspartate (NMDA) antagonists. Biochem Pharmacol 1998;56(5):553–9.

49. Taylor BF, Ramirez HE, Battles AH, et al. Analgesic activity of tramadol and buprenorphine after voluntary ingestion by rats (rattus norvegicus). J Am Assoc Lab Anim Sci 2016;55(1):74–82.

50. Curtin LI, Grakowsky JA, Suarez M, et al. Evaluation of buprenorphine in a postoperative pain model in rats. Comp Med 2009;59(1):60–71.

51. Fletcher D, Martinez V. Opioid-induced hyperalgesia in patients after surgery: A systematic review and a meta-analysis. Br J Anaesth 2014;112(6):991–1004.

52. Minville V, Fourcade O, Girolami JP, et al. Opioid-induced hyperalgesia in a mice model of orthopaedic pain: Preventive effect of ketamine. Br J Anaesth 2010;104(2):231–8.

53. Hayhurst CJ, Durieux ME. Differential opioid tolerance and opioid-induced hyperalgesia: A clinical reality. Anesthesiology 2016;124(2):483–8.

54. Wala EP, Holtman JR. Buprenorphine-induced hyperalgesia in the rat. Eur J Pharmacol 2011;651(1–3):89–95.

55. Zhou J, Ma R, Jin Y, et al. Molecular mechanisms of opioid tolerance: From opioid receptors to inflammatory mediators (Review). Exp Ther Med 2021;22(3):1–8.

56. Meert TF, Vermeirsch HA. A preclinical comparison between different opioids: antinociceptive versus adverse effects. Pharmacol Biochem Behav 2005;80(2):309–26.

57. Erichsen HK, Hao JX, Xu XJ, et al. Comparative actions of the opioid analgesics morphine, methadone and codeine in rat models of peripheral and central neuropathic pain. Pain 2005;116(3):347–58.

58. Allen M, Johnson RA. Evaluation of self-injurious behavior, thermal sensitivity, food intake, fecal output, and pica after injection of three buprenorphine formulations in rats (Rattus norvegicus). Am J Vet Res 2018;79(7):697–703.

59. Aung HH, Mehendale SR, Xie JT, et al. Methylnaltrexone prevents morphine-induced kaolin intake in the rat. Life Sci 2004;74(22):2685–91.

60. Greenwood-Van Meerveld B, Gardner CJ, Little PJ, et al. Preclinical studies of opioids and opioid antagonists on gastrointestinal function. Neurogastroenterol Motil 2004;16(SUPPL. 2):46–53.

61. Garner HR, Burke TF, Lawhorn CD, et al. Butorphanol-mediated antinociception in mice: partial agonist effects and mu receptor involvement. J Pharmacol Exp Ther 1997;282(3):1253–61.

62. Interlandi C, Leonardi F, Spadola F, et al. Evaluation of the paw withdrawal latency for the comparison between tramadol and butorphanol administered

locally, in the plantar surface of rat, preliminary study. PLoS One 2021;16(7): e0254497.

63. Abreu M, Aguado D, Benito J, et al. Reduction of the sevoflurane minimum alveolar concentration induced by methadone, tramadol, butorphanol and morphine in rats. Lab Anim 2012;46(3):200–6.

64. Gades NM, Danneman PJ, Wixson SKTE. The magnitude and duration of the analgesic effect of morphine, butorphanol, and buprenorphine in rats and mice. Contemp Top Lab Anim Sci 2000;39(2):8–13.

65. Kendall LV, Hansen RJ, Dorsey K, et al. Pharmacokinetics of sustained-release analgesics in mice. J Am Assoc Lab Anim Sci 2014;53(5):478–84.

66. Dahan A, Yassen A, Romberg R, et al. Buprenorphine induces ceiling in respiratory depression but not in analgesia. Br J Anaesth 2006;96(5):627–32.

67. Pergolizzi J, Aloisi AM, Dahan A, et al. Current knowledge of buprenorphine and its unique pharmacological profile. Pain Pract 2010;10(5):428–50.

68. DenHerder JM, Reed RL, Sargent JL, et al. Effects of time and storage conditions on the chemical and microbiologic stability of diluted buprenorphine for injection. J Am Assoc Lab Anim Sci 2017;56(4):457–61.

69. Doodnaught GM, Monteiro BP, Benito J, et al. Pharmacokinetic and pharmacodynamic modelling after subcutaneous, intravenous and buccal administration of a high-concentration formulation of buprenorphine in conscious cats. PLoS One 2017;12(4):e0176443.

70. Gehling AM, Kuszpit K, Bailey EJ, et al. Evaluation of volume of intramuscular injection into the caudal thigh muscles of female and male BALB/c mice (Mus musculus). J Am Assoc Lab Anim Sci 2018;57(1):35–43.

71. Myers PH, Goulding DR, Wiltshire RA, et al. Serum buprenorphine concentrations and behavioral activity in mice after a single subcutaneous injection of simbadol, buprenorphine SR-LAB, or standard buprenorphine. J Am Assoc Lab Anim Sci 2021;60(6):661–6.

72. Hestehave S, Munro G, Pedersen TB, et al. Antinociceptive effects of voluntarily ingested buprenorphine in the hot-plate test in laboratory rats. Lab Anim 2017; 51(3):264–72.

73. Flecknell PA, Roughan JV, Stewart R. Use of oral buprenorphine ('buprenorphine jello') for postoperative analgesia in rats - A clinical trial. Lab Anim 1999;33(2): 169–74.

74. Allen M, Nietlisbach N, Johnson RA. Evaluation of self-injurious behavior, food intake, fecal output, and thermal withdrawal latencies after injection of a high-concentration buprenorphine formulation in rats (Rattus norvegicus). Am J Vet Res 2018;79(2):154–62.

75. Jacobson C. Adverse effects on growth rates in rats caused by buprenorphine administration. Lab Anim 2000;34(2):202–6.

76. Sarabia-Estrada R, Cowan A, Tyler BM, et al. Association of nausea with buprenorphine analgesia for rats. Lab Anim 2017;46(6):242–4.

77. Jirkof P, Tourvieille A, Cinelli P, et al. Buprenorphine for pain relief in mice: repeated injections vs sustained-release depot formulation. Lab Anim 2015; 49(3):177–87.

78. Carbone ET, Lindstrom KE, Diep S, et al. Duration of action of sustained-release buprenorphine in 2 strains of mice. J Am Assoc Lab Anim Sci 2012;51(6):815–9.

79. Foley PL, Liang H, Crichlow AR. Evaluation of a sustained-release formulation of buprenorphine for analgesia in rats. J Am Assoc Lab Anim Sci 2011;50(2): 198–204.

80. Clark TS, Clark DD, Hoyt RF. Pharmacokinetic comparison of sustained-release and standard buprenorphine in mice. J Am Assoc Lab Anim Sci 2014;53(4).
81. Cary CD, Lukovsky-Akhsanov NL, Gallardo-Romero NF, et al. Pharmacokinetic profiles of meloxicam and sustained-release buprenorphine in prairie dogs (*Cynomys ludovicianus*). J Am Assoc Lab Anim Sci 2017;56(2):160–5.
82. Johnson RA. Voluntary running-wheel activity, arterial blood gases, and thermal antinociception in rats after 3 buprenorphine formulations. J Am Assoc Lab Anim Sci 2016;55(3):306–11.
83. Douglas Page C, Sarabia-Estrada R, Jay Hoffman R, et al. Lack of absorption of a sustained-release buprenorphine formulation administered subcutaneously to athymic nude rats. J Am Assoc Lab Anim Sci 2019;58(5):597–600.
84. Narver HL. Nalbuphine, a non-controlled opioid analgesic, and its potential use in research mice. Lab Anim 2015;44(3):106–10.
85. Jeger V, Arrigo M, Hildenbrand FF, et al. Improving animal welfare using continuous nalbuphine infusion in a long-term rat model of sepsis. Intensive Care Med Exp 2017;5(1):1–13.
86. Kick BL, Shu P, Wen B, et al. Pharmacokinetic profiles of nalbuphine after intraperitoneal and subcutaneous administration to C57BL/6 mice. J Am Assoc Lab Anim Sci 2017;56(5):534.
87. Criado AB, Gómez de Segura IA, Tendillo FJ, et al. Reduction of isoflurane MAC with buprenorphine and morphine in rats. Lab Anim 2000;34(3):252–9.
88. Thysman S, Preat V. In vivo iontophoresis of fentanyl and sufentanil in rats: Pharmacokinetics and acute antinociceptive effects. Anesth Analg 1993;77(1):61–6.
89. Deschamps JY, Gaulier JM, Podevin G, et al. Fatal overdose after ingestion of a transdermal fentanyl patch in two non-human primates. Vet Anaesth Analg 2012;39(6):653–6.
90. Sredenšek J, Bošnjak M, Lampreht Tratar U, et al. Case report: Intoxication in a pig (*Sus scrofa domesticus*) after transdermal fentanyl patch ingestion. Front Vet Sci 2020;7.
91. Martucci C, Panerai AE, Sacerdote P. Chronic fentanyl or buprenorphine infusion in the mouse: similar analgesic profile but different effects on immune responses. Pain 2004;110(1–2):385–92.
92. Evangelista-Vaz R, Bergadano A, Arras M, et al. Analgesic efficacy of subcutaneous-oral dosage of tramadol after surgery in C57BL/6J Mice. J Am Assoc Lab Anim Sci 2018;57(4):368–75.
93. Donati PA, Tarragona L, Franco JVA, et al. Efficacy of tramadol for postoperative pain management in dogs: Systematic review and meta-analysis. Vet Anaesth Analg 2021;48(3):283–96.
94. McKeon GP, Pacharinsak C, Long CT, et al. Analgesic effects of tramadol, tramadol-gabapentin, and buprenorphine in an incisional model of pain in rats (*Rattus norvegicus*). J Am Assoc Lab Anim Sci 2011;50(2):192–7.
95. Mills PO, Tansey CO, Genzer SC, et al. Pharmacokinetic profiles of gabapentin after oral and subcutaneous administration in black-Tailed prairie dogs (*Cynomys ludovicianus*). J Am Assoc Lab Anim Sci 2020;59(3):305–9.
96. Alles SRA, Cain SM, Snutch TP. Pregabalin as a pain therapeutic: Beyond calcium channels. Front Cell Neurosci 2020;14:83.
97. DEA. Drug Scheduling. Updated July 10, 2018. Available at: https://www.dea.gov/drug-information/drug-scheduling. Accessed April 20, 2022.
98. Tanabe M, Takasu K, Kasuya N, et al. Role of descending noradrenergic system and spinal α 2- adrenergic receptors in the effects of gabapentin on thermal and

mechanical nociception after partial nerve injury in the mouse. Br J Pharmacol 2005;144(5):703–14.

99. Zude BP, Jampachaisri K, Pacharinsak C. Use of flavored tablets of gabapentin and carprofen to attenuate postoperative hypersensitivity in an incisional pain model in rats (*Rattus norvegicus*). J Am Assoc Lab Anim Sci 2020;59(2):163–9.

100. Jones CK, Peters SC, Shannon HE. Efficacy of duloxetine, a potent and balanced serotonergic and noradrenergic reuptake inhibitor, in inflammatory and acute pain models in rodents. J Pharmacol Exp Ther 2005;312(2):726–32.

101. Meymandi MS, Keyhanfar F. Pregabalin antinociception and its interaction with tramadol in acute model of pain. Pharmacol Rep 2012;64(3):576–85.

102. Bookwalter T, Gitlin M. Gabapentin-induced neurologic toxicities. Pharmacotherapy 2005;25(12):1817–9.

103. Mlost J, Bryk M, Starowicz K. Cannabidiol for pain treatment: Focus on pharmacology and mechanism of action. Int J Mol Sci 2020;21(22):8870.

104. Thompson JM, Blanton HL, Pietrzak A, et al. Front and hind paw differential analgesic effects of amitriptyline, gabapentin, ibuprofen, and URB937 on mechanical and cold sensitivity in cisplatin-induced neuropathy. Mol Pain 2019;15.

105. Boehm CA, Carney EL, Tallarida RJ, et al. Midazolam enhances the analgesic properties of dexmedetomidine in the rat. Vet Anaesth Analg 2010;37(6):550–6.

106. Tajerian M, Millecamps M, Stone LS. Morphine and clonidine synergize to ameliorate low back pain in mice. Pain Res Treat 2012;2012:12.

107. Karna SR, Kongara K, Singh PM, et al. Evaluation of analgesic interaction between morphine, dexmedetomidine and maropitant using hot-plate and tail-flick tests in rats. Vet Anaesth Analg 2019;46(4):476–82.

108. Jang HS, Lee MG. Atipamezole changes the antinociceptive effects of butorphanol after medetomidine–ketamine anaesthesia in rats. Vet Anaesth Analg 2009;36(6):591–6.

109. Interlandi C, Calapai G, Nastasi B, et al. Effects of atipamezole on the analgesic activity of butorphanol in rats. J Exot Pet Med 2017;26(4):290–3.

110. Izer JM, Whitcomb TL, Wilson RP. Atipamezole reverses ketamine-dexmedetomidine anesthesia without altering the antinociceptive effects of butorphanol and buprenorphine in female C57BL/6J mice. J Am Assoc Lab Anim Sci 2014;53(6):675–83.

111. Tsukamoto A, Ohgoda M, Haruki N, et al. The anti-inflammatory action of maropitant in a mouse model of acute pancreatitis. J Vet Med Sci 2018;80(3): 17–0483.

112. Papich MG. Maropitant citrate. In: Papich MG, editor. Papich handbook of veterinary drugs. 5th edition. St. Louis, MO: Elsevier; 2021. p. 550–3.

113. IACUC. Analgesia (Guideline). Vertebrate Animal Research. Updated December 9, 2020. Available at: https://animal.research.uiowa.edu/iacuc-guidelines-analgesia. Accessed January 17, 2022.

114. Hawkins MG, Pascoe PJ. Anesthesia, analgesia, and sedation of small mammals. In: Quesenberry KE, Carpenter JW, editors. Ferrets, rabbits, and rodents. 3rd edition. St. Louis, MO: WB Saunders; 2012. p. 429–51.

115. Roughan JV, Flecknell PA. Behaviour-based assessment of the duration of laparotomy-induced abdominal pain and the analgesic effects of carprofen and buprenorphine in rats. Behav Pharmacol 2004;15(7):461–72.

116. Ingrao JC, Johnson R, Tor E, et al. Aqueous stability and oral pharmacokinetics of meloxicam and carprofen in male C57BL/6 mice. J Am Assoc Lab Anim Sci 2013;52(5):553–9.

117. Wright-Williams SL, Courade JP, Richardson CA, et al. Effects of vasectomy surgery and meloxicam treatment on faecal corticosterone levels and behaviour in two strains of laboratory mouse. Pain 2007;130(1–2):108–18.

118. Nunamaker EA, Goldman JL, Adams CR, et al. Evaluation of analgesic efficacy of meloxicam and 2 formulations of buprenorphine after laparotomy in female Sprague–Dawley rats. J Am Assoc Lab Anim Sci 2018;57(5):498–507.

119. Meloxicam SR. ZooPharm Veterinary Compounding Pharmacy. Available at: https://www.zoopharm.com/medication/meloxicam-sr-5ml-10ml-vial-2mg-ml/. Accessed March 1, 2022.

120. Wyatt J. Anesthesia and analgesia in other mammals. In: Fish RE, Brown MJ, Danneman PJ, et al, editors. Anesthesia and analgesia in laboratory animals. 2nd edition. San Francisco, CA: Academic Press; 2008. p. 457–80.

121. Franken ND, Van Oostrom H, Stienen PJ, et al. Evaluation of analgesic and sedative effects of continuous infusion of dexmedetomidine by measuring somatosensory- and auditory-evoked potentials in the rat. Vet Anaesth Analg 2008;35(5):424–31.

122. Kendall LV, Wegenast DJ, Smith BJ, et al. Efficacy of sustained-release buprenorphine in an experimental laparotomy model in female mice. J Am Assoc Lab Anim Sci 2016;55(1):66–73.

123. Healy JR, Tonkin JL, Kamarec SR, et al. Evaluation of an improved sustained-release buprenorphine formulation for use in mice. Am J Vet Res 2014;75(7):619–25.

124. Kendall LV, Singh B, Bailey AL, et al. Pharmacokinetics and efficacy of a long-lasting, highly concentrated buprenorphine solution in mice. J Am Assoc Lab Anim Sci 2021;60(1):64–71.

125. Chum HH, Jampachairsri K, McKeon GP, et al. Antinociceptive effects of sustained-release buprenorphine in a model of incisional pain in rats (Rattus norvegicus). J Am Assoc Lab Anim Sci 2014;53(2):193–7.

126. Levinson BL, Leary SL, Bassett BJ, et al. Pharmacokinetic and histopathologic study of an extended-release, injectable formulation of buprenorphine in Sprague-Dawley rats. J Am Assoc Lab Anim Sci 2021;60(4):462–9.

127. Houston ER, Tan SM, Thomas SM, et al. Pharmacokinetics and efficacy of a long-lasting, highly concentrated buprenorphine solution in rats. J Am Assoc Lab Anim Sci 2021;60(6):667–74.

128. Eshar D, Gardhouse SM. Prairie dogs. In: Quesenberry KE, Orcutt CJ, Mans C, et al, editors. Ferrets, rabbits, and rodents. 4th edition. St. Louis, MO: WB Saunders; 2020. p. 334–44.

129. Hutson CL, Gallardo-Romero N, Carroll DS, et al. Analgesia during monkeypox virus experimental challenge studies in prairie dogs (Cynomys ludovicianus). J Am Assoc Lab Anim Sci 2019;58(4):485–500.

Hystricomorph Rodent Analgesia

Miranda J. Sadar, DVM, DACZM[a],*, Christoph Mans, Dr med Vet, DACZM[b]

KEYWORDS

- Analgesia • Guinea pigs • Chinchillas • Rodent • Hystricomorph

KEY POINTS

- Buprenorphine doses are substantially higher in guinea pigs and chinchillas compared with other mammal species, but sedation may occur at effective analgesic doses in guinea pigs.
- In chinchillas, hydromorphone efficacy has been shown only at very high doses, and although no sedation occurs, a limited reduction in food intake and fecal output should be expected.
- Tramadol is not an effective analgesic in chinchillas, and at high doses, transient profound neurological adverse effects can occur. No information on tramadol in guinea pigs is available.
- Meloxicam is the most prescribed analgesic in guinea pigs and chinchillas, despite the paucity of information on effective dosing regimens and safety. In guinea pigs a dose of 1.5 mg/kg by mouth has been shown to reach therapeutic drug levels but has a short half-life.

INTRODUCTION

Guinea pigs (*Cavia porcellus*) and chinchillas *(Chinchilla lanigera)* are medium-sized South American hystricomorphic rodent species that are commonly kept as companion mammals and are used in biomedical research.[1] Surgical procedures, some diagnostic tests, and a variety of disease processes cause pain and inflammation, and analgesics should be administered to alleviate them.[1] Pain and inflammation can have far-reaching consequences due to potentially life-threatening complications, including anorexia, gastrointestinal stasis, and possible fatal dysbacteriosis.[2] Multiple pharmacologic agents are available to manage pain in hystricomorph rodents. To provide effective analgesia, it is vital to evaluate pain effectively and compare its presence

The authors do not have any commercial or financial conflicts of interest.
[a] Department of Clinical Sciences, College of Veterinary Medicine and Biomedical Sciences, Colorado State University, 300 West Drake Road, Fort Collins, CO 80523, USA; [b] Department of Surgical Sciences, School of Veterinary Medicine, University of Wisconsin-Madison, 2015 Linden Drive, Madison, WI 53706, USA
* Corresponding author.
E-mail address: miranda.sadar@colostate.edu

and intensity both before and after the administration of analgesic agents. Analgesic plans should include anticipation of pain, early treatment to minimize sensitization, and evaluation of individual animals for a response to therapy.[3] In cases in which objective scoring tools are not available or do not exist, observation of patient behavior is necessary and should be performed by trained personnel who are familiar with the species.

Pain response can differ between species, sexes, ages, and individuals, even if they are genetically similar.[4,5] Owing to this, each patient should be monitored closely to evaluate normal behaviors and postures, social interactions, grooming, general activity, and food and water intake. Guinea pigs are highly food motivated, and they eat continuously due to their high metabolism.[6] The lack of this behavior can be used as an indicator for pain in this species, and the unwillingness to consume a highly palatable treat may vary depending on the magnitude of pain that is being experienced. However, one should consider that systemic nonpainful disease processes (eg, dehydration, renal insufficiency), the use of sedative or anesthetic drugs, and even analgesic drugs can lead to changes in behavior and reduction in food intake.

Pain behaviors, as described in species-specific ethograms, strongly correlate with each other and have been evaluated in guinea pigs.[1,7] Pain-related behaviors that may be observed in guinea pigs include a change in posture from standing to recumbency; lying down with the pelvic limbs tucked under the body, positioned to the side, or extended behind the body; pelvic limb lifting; writhing; and flinching.[1] Behaviors that may be more variable include vocalization, abdominal contractions, back-arching, twitching, and weight shifting.[1,7] The use of facial grimace scales to assess pain has also gained popularity, and the attraction is that they may be both an easier, more rapid assessment to make and one that uses the human tendency to pay attention to faces.[8] Scales exist for multiple small mammal species. However, they have not been developed or adequately evaluated in hystricomorph rodents. Prey species, including rodents, often suppress spontaneous pain behavior in the presence of a human observer,[8,9] which can make it challenging to observe and effectively score pain cage side. The use of remote video evaluation can obtain more reliable information about pain behavior.[10]

Analgesic dosing regimens should consider pharmacokinetic and pharmacodynamic studies. The frequency of dosing ideally would be based on these and individual patient assessments of pain. However, due to hystricomorph rodents being prey animals, their ability to mask signs of pain should be considered. Most analgesic agents used to mitigate pain in hystricomorph rodents fall into the following classes: opioids (or opioidlike), non-steroidal anti-inflammatory drugs (NSAIDs), and local analgesics.

OPIOID DRUGS

Opioids are frequently used in veterinary medicine and are considered the most effective class of analgesic drugs for pain management.[11] Parenteral routes of administration are most common when providing opioids to hystricomorph rodents. Parenteral administration offers more reliable and consistent absorption and bioavailability rates than when the same drugs are administered orally or transmucosally. However, parenteral administration usually requires hospitalization and administration of the drugs by trained veterinary professionals, making outpatient management with opioid analgesics more challenging. Doses and routes of commonly used opioids are listed in **Table 1**.

Buprenorphine

Buprenorphine is a slow-onset, long-acting synthetic opiate derived from thebaine, an alkaloid of the poppy *Papaver somniferum*.[12] Buprenorphine has partial agonist

Table 1
Opioid analgesic drugs used in hystricomorph rodents

Opioids	Species	Dose, Route, Frequency	Comments
Buprenorphine	Guinea pig	0.05 mg/kg SC q < 6 h	PK and PD study, paw withdrawal pressure test; analgesic efficacy depleted by 6 h or less; may not be effective at this dose[37]
		0.2 mg/kg IV q 6 h	PK study, sedation noted[14]
		0.2 mg/kg OTM q 3–6 h	PK study, sedation noted[14]
	Chinchilla	0.05 and 0.1 mg/kg SC	PD study, paw thermal antinociception, no analgesic effects[16]
		0.2 mg/kg SC	PD study, paw thermal antinociception analgesic effects for 3 h[16]
Buprenorphine: sustained release	Guinea pig	0.15 mg/kg SC q 6 h	PK study, plasma concentrations dropped below 1 ng/mL at 6 h; weight loss and decreased fecal production occurred (Zoopharm, CO, USA)[15]
		0.3 mg/kg SC q 24–48 h	PK and PD study, paw withdrawal pressure test (1 mg/mL; Zoopharm)[37]
		0.3 mg/kg SC q 24–72 h	PK study, more frequent dosing (24 h) needed for females compared with males; weight loss and decreased fecal production occurred (Zoopharm)[15]
		0.48 mg/kg SC q 72–96 h	PD study, laparotomy and von Frey test (Manufacturer: Animalgesic Laboratories, Millersville MD)[10]
		0.6 mg/kg SC q 72 h	PK study, weight loss and decreased fecal production occurred (Zoopharm)[15]
Butorphanol	Guinea pig	0.2–0.4 mg/kg IV loading dose, followed by 0.2–0.4 mg/kg/h as a perioperative CRI	No controlled studies, anecdotal information[20]
		0.5–2 mg/kg IM, SC, IV q 4 h	No controlled studies, anecdotal information[20]

(continued on next page)

Table 1
(continued)

Opioids	Species	Dose, Route, Frequency	Comments
Fentanyl	Guinea pig	5–10 μg/kg IV loading dose, followed by 10–30 μg/kg/h as a perioperative CRI	No controlled studies, anecdotal information[20]
		1.25–5 μg/kg/h IV as a postoperative CRI	No controlled studies, anecdotal information[20]
Hydromorphone	Guinea pig	0.3 mg/kg IV q 2–3 h	PK study[11]
	Chinchilla	0.3 mg/kg IM q 4–5 h	PK study[11]
		0.5 and 1 mg/kg SC	PD study, paw thermal antinociception, no analgesic effects, no sedation, reduced food intake and fecal output (<30%)[19]
		2 mg/kg SC	PD study, paw thermal antinociception, analgesic effects for 2 h, no sedation, transient reduction in food intake and fecal output (<30%)[19]
Morphine	Guinea pig	0.1 mg/kg, preservative free as an epidural	No controlled studies, anecdotal information[20]
		2–5 mg/kg IM, SC q 2–4 h	No controlled studies, anecdotal information[38]
Nalbuphine hydrochloride	Guinea pig	1–2 mg/kg IM 1 2–4 h	No controlled studies, anecdotal only[39]
Oxymorphone	Guinea pig	1–2 mg/kg IM, SC q 6–8 h	No controlled studies, anecdotal information[20]

Abbreviations: CRI, Continuous rate infusion; IM, intramuscular; IV, intravenous; OTM, oral transmucosal; PD, pharmacodynamics; PK, pharmacokinetics; q, every; SC, subcutaneous.

activity at the mu receptor, whereas activity on the kappa and delta receptors is less known but appears to have antagonistic effects.[12] Buprenorphine is considered up to 30 times more potent than morphine and produces dose-dependent analgesic effects[13]; it has a high affinity for mu receptors in the central nervous system, which may contribute to its prolonged duration and increased potency relative to morphine.[13] The liver metabolizes buprenorphine through N-dealkylation and glucuronidation, and 70% of the metabolites are eliminated in feces through biliary excretion, with the remainder being excreted into the urine.[13]

Buprenorphine is prescribed as an injectable using the intravenous (IV), intramuscular (IM), and subcutaneous (SC) routes, or as an oral transmucosal (OTM) analgesic agent; it is commonly used for mild to moderate pain and in combination with other medications as part of preanesthetic protocols. Buprenorphine may not be advantageous for controlling acute pain due to its more prolonged onset of action than other opiates[13]; its efficacy appears to be species specific, mostly likely due to the variety of opioid receptors it affects.[12] In a pharmacokinetic study in guinea pigs at 0.2 mg/kg IV and OTM, sedation effects were variable, but all resolved within 6 hours.[14] Other adverse effects of using buprenorphine may include weight loss and decreased fecal output. In studies evaluating sustained-release buprenorphine in guinea pigs, significant changes in body weight (up to 10% or greater) were observed after dosing, and this change was independent of sex.[10,15] In the study by Zanetti and colleagues[15] in 2017 all animals regained the lost weight within 7 days after drug administration. Additional adverse effects include respiratory depression, which was reported after sustained-release buprenorphine administration in guinea pigs.[15]

In chinchillas, the analgesic efficacy and safety after single and repeated SC dosing have been investigated.[16] At 0.05 and 0.1 mg/kg, SC buprenorphine had no analgesic effects in a thermal nociception model. At 0.2 mg/kg, analgesia was induced for less than 4 hours. In contrast to studies in guinea pigs, no sedative effects were noted in chinchillas at 0.2 mg/kg. Inconsistent effects on food intake and fecal output were reported in chinchillas following single- and multiple-dose administration of buprenorphine. However, even after repeated administration of buprenorphine at 0.2 mg/kg SC every 6 hours for 3 doses, no change in food intake was reported and there was only a transient and mild decrease in fecal output.[16] The administration had no effects on body weight in chinchillas.

Utilizing a sustained-release formulation of buprenorphine has been evaluated in guinea pigs and may be advantageous due to decreased personnel time needed, reduced handling and stress for the patient, and more consistent and sustained drug levels compared with standard formulations if they are dosed too infrequently.[10,17] Disadvantages include variable absorption and high initial plasma concentrations. Sex differences were appreciated when sustained-release buprenorphine was evaluated in guinea pigs. Both sexes reached appropriate plasma concentrations at a high (0.6 mg/kg) dose, whereas only males reached target concentrations with a medium (0.3 mg/kg) dose.[15] Patients administered these sustained-release formulations should be monitored for the first 4 to 8 hours for signs of adverse effects, including sedation, respiratory depression, and/or pica. In addition, the delay between the administration of the drug and the onset of an analgesic response needs to be considered.

Hydromorphone

Hydromorphone is a semisynthetic full mu-opioid receptor agonist that is recommended as a first-choice option to treat moderate to severe pain in dogs and cats.[18] Hydromorphone has high bioavailability and rapid elimination in guinea pigs after

0.3 mg/kg IM administration.[11] Adverse effects that have been reported in other species that may be relevant to hystricomorph rodents include respiratory depression, central nervous system depression, and bradycardia. No sedation or clinically apparent adverse effects were reported after hydromorphone administration in guinea pigs.[11]

In chinchillas, hydromorphone has been evaluated for its analgesic efficacy and safety after SC administration at 0.5, 1, and 2 mg/kg.[19] Only at 2 mg/kg, but not at lower doses, could an analgesic effect be measured in a thermal nociception model. The duration of analgesic effects was less than 4 hours. Food intake was significantly reduced in a dose-dependent manner following the administration of hydromorphone at the doses evaluated, but food intake reduction was less than 30% when compared with the control treatment. Fecal output was reduced by less than 30% for the 1 and 2 mg/kg doses.

Other Opioids

Other opioids used in hystricomorph rodents include butorphanol, nalbuphine, morphine, and oxymorphone. Butorphanol is a mixed agonist/antagonist with low intrinsic activity at the mu receptor, and it has strong agonist activity at the kappa receptor.[20] It is used for mild pain and as a sedative agent, but it has been minimally evaluated in hystricomorph rodents. Butorphanol can be used as a partial reversal agent for mu agonists, but it is a weak antagonist and may increase sedation.[20] Alternatively, nalbuphine is a kappa agonist that can be a more potent antagonist, and there may be residual analgesic effect via the kappa receptors with its use.[20]

TRAMADOL

Tramadol and its major active metabolite, O-desmethyl-tramadol (M1), are centrally acting analgesics that have mu-opioid receptor activity and inhibit the reuptake of norepinephrine and serotonin reuptake centrally.[21] Significant interspecies differences in drug metabolism exist, making it challenging to extrapolate from one species to another. Limited research on the analgesic efficacy and safety of tramadol is available in rodents, and the information is mostly limited to mice and rats with mixed results on analgesic efficacy. The recommended dosages range from 5-40 mg/kg orally or parenterally for rodents.[22–24] However, a safety and efficacy study in chinchillas showed that the SC administration of tramadol between 10-40 mg/kg did not have any analgesic efficacy in a thermal nociception model.[19]

Tramadol's main analgesic effects are due to its action on mu-opioid receptors of its major metabolite O-desmethyltramadol (M1), and differences in metabolism of tramadol have been suggested to be responsible for the variable analgesic effects of tramadol across species. In dogs and horses, limited amounts of M1 are produced, and therefore tramadol is considered to have limited analgesic properties in these species.[25,26] In tramadol-treated rats, M1 plays a significant role in the induced antinociception, whereas tramadol itself has limited effects.[27] No information on the metabolism of tramadol to M1 in chinchillas is available, but limited metabolism to M1 may be a possible explanation why tramadol has no analgesic effects in chinchillas.

At doses greater than 40 mg/kg, SC tramadol showed clinically unacceptable adverse effects in chinchillas. At 60 mg/kg, SC tramadol caused transient severe neurologic adverse effects, consistent with the clinical signs of serotonin syndrome in other species.[28] Therefore, tramadol is not recommended as an analgesic drug in chinchillas. No studies investigating the efficacy or safety of tramadol in guinea pigs have been published. Therefore, tramadol dosages for guinea pigs currently recommended in the literature and used by clinicians are anecdotal and have no proven efficacy.

NON-STEROIDAL ANTI-INFLAMMATORY DRUGS

NSAIDs are commonly used to relieve pain and inflammation in small mammals due to their distinct analgesic, antipyretic, and/or anti-inflammatory properties.[2] Data on the use of NSAIDs for acute postoperative pain are available for a restricted range of agents, including meloxicam and carprofen. Some NSAIDs have been associated with adverse effects. However, these reports appear anecdotal and uncommon for the 2 drugs mentioned (**Table 2**).

Meloxicam

Meloxicam is a drug in the oxicam group that preferentially inhibits the cyclooxygenase (COX)-2 enzyme, and as a result, it has a greater therapeutic range than non- or less-selective COX inhibitors.[29] Meloxicam is widely used in hystricomorphic rodents; however, there are minimal data on its efficacy and safety. It is considered to have potent anti-inflammatory effects, and is well tolerated with fewer adverse effects on the stomach mucosa and renal blood flow, although controlled studies evaluating the adverse effects of meloxicam are lacking.[2] The pharmacokinetics of meloxicam has been evaluated in guinea pigs, and at 1.5 mg/kg PO or IV, the peak plasma concentrations achieved were similar to those in rabbits administered 1 mg/kg PO.[2] Conversely, the terminal elimination half-life was reported to be shorter (3.51 ± 1.11 hours) in guinea pigs compared with rabbits (6–9 hours). This report may suggest that dosing more frequent than every 24 hours is required when administering this drug to guinea pigs; however, further research on the safety of multiple dosing in this species is needed. Meloxicam has a low absolute oral bioavailability (54%) in guinea pigs, which may affect the dose of this drug when administered by this route.[2]

For chinchillas, no evidence-based information on the efficacy and safety of NSAIDs is available. Meloxicam is the most commonly used NSAID in this species.

Other Non-Steroidal Anti-Inflammatory Drugs

Other less-selective COX inhibitors include carprofen and ketoprofen. Carprofen is a weakly nonspecific COX inhibitor that may achieve its therapeutic effects through different pathways, at least in part.[20] Carprofen has been evaluated in a surgical model in guinea pigs. At 4 mg/kg SC every 24 hours for 3 doses, it failed to effectively induce analgesia. Still, this dose was found to enhance buprenorphine's analgesic properties when administered together in a multimodel protocol to guinea pigs.[10] Ketoprofen is a potent, nonselective COX inhibitor with limited pharmacokinetics data in small mammals; it is typically administered parenterally due to challenges in accurately dosing oral formulations.[20]

GABAPENTIN

Gabapentin is a chemical analogue of γ-aminobutyric acid that is most commonly used to treat chronic pain and as an adjunctive therapy for seizures. It is reported to be poorly active against mechanical hyperalgesia in guinea pigs after a single oral dose; however, it was more effective with repeated administration.[30] At the highest dose evaluated, 100 mg/kg by mouth once, administration was associated with flaccidity. Gabapentin's effects appear significantly enhanced when used as part of a multimodal analgesic plan.[31] There is no information on the analgesic efficacy of gabapentin in chinchillas (see **Table 2**).

Table 2
Nonopioid analgesic drugs used in hystricomorph rodents

Drug	Species	Dose, Route, Frequency	Comments
Carprofen	Guinea pig	1 mg/kg SC 4 mg/kg SC q 24 h for 3 days	PD study, ineffective in surgical laparotomy study[7] PD study, castration model; partially effective, more effective if combined with buprenorphine[10]
Meloxicam	Guinea pig	0.3–0.5 mg/kg SC, PO q 24 h 0.2 mg/kg SC q 24 h for 2 days 0.3 mg/kg PO 1.5 mg/kg IV, PO q 12 h	PD study, ineffective[40] PD, study, ineffective when combined with bupivacaine and/or lidocaine[1] PK pilot study, ineffective[2] PK study; when administered PO for 5 d there was no bioaccumulation[2]
Ketoprofen	Guinea pig	1–2 mg/kg SC, IM q 12–24 h	No controlled studies, anecdotal information[20]
Bupivacaine	Guinea pig	1 mg/kg, preservative free as an epidural	No controlled studies, anecdotal information[20]
Gabapentin	Guinea pig	10, 30, 100 mg/kg PO q 12 h × 5 d	PD study, reversed experimentally induced hyperalgesia after multiple doses; 100 mg/kg dose associated with flaccidity; no long-term studies evaluating this drug[30]
Ketamine	Guinea pig	2–5 mg/kg IV loading dose, followed by 1–2 mg/kg/h as a perioperative CRI 0.25–1 mg/kg/h IV as a postoperative CRI	No controlled studies, anecdotal information[20] No controlled studies, anecdotal information[20]
Tramadol	Chinchilla	10, 20, and 40 mg/kg SC 60 mg/kg SC	PD study, paw thermal antinociception no analgesic effects[19] Transient neurological adverse effects, do not use[19]

Abbreviations: IM, intramuscular; IV, intravenous; PD, pharmacodynamics; PK, pharmacokinetics; q, every; SC, subcutaneous.

CANNABIDIOL

Cannabidiol (CBD) is the nonpsychotropic component of the cannabis plant, and it has gained popularity in recent years for its anti-inflammatory and pain-modulating effects.[32] CBD exhibits these effects by acting on the endocannabinoid system, and this biochemical signaling system is thought to play a role in osteoarthritis pathogenesis and analgesia.[33] A pharmacokinetic study by Spittler and colleagues[32] in 2021 evaluating 2 doses (25 and 50 mg/kg) of CBD in an almond oil suspension revealed that parameters increased in a dose-dependent manner in guinea pigs. Based on the pharmacokinetic data, guinea pigs had poor absorption rates of CBD.[32] No changes were noted in behavior, activity parameters, complete blood cell counts, or serum biochemistry panels in the guinea pigs.[32] This was a single dose, single-sex study evaluating young male guinea pigs, and further evaluation, including pharmacodynamics, is necessary in this species.

LOCAL ANESTHETICS

Local anesthetics are used to provide analgesia during, and following, painful procedures; they can be administered as splash blocks, by local infiltration, by blocking specific sensory nerves, and by the epidural or intrathecal routes.[34] Small mammals can be administered small volumes of commercially available formulations, and both lidocaine and bupivacaine can be diluted up to 1:4 with only moderate effects on the duration of action.[35] Local anesthetic agents have a short duration of action, with lidocaine up to 30 minutes and bupivacaine up to 60 minutes.[3] However, sustained-release formulations of bupivacaine are commercially available and can be successfully used in hystricomorphic rodents to achieve a longer duration of analgesic effects. Additional information and a succinct summary on the use of local anesthetics can be found elsewhere.[36]

MULTIMODAL ANALGESIA

Multimodal analgesia combines multiple agents with different mechanisms of action into a treatment plan, which often results in increased efficacy while using lower doses of the individual agents. Unfortunately, studies using multimodal analgesia are lacking in hystricomorph rodents. One study performed in guinea pigs undergoing ovariohysterectomy procedures was treated at induction with an extended-release formulation of buprenorphine, carprofen, or multimodal treatment.[10] The frequency of pain-related behaviors was reduced in the multimodal group compared with buprenorphine or carprofen alone. Evaluating analgesic efficacy can be complicated by species, pain model used, and environment where the patient is being assessed. Further studies evaluating multimodal therapies and alternative doses and dosing frequencies are needed to provide better options for analgesia.

SUMMARY

Pain in hystricomorph rodents can be managed effectively, as in other species. There is a need for further evaluation of available analgesic medications, both pharmacokinetically evaluating routes and doses and pharmacodynamically to determine clinical effectiveness. The use of multimodal approaches to analgesia has been underreported in hystricomorph rodents, and the expansion of data in this area will lead to significant advances in preventing and alleviating pain in these species.

CLINICS CARE POINTS

- Multimodal analgesic studies are lacking in hystricomorph rodents, and are an area that should be focused on in future research.

- Cannabidiol studies have been minimal in guinea pigs, and no information on cannabidiol in chinchillas is available.

- There is a lack of pharmacokinetic and pharmacodynamic studies for multiple analgesic medications in guinea pigs and chinchillas, including butorphanol, fentanyl, morphine, nalbuphine hydrochloride, oxymorphone, ketoprofen, bupivicaine, and ketamine.

REFERENCES

1. Ellen Y, Flecknell P, Leach M. Evaluation of using behavioural changes to assess postoperative pain in the guinea pig (Cavia Porcellus). PLoS One 2016;11:1–20.
2. Moeremans I, Devreese M, De Baere S, et al. Pharmacokinetics and absolute oral bioavailability of meloxicam in guinea pigs (Cavia porcellus). Vet Anal Anesth 2019;46:548–55.
3. Foley PL, Kendall LV, Turner PV. Clinical Management of Pain in Rodents. J Am Assoc Lab Anim Sci 2019;69:468–89.
4. Kest B, Wilson SG, Mogil JS. Sex differences in supraspinal morphine analgesia are dependent on genotype. J Pharmacol Exp Ther 1999;289:1370–5.
5. Mogil JS, Wilson SG, Bon K, et al. Heritability of nociception I: responses of 11 inbred mouse strains on 12 measures of nociception. Pain 1999;80:67–82.
6. Bays TB. Guinea pig behavior. In: Bays TB, Lightfoot T, Mayer J, editors. Exotic pet behavior: birds, reptiles, and small animals. St Louis: Saunders Elsevier; 2006. p. 207–38.
7. Dunbar ML, David EM, Aline MR, et al. Validation of a behavioral ethogram for assessing postoperative pain in guinea pigs (Cavia porcellus). J Am Assoc Lab Anim Sci 2016;55:29–34.
8. Leach MC, Coulter CA, Richardson CA, et al. Are we looking in the wrong place? Implications for behavioral-based pain assessment in rabbits (Oryctolagus cuniculi) and beyond? PLoS One 2011;6:e13347.
9. Leach MC, Allweiler S, Richardson C, et al. Behavioural effects of ovariohysterectomy and oral administration of meloxicam in laboratory-housed rabbits. Res Vet Sci 2009;87:336–47.
10. Oliver VL, Athavale S, Simon KE, et al. Evaluation of pain assessment techniques and analgesia efficacy in a female guinea pig (Cavia porcellus) model of surgical pain. J Am Assoc Lab Anim Sci 2017;56:425–35.
11. Ambros B, Knych HK, Sadar MJ. Pharmacokinetics of hydromorphone hydrochloride after intravenous and intramuscular administration in guinea pigs (Cavia porcellus). Am J Vet Res 2020;81:361–6.
12. Rockwell K. Therapeutic review: buprenorphine. J Exot Pet Med 2019;30:12–6.
13. Plumb DC. Buprenorphine. In: Plumb's veterinary drug handbook. Stockholm: PharmaVet; 2017. p. 181–3.
14. Sadar MJ, Knych HK, Drazenovich TL, et al. Pharmacokinetics of buprenorphine after intravenous and oral transmucosal administration in guinea pigs (Cavia porcellus). Am J Vet Res 2018;79:260–6.

15. Zanetti AS, Putta SK, Casebolt DB, et al. Pharmacokinetics and adverse effects of 3 sustained-release buprenorphine dosages in healthy guinea pigs (Cavia porcellus). J Am Assoc Lab Anim Sci 2017;56:768–78.
16. Fox L, Mans C. Analgesic efficacy and safety of buprenorphine in chinchillas (Chinchilla lanigera). J Am Assoc Lab Anim Sci 2018;57:286–90.
17. Foley PL. Current options for providing sustained analgesia to laboratory animals. Lab Anim (NY) 2014;43:364–71.
18. Pettifer G, Hydromorphone DD. A cost-effective alternative to the use of oxymorphone. Can Vet J 2000;41:135–7.
19. Evenson EA, Mans C. Analgesic efficacy and safety of hydromorphone in chinchillas (Chinchilla lanigera). J Am Assoc Lab Anim Sci 2018;57:282–5.
20. Hawkins M, Pascoe PJ. Anesthesia, analgesia, and sedation of small mammals. In: Quesenberry KE, Orcutt CJ, Mans C, et al, editors. Ferrets, rabbits, and rodents: clinical medicine and surgery. 4th edition. St. Louis: Elsevier; 2020. p. 536–58.
21. Lewis KS, Han NH. Tramadol: a new centrally acting analgesic. Am J Health Syst Pharm 1997;54:643–52.
22. Mayer J. Rodents. In: Carpenter JW, editor. Exotic animal formulary. 2nd edition. St. Louis: Elsevier; 2013. p. 494.
23. Guzman-Silva MA, Pollastri CE, Pantaleao JAS, et al. Tramadol minimizes potential pain during post-oophorectomy in Wistar rats. Altern Anim Exp 2007;14:91–2.
24. Tsai YC, Sung YH, Chang PJ, et al. Tramadol relieves thermal hyperalgesia in rats with chronic constriction injury of the sciatic nerve. Fundam Clin Pharmacol 2000; 14:335–40.
25. KuKanich B, Wiese AJ. Opioids. In: Grimm KA, Lamont LA, TRanquillie WJ, editors. Lumb & jones' veterinary anesthesia and analgesia. 5th edition. Ames: Wiley; 2015. p. 207–26.
26. Delgado C, Bentley E, Hetzel S, et al. Comparison of carprofen and tramadol for postoperative analgesia in dogs undergoing enucleation. J Am Vet Med Assoc 2015;245:1375–81.
27. Garrido MJ, Sayar O, Segura C, et al. Pharmacokinetic/pharmacodynamic modeling of the antinociceptive effects of (+)-tramadol in the rat: role of cytochrome P450 2D activity. J Pharmacol Exp Ther 2003;305:710–8.
28. Beakley BD, Kaye AM, Kaye AD. Tramadol, Pharmacology, Side Effects, and Serotonin Syndrome: A Review. Pain Physician 2015;18:395–400.
29. Ogino K, Hatanaka K, Kawamura M, et al. Evaluation of pharmacological profile of meloxicam as an anti-inflammatory agent, with particular reference to its relative selectivity for cyclooxygenase-2 over cyclooxygenase-1. Pharmacology 1997;55:44–53.
30. Fox A, Gentry C, Patel S, et al. Comparative activity of the anticonvulsants oxcarbazepine, carbamazepine, lamotrigine and gabapentin in a model of neuropathic pain in the rat and guinea pig. Pain 2003;105:355–62.
31. Corona-Ramos J, De la O-Arciniega M, Déciga-Campos M, et al. The antinociceptive effects of tramadol and/or gabapentin on rat neuropathic pain induced by a chronic constriction injury. Drug Dev Res 2016;77:217–26.
32. Spittler AP, Helbling JE, McGrath S, et al. Plasma and joint tissue pharmacokinetics of two doses of oral cannabidiol oil in guinea pigs (Cavia porcellus). J Vet Pharmacol Ther 2021;44:967–74.
33. O'Brien M, McDougall JJ. Cannabis and joints: Scientific evidence for the alleviation of osteoarthritis pain by cannabinoids. Curr Opin Pharmacol 2018;40: 104–9.

34. Flecknell PA. Rodent analgesia: Assessment and therapeutics. Vet J 2018; 232:70–7.
35. Grant GJ, Piskoun B, Lin A, et al. An in vivo method for the quantitative evaluation of local anesthetics. J Pharmacol Toxicol Methods 2000;43:69–72.
36. DiGeronimo PM, da Cunha AF. Local and regional anesthesia in zoological companion animal practice. Vet Clin Exot Anim Pract 2022;25:321–36.
37. Smith BJ, Wegenast DJ, Hansen RJ, et al. Pharmacokinetics and paw withdrawal pressure in female guinea pigs (Cavia porcellus) treated with sustained-release buprenorphine and buprenorphine hydrochloride. J Am Assoc Lab Anim Sci 2016;55:789–93.
38. Flecknell PA. Guinea pigs. In: Meredith A, Redrobe S, editors. BSAVA manual of exotic pets. 4th ed. Gloucester: BSAVA; 2002. p. 52–64.
39. Flecknell PA. Analgesia and post-operative care. In: Flecknell PA, editor. Laboratory animal anaesthesia. 3rd edition. London: Academic Press, Elsevier; 2009. p. 139–79.
40. Gleeson M, Hawkins MG, Howerton CL, et al. Evaluating postoperative parameters in guinea pigs (Cavia porcellus) following routine orchiectomy. J Exot Pet Med 2016;25:242–52.

Pain Recognition in Rabbits

Amy L. Miller, PhD[a],*, Matthew C. Leach, MSc, PhD[b]

KEYWORDS

- Rabbit • Pain assessment • Behavior • Rabbit grimace scale

KEY POINTS

- The use of a one-way viewing screen or video link should be considered when carrying out observational pain assessment of rabbits to avoid freezing behavior in the presence of an unfamiliar caregiver.
- Even where possible a multi-modal approach to the assessment of rabbit pain should be employed, which should include:
  - Observations to determine the presence of key pain-associated behaviors such as wincing, flinching and staggering.
  - The Rabbit Grimace scale (RbtGS) to determine the presence of pain and the effectiveness of analgesia administered.
- Whenever possible, baseline scores (i.e., when the animal is not painful) should be recorded as a comparator for postprocedure scores. If this is not possible, the implementation of the multi-modal assessment approach is strongly advised.

INTRODUCTION

Rabbits are popular companion animals, common laboratory animal, and farmed species globally. In the UK, 1 million rabbits are kept as companion animals[1] due to their small size and temperament. Additionally, over 11,000 are used in regulated scientific procedures each year.[2] In 2007, it was estimated that in the USA there were 6 million pet rabbits,[3] although this estimate has reduced to around 2.2 million in 2016.[4] As a consequence of their popularity, rabbits undergo a significant number of both advanced and routine surgical procedures in veterinary clinics and therefore, the requirement for appropriate pain assessment and alleviation is greater than ever. Most rabbits will undergo at least one potentially painful procedure during their lifetime, with routine neutering being one of the most common. Historically, pain relief has been administered less frequently to rabbits than other popular companion species such as cats and dogs[5,6] and has also been administered suboptimally in laboratory rabbits.[7,8] This lack of provision of appropriate analgesia may be in part linked to

[a] School of Health and Life Sciences, Teesside University, Middlesbrough Tower, Middlesbrough, TS1 3BX, United Kingdom; [b] School of Natural and Environmental Sciences, Newcastle University, Agriculture Building, Newcastle Upon Tyne, NE1 7RU
* Corresponding author.
E-mail address: a.miller@tees.ac.uk

Vet Clin Exot Anim 26 (2023) 187–199
https://doi.org/10.1016/j.cvex.2022.07.007
1094-9194/23/© 2022 Elsevier Inc. All rights reserved.

the limited amount of research that has been carried out to develop and validate methods of pain assessment in this species.[9] Without an accurate method of pain assessment, the efficacy of any analgesia provided cannot be determined and suboptimal care may result. This unalleviated pain in companion rabbits' compromises welfare, impedes recovery[10,11] and could result in significant stress for owners and care providers.[12]

RECOGNIZING PAIN IN RABBITS

In a familiar low-stress environment, normal rabbits are typically alert, active, and inquisitive.[13] When in pain, they may appear apprehensive, anxious, or dull.[14] Conversely, it has also been noted that when painful they may show aggressive behavior, whereas activity may be increased alongside increased scratching or licking.[14] Rabbits will frequently scan their environment and will attempt to flee or hide if any danger is perceived[15] e.g., in the presence of an unfamiliar caregiver. In a clinical scenario where escape is not possible, rabbits may freeze thus masking signs of pain or discomfort.[16] Freezing is thought to be a behavioral adaption to avoid attracting the attention of predators.[15] This type of behavior poses a significant challenge when assessing pain in rabbits as direct observation is difficult. It can result in masking of pain-specific behaviors or changes in general activity levels.[17] To ensure pain is appropriately assessed and treated in rabbits, the absence of clear signs should not be taken to indicate the absence of pain or distress and further observations should be made.

Effective recognition and assessment of pain in any species are challenging; however, in prey species such as rabbits, the challenge is even greater.[18] When considering companion rabbits, much can be taken from methods developed to assess pain in laboratory rabbits, where research staff have an ethical, and in many countries, a legal requirement to reduce to an absolute minimum any pain experienced by rabbits enrolled on studies e.g. Animals (Scientific Procedures) Act 1986 (UK), European Directive 2010/63 (EU), Animal Welfare Act (USA). There have been various studies carried out that have aimed to determine the most effective means of assessing pain in rabbits in a controlled environment and key studies are discussed here. By having a validated means of assessing pain, we can then determine if any analgesic administered to an individual rabbit is effective in preventing, or at least reducing any pain experienced.

SUBJECTIVE AND OBJECTIVE CLINICAL SIGNS

Various indicators can be of value when assessing pain in rabbits, although they should be used with caution as they may not be pain specific and could be the results of e.g. stress or fear.

In rabbits, the presence of pain can result in decreased gastrointestinal motility,[19] potentially leading to life-threatening condition, if not detected quickly. Rabbits with reduced gastrointestinal motility often reduce their food intake, thus further exacerbating the situation and can lead to enterotoxemia. Reductions in food intake can go undetected if animals are fed *ad libitum* and changes in their intake may be subsequently detected as a reduction in body weight. While important to monitor food and water consumption, relying on this measure to assess pain is not recommended in isolation due to its retrospective nature and could result in a significant period when a rabbit goes untreated. Linked to a decrease in food consumption, fecal output has also been observed to sharply decrease in the 2 days immediately following surgery.[20] In this study rabbits were provided with hay and this practice is recommended during the postoperative period to help maintain gastrointestinal motility.[20] While it is possible to manually weigh fecal matter to quantify the level of waste produced, Weaver and colleagues[20] developed a fecal output scoring system which is designed to be used by all staff in the clinic, irrespective of the level of experience, to rapidly quantify fecal output. Scoring is on a 5-point scale and accounts for both the amount and formation of the droppings present in the pen/cage (For full details of the scoring system, see Weaver and colleagues[20]). While again retrospective, it is a useful tool to provide additional evidence of welfare status in rabbits following surgery or injury and can be used, following a short period of training, by various staff members to monitor the rabbits when pain is likely to be present and determine if further intervention is required.

Vocalizations have been observed to occur in rabbits when they are in significant acute pain,[15] and although teeth grinding may occur when experiencing discomfort,[11] this can be difficult to differentiate from quiet grinding that can occur when the rabbit is content.[15] Further research is required to determine how clinically useful these are as indicators of pain in rabbits and how such measures could be used effectively in a clinical setting.

In a clinical setting, rabbits may often be housed individually, but in some cases, they may be kept in groups with litter mates or household companions. When housed in a group, an animal in pain may move away from companions and remain isolated at the rear of the cage or in an enclosed space within a pen if one is available. Any change in the typical level or type of interaction between familiar conspecifics should be noted as an indicator of a change in welfare status and could indicate that the rabbit is painful.

BEHAVIORAL ASSESSMENT

Observing and quantifying spontaneous behavior has been used successfully in pain assessment following surgery in various laboratory species such as rats,[21] guinea pigs[22] and also companion species including cats[23] and dogs.[24] Typically, when an animal is in pain, we see a reduction in exploratory and locomotory behaviors along with the exhibition of new, abnormal behaviors that are not usually observed in pain-free animals. These new behaviors have been termed "pain behaviors" and typically occur only when an animal is presumed to be experiencing pain, occur at a relatively low frequency, and are often subtle in nature.

Leach and colleagues carried out one of the first studies to develop a behavioral pain assessment system for rabbits following a routine surgical procedure, ovariohysterectomy. This study demonstrated that a range of spontaneous behavioral changes occurred in the immediate hours following surgery, including increased periods of inactivity coupled with the presence of abnormal behaviors such as twitching, wincing, and staggering (**Table 1** for full definitions of these behaviors)16. These pain behaviors are not observed in pain-free animals, are typically very short in duration and only observed in the hours immediately following surgery and seem to occur relatively infrequently e.g. around 10–14 instances in a 20-minute period.[16] This demonstrates both the importance of being familiar with these abnormal behaviors, but also ensuring that the rabbits are observed for long enough to ensure that these subtle changes in their behavior are detected. Viewing for too short a period could lead to these key indicators being missed and the assumption that the rabbit is not experiencing discomfort. A similar study, which also aimed to identify behaviors that could be used to assess pain in male rabbits being neutered[25] concluded that key indicators of pain in rabbits include a reduction in levels of normal locomotory behaviors such as searching and

Table 1
Specific behaviors that have been shown to significantly change, in a research setting, following abdominal surgery or tattooing

Behavior	Definition	Direction of Change When in Pain	References
Twitching	Rapid contraction back muscles/movement fur	Increase	Leach et al,[16] 2009 Miller et al,[27] 2022 Roughan et al[39] 2004
Flinching	Body jerks upwards	Increase	Leach et al,[16] 2009 Miller et al,[27] 2022 Roughan et al,[39] 2004 Farnworth et al,[25] 2011
Wincing	Rapid movement of body backwards plus eye closing & swallowing action	Increase	Leach et al,[16] 2009 Miller et al,[27] 2022 Farnworth et al,[25] 2011
Staggering	Partial loss of balance	Increase	Leach et al,[16] 2009 Miller et al,[27] 2022 Farnworth et al,[25] 2011
Belly press	Abdomen pushed toward the floor	Increase	Leach et al,[16] 2009 Miller et al,[27] 2022 NRC[14] 2009
Back arching	Upwards arch of the back	Increase	Leach et al,[16] 2009 Miller et al,[27] 2022 Farnworth et al,[25] NRC[14]
Searching	Explore pen with nose	Decrease	Leach et al,[16] 2009 Farnworth et al,[25] 2011
Movement duration	Locomotion around pen	Decrease	Leach et al,[16] 2009 Keating et al,[32] Weaver et al[20]
Consumption	Food & drink consumption	Decrease	Leach et al,[16] 2009 Farnworth et al,[25] 2011
Rearing	On hind limbs with forelimbs raised from the ground	Decrease	Leach et al,[16] Keating et al,[32] Weaver et al,[20] Farnworth et al[25]
Inactive	Still with the exhibition of no distinct behavior	Increase	Leach et al,[16] 2009 Kohn et al,[11] 2007 Goldschlager et al,[40] 2013
Grooming	Directed maintenance of fur	Increase or decrease	Keating et al,[32] 2012 Farnworth et al,[25] 2011 NRC[14] 2009
Shuffle	Slow shuffle movement of hind limbs one at a time	Increase	Farnworth et al,[25] 2011
Writhing	Contraction of abdominal muscles	Increase	Flecknell & Waterman-Pearson,[41] 2000 NRC[14] 2009

Note: Miller et al (2022) combined back arching, belly press, twitching, flinching, wincing, and staggering into a combined composite behavioral score for analysis rather than comparing the changes in individual behaviors over time.

rearing and an increase in typically unseen behaviors/"pain behaviors" such as flinching, wincing and back arching.

A drawback associated with behavioral pain assessment is that it can be highly labor intensive and time-consuming, posing a significant limitation, in particular when the animal is not familiar to the caregiver. Ensuring enough time has been spent to detect the presence of these abnormal pain behaviors, if they are present is critical. An additional problem associated with behavioral assessment in rabbits is the freezing response. While this reduced locomotion can be associated with pain,[16] it can also occur due to distress or discomfort and is commonly displayed in the presence of an observer or unfamiliar environment.[26] This can be overcome by remote viewing of animals. Many research studies where pain assessment and analgesic efficacy have been studied in rabbits have made use of a remote viewing setup[e.g.16,27] A typical setup consists of rabbits housed individually in floor pens to allow clear observations. While not always possible in a clinical environment, the use of one-way glass (or film) offers a viable alternative and the use of high-definition video cameras can also be implemented for remote viewing. Research studies have also demonstrated that providing a familiar companion rabbit to be located next to or with the rabbit (if a pen mate) being assessed, to further promote the exhibition and reduce incidences of freezing.

Weaver and colleagues[20] also aimed to determine relevant indicators of postsurgical pain in rabbits, but rather than focus specifically on "pain behaviors," opted to document changes in normal active behaviors. Their study focused on female New Zealand White rabbits, a common laboratory breed. Blinded observers scored behavior and food consumption in the days immediately prior to and after surgery. As with other studies, a significant reduction in activity and inappetence were seen following surgery. Rearing and distance traveled were still below baseline levels at 7 days postsurgery, while other indicators such as water consumption had returned to presurgery levels by day 5 following surgery. This highlights the importance of having a good knowledge of the usual activity levels of the individual, and the need to liaise with owners to ascertain any changes in the activity levels of their rabbits either following surgery or at other times when the animal is potentially experiencing pain. Monitoring food and water consumption is important but is also retrospective meaning that they have reduced value as a means of pain immediately at the cage or pen side, as by the time you identify a change in these parameters then several hours will have passed. Consequently, earlier indications of compromises to welfare, such as those provided by monitoring of activity levels, offer a significant advantage.

In these controlled research studies, various key behaviors have been identified as being of importance when assessing pain, postpainful procedures in rabbits. A summary of these key changes is shown in **Table 1**.

To be able to able to successfully use spontaneous behavior to assess pain in rabbits, training staff to be confident in identifying these key pain behaviors and also focus on the correct area of the body when observing the rabbits is essential.[28] Most of the subtle pain behaviors identified thus far occur on the back, abdomen or hindquarters of the animal so viewing these particular locations on the body is imperative. A study by Leach and colleagues[28] used eye-tracking software to determine exactly where observers were looking when viewing video footage of rabbits to assess pain. Interestingly, irrespective of the level of experience in working with rabbits, overwhelmingly observers focused first, more frequently, and for longer on the face of the rabbit than on other areas of the body.[28] This has the potential to result in some of these more subtle and infrequent pain behaviors that have been described, being missed during periods of observation, and introduces the potential for rabbits in pain to go undetected. Time spent focusing on the face is unlikely to be effective if observers are intending to score behaviors such as those identified in **Table 1**. Therefore, making observers aware of where they are looking can support the successful implementation of behaviors based on scoring in the clinical, pen-side environment.

THE RABBIT GRIMACE SCALE

As already noted, Leach and colleagues[28] found that when observing rabbits, assessors typically spend significant amounts of time focused on the face of the animal. While this may impede the detection of subtle changes in the behavior such as twitches or writhes, it may offer an advantage when assessing pain using a grimace scale. Historically, grimace scales have been used as the "gold standard" when assessing pain in nonverbal humans, including the very young.[29] When assessing pain in humans, a characteristic "pain face" has been described, consisting of specific musculature movements in the face when a noxious stimulus is applied.[30] Each individual muscular movement on the face is termed a "facial action unit" (FAUs) and facial expressions are comprised of one or more action units. A subset of action units has been shown to be associated with pain, and changes in each of these individual action units can be quantified. When presented with a face or image of a face, by scoring each of these FAUs, the presence of pain can be scored.[30] In 2010, the first example of this type of work in nonhuman animals was published. The mouse grimace scale (MGS) a novel method of pain assessment in mice was first described.[31] This scale was found to be effective in detecting acute pain in laboratory mice following a range of procedures, including surgery. Since then, grimace scales have been developed for a number of species, including rabbits (RbtGS).[32] The Rabbit Grimace Scale (RbtGS) consists of 5 Facial Action Units (FAUs); orbital tightening, cheek flattening, nostril shape, whisker shape, and position and ear shape and position. A 3-point scale is used to score the intensity that each of these FAUs exhibited, i.e. each action unit is scored as either "Not present" (score of 0), "Moderately present" (score of 1), or "Obviously present" (score of 2). Animals are scored for each action unit and then a summary score is calculated and used to assess the level of pain experienced by a rabbit and changes over time can be determined, with higher scores being associated with pain. The summary score is either [1] the sum of all the FAUs or the average of all of the FAUs. The former is easier to use on the cage side and the latter is less sensitive when a particular action cannot be scored. **Fig. 1** shows the 5 FAUs that make up the RbtGS and provides guidance on how each FAU is scored on the 3-point scale.

One of the benefits of grimace scale scoring is that it is significantly less time-consuming than standard behavioral analysis, therefore, has the potential to allow more rapid means of assessing pain and is potentially more practical in a clinical scenario. Since humans have a natural tendency to look at the faces of animals, rather than their body,[28] assessing facial expressions may also be an easier method to implement. It has also been noted that staff can be trained to accurately implement grimace scales in pain assessment with interrater reliability being high in various species, including rabbits.[31,33]

Ear tattooing is a commonly used method of permanent identification for laboratory and companion rabbits around the world and is likely to be a painful procedure.[32] Keating and colleagues[32] used ear tattooing to develop and then validate the RbtGS and demonstrated that immediately following ear tattooing, RbtGS scores in New Zealand White rabbits increased, alongside changes in blood pressure and vocalizations. The application of the local anesthetic cream EMLA to the ears of the rabbits in advance of tattooing mitigated these changes further validating the RbtGS as a means

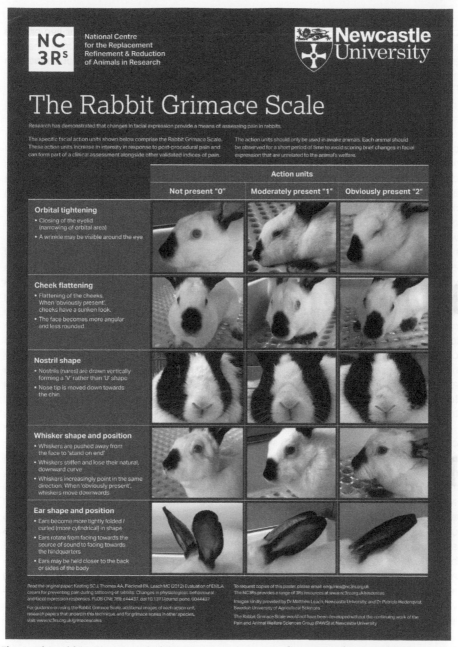

Fig. 1. The rabbit grimace scale (RbtGS), example images for scores of 0, 1, and 2 for each of the 5 facial action units. From Keating and colleagues.[32] (The Rabbit Grimace Scale. Poster designed and produced by NC3Rs.)

of assessing pain. A recent study by Miller and colleagues[27] aimed to evaluate pain following routine castration in 2 breeds of rabbit (Dutch Belted & New Zealand White) and to determine if the RbtGS provided an effective and rapid means of assessing pain following a routine surgical procedure. This study also evaluated if there was variation between 2 methods of applying the RbtGS: 1. scoring from video, akin to a live clinical situation using a remote viewing technique and 2. retrospectively from still images, akin to the majority of studies that have been used to assess analgesia in laboratory animals. One hour following surgery, both breeds of rabbits showed increases in RbtGS scores that closely correlated with changes in spontaneous pain behaviors, indicating the utility of the RbtGS in pain assessment which could be used in a clinical scenario.

However, the evidence supporting the clinical utility of grimace scales in many species remains mixed. For example, live grimace scale scoring has been compared to retrospective scoring of images in laboratory mice[34] where live scores were significantly lower than retrospective scores from images at baseline. In contrast, Leung and colleagues[35] compared the rat grimace scale scores in a live vs retrospective manner and found that both methods could successfully discriminate between analgesia treated vs control rats following intraplantar carrageenan injection and scores were reflective of each other. In mice, it has been noted that MGS scores do vary between strains of mice when no pain is present[34] i.e., baseline scores are not always zero. This variation in baseline score has not to date been studied in rabbits. While variation has been described between methods of grimace scale data collection and between baseline scores within a species, what these studies do all demonstrate is that when a consistent method of assessment is used, grimace scale scores do increase when animals are presumed to be painful. While not always possible in a clinical situation, the ability to collect preprocedure RbtGS scores to act as a direct comparator following a painful procedure would be a significant advantage in determining the level of pain experienced and the benefit of any analgesic intervention administered. Where this type of preprocedure scoring is not possible, comparison to scores of another individual of the same sex and breed could be made with caution, to support other indices of pain such as behavior and clinical signs.

To date, the RbtGS has only been assessed in a very limited number of acute procedures. Consequently, further research into the use of the RBtGS in a clinical scenario where other procedures leading to acute and chronic pain are studied is needed. Breeds of rabbits with lop ears poise a further potential issue for this scale, in the FAU ear shape and position are more difficult to assess. This can be dealt with in 2 ways. [1] These breeds should only be scored using the 4 remaining FAUs and the summary score adjusted accordingly, e.g. use the mean across the FAUs or a reduced total (8 rather than 10). (2) Although the movement and shape of the ears are compromised by the lop trait, the position of the ears can still be judged based on the tension in the muscles at the base of the ears. Where baseline or preanalgesia assessment of the RbtGS is not possible, a multi-modal approach (i.e., using multiple indices) is highly recommended, such as a composite pain scale where various parameters are considered and the requirement for a comparator score is less important.

COMPOSITE PAIN SCALES

Composite pain scales take into account various behavioral and physiological parameters when assessing pain. The first composite pain scale, developed specifically for rabbits was the CANCRS which was designed specifically for the clinical environment and appropriate to be used with various breeds.[33] CANCRS merged the RbtGS and behavior with various clinical parameters to produce a multidimensional pain scale. Interrater reliability between veterinarians and veterinary medicine students were found to be very good and demonstrates the potential utility of this scale in the clinical environment. In the development of this composite pain scale, time to implement was also considered and the mean length of time to assess a rabbit using CANCRS was 3.4 minutes[33]—thus potentially a more rapid means of assessment than full remote behavioral observation provided a suitably trained caregiver is present to accurately assess the rabbit. Full details of the parameters and scoring system are shown in **Table 2**. Following assessment, the sum of all scored parameters is used to inform on pain assessment. Final scores of 0–5 were classified as "no pain," scores of 6–11 were classified as "discomfort," scores of 12–17 were classified as "moderate pain" and scores of >18 were classified as "severe pain." The CANCRS was further evaluated to determine its responsiveness into detecting a change in pain scores following analgesic treatment in rabbits with abdominal pain.[36] Here, they weighted each of the parameters from their original CANCRS scale and eliminated those with low sensitivity in this particular clinical situation. It was concluded that "respiratory pattern" and vocalization should not be used when assessing abdominal pain in rabbits, but should be considered, with additional research required, for assessing other specific conditions.[36]

Recently a further composite pain scale has been developed: the Bristol rabbit pain scale (BRPS),[18] a similar scale to that available for cats[37] and horses.[38] Through specialist focus groups, key descriptors thought to be associated with pain were listed and then used direct observation of rabbits following ovariohysterectomy or orchidectomy, these descriptors were confirmed to occur more frequently postprocedure compared to preprocedure. Equally, behaviors thought not to be associated with pain were assessed to confirm that they occurred more frequently presurgical procedure compared to postsurgical procedure. The final list of behaviors that were deemed to change in response to pain, had a definition that was not deemed to be ambiguous and could be assessed over a relatively short period of time were taken forward to form the BRPS. Internal consistency of observers was also assessed to confirm the utility of this new scale. The BRPS is shown in **Table 3** and consists of 6 categories, each of which can be scored on a 4-point scale and used in the assessment of rabbits following ovariohysterectomy or orchidectomy surgery. The rabbit to be assessed is observed for 3 minutes and then the cage/pen is quietly approached, and a score (0–3) is determined for each of the 6 categories. The score is based on what the rabbit is observed to do for most of the assessment period. A score between 0 and 21 will then be recorded.

Table 2
CANCRS composite rabbit pain scale–adapted from Banchi et al[33]

Category	Parameter to Score	Score Range
Rabbit Grimace Scale	Orbital tightening	0–2
	Cheek flattening	0–2
	Nostril shape	0–2
	Whisker shape and position	0–2
	Ear shape and position	0–2
Clinical Parameters	Pupil dilation	0–1
	Heart rate % increase (based on 250bpm)	0–2
	Respiratory rate (based on 60 breaths per min)	0–2
	Respiratory pattern	0–1
	Palpation of the painful area	0–2
	Mental status	0–2
	Vocalizations	0–3

Table 3
Final version of the Bristol Rabbit pain scale–adapted from Benato et al[18]

Category	Score 0	Score 1	Score 2	Score 3
Demeanor	Looking around, alert and responsive to surrounding environment OR is asleep	Awake but shows little interest in the surrounding environment	Dull and is not responsive to the observer or surrounding environment	Unresponsive to observer or surrounding environment, even if approached
Locomotion	Active and hopping around the area OR is asleep	Appears hesitant to move and shows little activity	Inactive and does not move during the observation period, except when approached	Inactive and does not move at all, even when approached
Posture	Resting in a relaxed and comfortable posture e.g., lying on a flank or on its front with hind legs to the side OR is moving freely OR is asleep	Sitting or lying on its front with visible forelegs	Sitting or lying on its front with its legs under the body and appears hunched	Sitting or lying in front with legs under body. The body looks tense, stiff, and hunched OR pressing the abdomen to the ground.
Ears Note: lop eared rabbits may show less pronounced changed	Moves ears freely and turns them toward sounds OR is asleep	Moves and slightly turns ears toward sound	No obvious movement of ears reacts slightly to sounds e.g. with a heard turn	Does not move ears at all and does not react to sounds OR ears are flattened against the back
Eyes	Has eyes open OR is asleep	Eyes remain semiclosed	Eyes remain closed	Eyes remain closed and tightened
Grooming	Meticulous grooming OR is asleep	Grooming but gets distracted easily	Attempting to groom, but with little energy	No grooming at all

The development of this species-specific scale, incorporating a range of relevant and expert informed indices provides a tool that has the potential to improve acute pain assessment in rabbits following further work to validate in a clinical environment and also for its use following other routine surgical procedures.[18]

SUMMARY

The nature of rabbits as a prey species makes pain assessment particularly challenging as they are reluctant to show any signs of weakness/abnormal behavior in the presence of an unfamiliar observer. The presence of pain in rabbits leads to significant compromises to welfare, increased recovery times, secondary complications such as ileus and also stress for caregivers. Fewer research studies have been undertaken to date to assess and validate appropriate means of pain assessment in rabbits than found in other companion or laboratory species. In the last few years, increasing research priority has been given to rabbits due to their popularity as companion species and also the ethical and legal responsibilities of researchers who work with rabbits e.g.[17,27] Hopefully this work can be further built upon to further validate and establish key pain indices in several rabbit breeds for a range of common painful procedures/injuries. In scenarios where rabbits are enrolled on scientific projects, the presence of pain can also lead to increased variability within the data set, compromising data quality. Appropriate steps should be taken to implement validated pain assessment techniques that we do have, alongside continual monitoring, to determine when rabbits are experiencing pain and if measures to alleviate this pain are effective.

CLINICS CARE POINTS

- Provide a quiet area for the rabbits which has a remote viewing set up (e.g., cameras, one-way window, and so forth) to reduce the likelihood of freezing behavior if an unfamiliar caregiver is assessing the animal. Where possible, the use of high-definition video cameras (readily available and low cost now), in multiple locations to allow subtle changes in behavior to be detected and allow for rabbit grimace scale scoring to be carried out effectively.

- When rabbits are undergoing elective procedures and/or prior to analgesia administration, collect baseline behavioral and facial expression scores to allow changes to be quantified. Note: analgesia should not be withheld to allow scoring when it is thought a rabbit is experiencing pain.

- Where baseline assessment and remote viewing of rabbits is not possible, the use of a composite pain scale should be considered to incorporate a range of relevant information in the clinical environment.

REFERENCES

1. Pet Population report PFMA. Pet Population report 2022. https://www.pfma.org.uk/pet-population-2022. Accessed August 15, 2022.
2. Home Office. Statistics of Scientific Procedures on living animals, Great Britain 2018. UK government document publised by the Home Office. Available at: https://www.gov.uk/government/statistics/statistics-of-scientific-procedures-on-living-animals-great-britain-2018. Accessed August 15, 2022.
3. American Veterinary Medical Association (AVMA) U.S. Pet ownership & demographics sourcebook. 2007. Available at: https://www.avma.org/resources/reports-statistics/market-research-statistics-us-pet-ownership-2007. Accessed August 15, 2022.
4. American Veterinary Medical Association (AVMA) U.S. Pet ownership & demographics sourcebook. 2018. Available at: https://www.avma.org/resources-tools/reports-statistics/us-pet-ownership-statistics. Accessed August 15, 2022.
5. Lascelles BD, Capner CA, Waterman-Pearson. Current British attitudes to perioperative analgesia for cats and small mammals. Vet Rec 1999;145:601–4.
6. Capner CA, Lascelles BD, Waterman-Pearson AE. Current British attitudes to perioperative analgesia for dogs. Vet Rec 1999;145(4):95–9.

7. Coulter CA, Flecknell PA, Richardson CA. Reported analgesic administration to rabbits, pigs, sheep, dogs and non-human primates undergoing experimental surgical procedures. Lab Anim 2009;43:232–8.
8. Coulter CA, Flecknell PA, Leach MC, Richardson CA. Reported analgesic administration to rabbits undergoing experimental surgical procedures. BMC Vet Res 2011;7:12.
9. Benato L, Rooney NJ, Murrell JC. Pain and analgesia in pet rabbits within the veterinary environment: a review. Vet Anaesth Analgesia 2019;46(2):151–62.
10. Jirkof P. Side effects of pain and analgesia in animal experimentation. Lab Animal 2017;46:123–8.
11. Kohn DF, Martin TE, Foley PL, Morris TH, Swindle MM, Vogler GA, Wixson SA. Guidelines for the assessment and management of pain in rodents and rabbits. J America Assoc Lab Anim Sci 2007;46(2):97–108.
12. Spitzagel MB, Jacobson DM, Cox MD, et al. Predicting caregiver burden in general veterinary clients: Contribution of companion animal clinical signs and problem behaviors. Vet J 2018;236:23–30.
13. Barter, L. Rabbit Analgesia. Vet Clin North Am Exot Anim Pract, 14, 2011, 93–104.
14. National Research Council. Recognition and alleviation of pain in laboratory animals. Washington, DC: The National Academies Press; 2009. p. 47–69.
15. Varga M. Analgesia and pain management in rabbits. Vet Nurs J 2016;31(5):149–53.
16. Leach MC, Allweiler S, Richardson CA, et al. Behavioural effect of ovariohysterectomy and oral administration of meloxicam in laboratory housed rabbits. Res Vet Sci 2009;87(2):336–47.
17. Pinho RH, Leach MC, Minto BW, et al. Postoperative pain behaviours in rabbits following orthopedic surgery and effect of observer presence. PLoS One 2020;15(10):e0240605.
18. Benato L, Murrell J, Knowles TJ, Rooney NJ. Development of the Bristol rabbit pain scale (BRPS): a multidimensional composite pain scale specific to rabbits (Oryctolagus cuniculus). PLoS One 2021;16(6):e0252417.
19. Oglesbee BL, Lord B. Gastrointestinal Diseases of Rabbits. Ferrets, Rabbits, and Rodents 2020:174–87. doi: 10.1016/B978-0-323-48435-0.00014-9.
20. Weaver LA, Blaze CA, Linda DE, Andrutis KA, Karas AZ. A model for clinical evaluation of perioperative analgesia in rabbits (Oryctolagus cuniculus). J Am Assoc Lab Anim Sci 2010;49(6):845–51.
21. Roughan JV, Flecknell PA. Evaluation of a short duration behaviour-based postoperative pain scoring system in rats. Eur J Pain 2003;7(5):397–406.
22. Ellen Y, Flecknell PA, Leach MC. Evaluation of using behavioural changes to assess post-operative pain in the guinea pig (Cavia porcellus). PLoS One 2016;11(9):e0161941.
23. Vaisanen MAM, Tuomikoski SK, Vainio OM. Behavioural alterations and severity of pain in cats recovering at home following elective ovariohysterectomy or castration. J Am Vet Med Assoc 2007;231(2):236–42.
24. Holton L, Reid J, Scott EM, et al. Development of a behaviour based scale to measure acute pain in dogs. Vet Rec 2001;148(17):525–31.
25. Farnworth MJ, Walker JK, Schweizer KA, Chuang CL, Guild SJ, Barrett CJ, Leach MC, Waran NK. . Potential behavioural indicators of post-operative pain in male laboratory rabbits following abdominal surgery. Anim Welfare 2011;20:225–37.
26. Turner PV, Chen CH, Taylor MW. Pharmacokinetics of meloxicam in rabbits after single and repeat oral dosing. Comp Med 2006;56(1):63–7.

27. Miller AL, Clarkson JM, Quigley C, Neville V, Krall C, Geijer-Simpson A, Flecknell PA, Leach MC. Evaluating pain and analgesia effectiveness following routine castration in rabbits using behavior and facial expressions. Frontieres Vet Sci 2022;9:782486.
28. Leach MC, Coulter CA, Richardson CA, Flecknell PA. Are we looking in the wrong place? Implications for behavioural based pain assessment in rabbits (Oryctolagus Cuniculi) and beyond. PLoS One 2011;6(3):e13347.
29. Peters JWB, Koot HM, Grunau RE, de Boer J, Druenen HJ, et al. Neonatal facial coding system for assessing post operative pain in infants: Item reduction is valid and feasible. The Clin J Pain 2003;19:353–63.
30. Prkachin KM. The consistency of facial expressions of pain: a comparison across modalities. Pain 1992;51(3):297–306.
31. Langford DJ, Bailey AL, Chanda ML, et al. Coding facial expressions of pain in the laboratory mouse. Nat Methods 2010;7(6):447–9.
32. Keating S, Thomas AA, Flecknell PA, Leach MC. Evaluation of EMLA cream for preventing pain during tattooing in rabbits: Changes in physiological, behavioural and facial expression responses. PLoS One 2012;7(9):e44437.
33. Banchi P, Quaranta G, Ricci A, von Degerfeld MM. Reliability and construct validity of a composite pain scale for rabbits (CANCRS) in a clinical environment. PLoS One 2020;15(4):e0221377.
34. Miller AL, Leach MC. The mouse grimace scale: a clinically useful tool? PLoS One 2015;10(9):e0136000.
35. Leung V, Zhang E, Pang DSJ. Real-time application of the Rat Grimace Scale as a welfare refinement in laboratory rats. Scientific Rep 2016;6:31667.
36. Banchi P, Quaranta G, Ricci A, von Degerfeld MM. A composite pain scale to recognize abdominal pain and its variation over time in response to analgesia in rabbits. Vet Anaesth Analgesia 2022;49(3):323–8.
37. Calvo G, Holden E, Reid J, Scott EM, Firth A, Bell A, Robertson S, Nolan AM. Development of a behaviour based measurement tool with defined intervention level for assessing acute pain in cats. J Small Anim Pract 2014;55:622–9.
38. Lawson AL, Opie RR, Stevens KB, Knowles EJ, Mair TS. Application of an equine composite pain scale and its association with plasma adrenocorticotrophic hormone concentrations and serum cortisol concentrations in horses with colic. Equine Vet Educ 2020;32(11):20–7.
39. Roughan JV, Flecknell PA, Orr H. Behavioural assessment of post-operative pain and analgesic effects of carprofen in the domestic rabbit. Proc 8th World congress Vet Anaesth 2004;31:1–71.
40. Goldschlager GH, Gillespie VL, Palme R, Baxter MG. Effects of multimodal analgesia with low dose buprenorphine and meloxicam on fecal glucocorticoid metabolites after surgery in New Zealand White Rabbits (Oryctolagus cuniculus). J Am Assoc Lab Anim Sci 2013;52(5):571–6.
41. Flecknell PA, Waterman-Pearson A. Pain management in animals. London, UK: Harcourt Publishers Ltd; 2000. p. 53–79.

Treatment of Pain in Rabbits

Sarah Ozawa, DVM, DACZM[a],*, Alessia Cenani, DVM, MS, DACVAA[b],
David Sanchez-Migallon Guzman LV, MS, DECZM (Avian, Small Mammal), DACZM[c]

KEYWORDS

- Rabbit • *Oryctolagus cuniculus* • Analgesia • Opioid • Multi-modal
- Nonsteroidal anti-inflammatory • Regional analgesia • Epidural

KEY POINTS

- Pain management is an essential component of veterinary care of companion, laboratory, wildlife and zoologic rabbit species, and is likely underutilized.
- Although there are many similarities to pharmacologic drugs and techniques to dog and cat medicine, rabbit-specific knowledge of the current literature is essential for appropriate pain management.
- Given that rabbits are prey species, they are sensitive to catecholamine-induced stress responses. Appropriate analgesics may blunt those effects and contribute to appropriate patient care.
- Locoregional techniques should be considered in a multimodal pain management plan. Important considerations include rigorous asepsis, knowledge of toxic doses, and total volume of the drug that is administered.
- The efficacy and safety of many locoregional techniques have not been evaluated in clinical studies in rabbits and the information is often extrapolated from other species.

INTRODUCTION

According to the American Veterinary Medical Association (AVMA) demographics, rabbits are the third most common companion mammal in the United States.[1] In addition, rabbits are highly used in research, present in zoologic collections and native wildlife species are present in many countries. Therefore, veterinarians in a wide capacity of roles may need to use analgesics in rabbits.

A study evaluating analgesia used in rabbits undergoing experimental surgical procedures found that the reporting of the use of systemic analgesia significantly increased from 16% in the years 1995 to 1997 to 50% in 2005 to 2007.[2] However,

a Department of Clinical Sciences, College of Veterinary Medicine, North Carolina State University, 1060 Williams Moore Dr, Raleigh, NC 27606, USA; b Department of Surgical and Radiographical Sciences, School of Veterinary Medicine University of California Davis, One Shields Avenue, Davis, CA 95616, USA; c Department of Medicine and Epidemiology, School of Veterinary Medicine University of California Davis, One Shields Avenue, Davis, CA 95616, USA
* Corresponding author.
E-mail address: sozawa@ncsu.edu

Vet Clin Exot Anim 26 (2023) 201–227
https://doi.org/10.1016/j.cvex.2022.09.001
1094-9194/23/© 2022 Elsevier Inc. All rights reserved.

the overall proportion of rabbits that received analgesics did not differ between the two time periods. This likely means that pain is still being undertreated in rabbit species, potentially due to concerns for adverse effects and lack of familiarity with appropriate drugs, dosage, and routes of administration in this species. Untreated pain however can result in activation of the sympathetic nervous system and resulting negative effects on tissue perfusion, appetite, and gastrointestinal motility, immune response, and wound healing that can all increase morbidity and mortality.

There are several considerations when selecting what analgesic drugs are most appropriate to use in rabbits. Many of these drugs can be used together to target the pain pathways at different levels, a strategy also called multimodal pain management. In other species, multimodal pain management provides better pain relief compared with the use of a single analgesic drug.[3] In rabbits, when buprenorphine and meloxicam were used together, they gained body weight as opposed to those that received meloxicam or buprenorphine alone.[4] Although not synonymous with analgesia, in general rabbits that are less painful may be more likely to eat more and therefore gain weight. In addition, when drugs with synergistic action are used in combination, a lower dose of each drug can be used compared with the amount required when these agents are administered alone, minimizing potential dose-dependent adverse effects.

Timing of the administration of analgesics drugs is also important. Proving pain management before a painful stimulus, or preemptive pain management, prevents the establishment of central sensitization induced by sustained afferent input to the central nervous system during noxious stimulation, thereby reducing post-procedural pain.[5] Buprenorphine administered to rabbits before colorectal distension attenuated cardiovascular responses. However, if buprenorphine was administered during distension, the same effect was not seen.[6] In addition, analgesic therapy is also needed intra and postoperatively in patients undergoing painful procedures or surgery. Alongside pharmacologic treatment, nonpharmacological strategies, and husbandry interventions, which are discussed elsewhere, play a crucial role in pain management.

Rabbits are a common laboratory model for both human and animal medicine. Therefore, there is a reasonable body of literature evaluating analgesic drugs in this species. However, the reader should cautiously interpret some of these studies. Most research is performed on a single breed of rabbit, the New Zealand White rabbit. In other species, there are breed-related differences that may impact drug metabolism and pharmacokinetics.[7] In addition, most of these studies are performed on healthy, young rabbits. Therefore, the effects of systemic illness, organ dysfunction, and metabolism on the drug are often unknown and dose adjustments may be required in clinical patients depending on many patient specific factors. Clinical dosing of analgesic drugs in companion rabbits therefore may be different than the recommendations from laboratory animal resources. In addition, literature recommendations are not available for all analgesic drugs. Many studies in rabbits have evaluated the pharmacokinetics of the drug, but not the pharmacodynamic effect. Therefore, therapeutic plasma concentrations may be extrapolated from other species. In addition, many studies have evaluated the minimum alveolar concentration (MAC)-reduction following the administration of a drug. Although a reduction in MAC can be indicative of analgesia, it is not synonymous with analgesia and other variables can produce an MAC reduction unrelated to analgesic properties. Extrapolation from small animal medicine is often elected if no rabbit-specific studies are available. However, rabbits possess unique gastrointestinal anatomy and physiology that may affect the pharmacokinetics and pharmacodynamics of a drug and therefore direct inferences from small animal medicine is not always appropriate.

PHARMACOLOGIC PAIN MANAGEMENT

Pharmacologic pain management is indicated for acute and chronic pain. Selection of an analgesic drug can be influenced by the severity of pain, available literature, and selected route of administration. The ability to obtain intravenous (IV) access, access to injectable medications, and owners' ability to medicate play a crucial role in this process. In addition, we must consider the legalities of controlled drugs and the judicious use of scheduled drugs with the potential for abuse. The main classes of medications for pain management in rabbits include opioids, nonsteroidal anti-inflammatory drugs (NSAIDs), α2-adrenergic agonists, N-methyl-D-aspartate (NMDA) antagonists, local analgesics, and other miscellaneous drugs. Reported dosages and route of administration are listed in **Table 1**.

Table 1
Analgesic drug dosages published in rabbits based on pharmacokinetic, pharmacodynamic, and or empirical used

Drug	Dose	Route	Frequency	References
Opioids				
Buprenorphine	0.03 to 0.1 mg/kg	IV, SC, and IM	q 4 to 6 h	28,29,34
Buprenorphine high concentration	0.24 mg/kg	SC	q 42 h	29
Buprenorphine sustained-release	0.12 mg/kg	SC	q 72 to 96 h	29
Butorphanol	0.1 to 1 mg/kg	IV, SC, and IM	q 2 to 4 h	31,116,117,a
Fentanyl	12.5 to 25 µg/h	Dermal	q 72 to 96 h	12,13
	15 to 60 µg/kg/h	IV	Intraoperative	10,a
	1.25 to 5 µg/kg/h	IV	Postoperative	a
Hydromorphone	0.1 to 0.4 mg/kg	IV, SC, and IM	q 4 to 6 h	a
Methadone	0.2 mg/kg	IV, SC, and IM	q 4 to 6 h	38,a
Morphine	2 to 5 mg/kg	IM and SC	q 2 to 4 h	117
Tramadol	4.4 mg/kg	IV	q 8 to 12 h	49,
	10 to 20 mg/kg	SC	q 8 to 12	48
	10 to 15 mg/kg	PO		46,a
NSAIDs				
Carprofen	2 to 5 mg/kg	SC and PO	q 12 to 24 h	61,86,a
Grapiprant	2 mg/kg	IV	q 10 h	64
Meloxicam	1 mg/kg	SC and PO	q 24 h	54–56,a
	0.5 mg/kg		q 12 h	a
Local anesthetics				
Lidocaine	50 to 100 µg/kg/min Loading dose 1 to 2 mg/kg	IV		22
Other drugs				
Gabapentin	15 to 30 mg/kg	PO	q 8 to 12 h	69,a
	25 mg/kg	SC		67
Ketamine	0.25 to 5 mg/kg/h	IV		75,a
Maropitant	1 to 10 mg/kg	SC and IV	q 24 h	78,80

[a]Doses based on clinical experience and anecdotal reports.

OPIOID DRUGS

Opioids are effective analgesics used to treat moderate to severe acute pain. Opioids can be classified by their ability to bind to mu-, delta-, or kappa-opioid receptors, as well as the effect elicited upon binding. A full agonist produces a dose-dependent increase in effect until full stimulation of the receptor occurs, as opposed to a partial agonist that produces a plateau effect lower than the effect of a full agonist.[8] Both mu- and kappa-opioid receptors play a crucial role in pain in mammals, although species-specific variations in the mu-opioid receptor exist and may explain differing species sensitivities and response to opioids. Opioids are primarily administered parenterally to target centrally located opioid receptors; however, peripheral opioid receptors seem to be activated and upregulated by trauma or inflammation and local administration of opioids can be considered. In addition, many of these drugs are reversible. Oral use of opioids has not been well studied in rabbits.

Examples of full mu-opioids include morphine, hydromorphone, methadone, and fentanyl. These drugs differ in their potency, or amount of drug required to elicit equipotent analgesia, as well as onset and duration of action.

Fentanyl is a rapid and potent full mu-opioid agonist. IV fentanyl has been shown to decrease response to forepaw clamp in a dose-dependent manner in anesthetized rabbits,[9] and to reduce isoflurane MAC by 63% at the highest plasma concentrations[10] when administered as a continuous infusion in anesthetized New Zealand White rabbits. In addition, the administration of fentanyl improved mean arterial pressure and cardiac output compared with isoflurane alone.[11] These studies however were performed in anesthetized intubated and ventilated rabbits, and the dosages of fentanyl used are not recommended to treat pain in awake rabbits.

Transdermal administration of fentanyl has been investigated in rabbits. Fentanyl pharmacokinetic differed in rabbits that had fentanyl patches placed on shaved skin compared with those with depilated skin.[12] Hair regrowth was rapid in several rabbits that were shaved before application resulting in undetectable plasma concentrations. Two rabbits from the depilatory group showed moderate sedation and a decreased respiratory rate.[12] In addition, the site of fentanyl patch placement may affect plasma concentrations. In rabbits application of a 12 μg/h fentanyl patch on the neck and on the outer surface of the ear produced plasma concentrations that were analgesic in other species for 6 to 72 and 9 to 48 h, respectively.[13] Conversely, analgesic concentrations were not reached when the patch was placed on the inner ear surface. This may be due to drug absorption from this site or challenges with maintenance as patches detached from several rabbits when placed on the inner ear location. Rabbits with patches placed on the outer ear and neck developed diffuse erythema underlying the patch following removal.[13] Whether these concentrations are analgesic in rabbits is unknown as neither study evaluated analgesic properties of fentanyl patches. In a study evaluating analgesic drugs following a surgical procedure, there was no difference in activity level, body weight or fecal output between the control group (no analgesia) and 3.0 to 3.5 kg rabbits that received a 25 μg/h fentanyl patch.[14] Although there are no reports of accidental ingestion, rabbits naturally groom and therefore consumption of the patch is considered a potential complication.

Fewer clinically relevant studies are available on other full mu-opioids. IV morphine in rabbits at 4 mg/kg resulted in decreased reaction and withdrawal response to tail clamping starting at 30 min after injection compared with predrug measurements that lasted 2 to 3 h.[15] Remifentanil at 0.3 μg/kg/min was shown to induce an acute tolerance for analgesic and depression of cardiovascular variables. After 120 min of starting the infusion, subcutaneous (SC) electrical stimulation thresholds, escape movement response and cardiorespiratory parameters returned to pre-infusion levels.[16] This may be due to opioid drug tolerance due to desensitization of pain signaling pathways to opioids. Alternatively, this could be due to hyperalgesia, or a state of nociceptive sensitization.[17] However, no control group was present in this study and the results may be due to temporal adaptation as well.

Although pharmacokinetic studies have been performed evaluating plasma concentrations and the metabolism of hydromorphone and oxymorphone in rabbits, there are few studies evaluating the analgesic efficacy of this drug.[18-20] Following the administration of 5 mg/kg of hydromorphone IV, the drug was rapidly absorbed and cleared.[18] Unfortunately, full pharmacokinetic parameters are not described, but the maximum plasma concentrations were 3000 to 4000 ng/mL. This is > 1000× the plasma concentrations that have antinociceptive effects in dogs.[21] Clinical dosing recommendations for hydromorphone (0.1 to 0.4 mg/kg) are much lower than the dose used in this study and more similar to dosages used in dogs and cats. The oral bioavailability of hydromorphone in rabbits was only 20.4% and is therefore not a recommended route of administration.[18]

Buprenorphine is one of the most commonly used analgesics in rabbits,[2] both because it has been shown to have moderate analgesic properties in rabbits[22,23] and its suggested long duration of action, with increasing doses of buprenorphine leading to an increased duration of analgesic effects.[24] Buprenorphine has been historically classified as a partial mu agonist and is most appropriate for moderate pain; however, in some species such as cats, buprenorphine has been suggested to be as effective as full opioid agonists for certain types of pain.[8,25] When buprenorphine was used in combination with ketamine and medetomidine, the duration of anesthesia was longer compared with ketamine and medetomidine alone which may be due in part to its analgesic properties.[26]

Buprenorphine can be administered intravenously, subcutaneously or intramuscularly. The onset of analgesic effects is about 30 min following IV administration.[24] Buprenorphine administered every 6 to 77 h may be appropriate for pain relief, depending on the dose, formulation, and route of administration. In a study that compared buprenorphine hydrochloride (HCl) 0.2 mg/kg SC every 12 h to sustained release buprenorphine (Buprenorphine SR, ZooPharm, Windsor, CO, 0.12 mg/kg SC), rabbits that received the standard buprenorphine HCl formulation had pain scores indicative of moderate to severe pain at 12 h, before the next dose was administered, following placement of titanium implants in the tibia.[27] Plasma concentrations of buprenorphine remained above concentrations considered analgesic in other species for only 4 h following administration of 0.05 mg/kg SC of buprenorphine HCl in another study, confirming the duration of buprenorphine may be shorter than previously thought. A study comparing pharmacokinetics of buprenorphine intramuscular (IM) or SC in rabbits found that serum concentrations following SC administration were lower than following IM administration and resulted in a longer elimination half-life. The bioavailability of SC buprenorphine was approximately 50% of IM buprenorphine. According to this study and those above-mentioned, whereas the SC route may decrease stress and pain associated with injection, it may not result in adequate plasma concentrations at the doses studied.[28] There are several formulations of buprenorphine that may increase its duration of action. High concentration buprenorphine allows for higher dosages of the drug to be given without a concurrent increase in injection volume. This is in contrast to a sustained-release formulation that slowly released buprenorphine from a carrier compound. In rabbits, following administration of a high concentration formulation of buprenorphine (Simbadol Zoetis Parsippany, NJ) at 0.24 mg/kg SC and sustained-release buprenorphine (Buprenorphine-SR Zoo

Pharm, Windsor, CO) at 0.15 mg/kg SC, plasma concentrations above those effective in other species were maintained for up to 42 and 77 h, respectively.[29] After sustained-release buprenorphine, effective plasma concentrations were not achieved until 15 h after its administration, and therefore its use may not be appropriate to provide immediate analgesia.[29] High-concentration buprenorphine and buprenorphine HCl reached plasma concentrations shortly after administration. The analgesic efficacy of these formulations was not evaluated in this study.

Following bone replacement in New Zealand White rabbits, buprenorphine HCl was administered at 0.05 mg/kg SC or transmucosally at 0.15 mg/kg every 8 h.[30] The oral transmucosal route required large volumes, achieved lower plasma concentrations compared with the SC route, and is therefore not recommended in rabbits.[30] Postoperative pain scores were increased in both treatment groups compared with preoperative pain scores indicating that neither was likely an effective analgesic for this surgery.

Butorphanol is a mu-opioid receptor antagonist and kappa agonist. It can be a mild analgesic in other species and has a short duration of action. Studies in rabbits investigating the analgesic properties of butorphanol are lacking and overall butorphanol is not recommended for overtly painful conditions in rabbits. Butorphanol half-life is only 1.64 h after IV administration in rabbits,[31] and increasing doses of butorphanol (up to 1.5 mg/kg) decreased nociceptive response to a thermal stimulus to a lower extent compared with other opioids in awake rabbits by 7.63%.[24] The same was true for nalbuphine (5 to 10 mg/kg).

Opioid drugs are considered relatively safe, but adverse effects can occur, especially at higher doses or with long-term administration. Gastrointestinal motility in isolated rabbit intestines has been experimentally decreased by mu- and kappa-opioid receptor agonists.[32,33] Studies however have produced conflicting evidence on the effect of buprenorphine on gastrointestinal transit in rabbits. One study found that following a single dose of buprenorphine (0.1 mg/kg IM), rabbits had a higher number of pyloric and duodenal contractions and no difference in feces production compared with control rabbits.[34] Another study found that the time to appearance of feces and daily fecal output was lower for rabbits receiving buprenorphine (30 h) at 0.05 mg/kg SC every 12 h for 2 days compared with control rabbits (18 h), and this was not ameliorated by the addition of methylanlrexone.[35] Reduction in daily fecal output was likely secondary to a reduction in food intake. Additional studies have found a negative effect of buprenorphine administered at 0.03 mg/kg SC every 8 h on gastrointestinal transit in rabbits.[36] Sustained-release buprenorphine has also been shown to reduce fecal output compared with control rabbits.[29] Following administration of a single dose of morphine (10 mg/kg IM) or butorphanol (5 mg/kg) gastrointestinal transit time was decreased on ultrasound examination in healthy rabbits.[37] These dosages are however higher than that is clinically recommended or commonly used. Methadone at 0.2 mg/kg SC did not result in a negative effect on food intake or fecal output in rabbits compared with buprenorphine (0.1 mg/kg) and hydromorphone (0.2 mg/kg).[38] It is important to note that most of these studies were performed in healthy rabbits; therefore, the effects of opioids on gastrointestinal motility when compared with painful rabbits are unknown. It is entirely possible that pain may also result in ileus in rabbits which supports the recommendation for opioid administration in painful rabbits if food intake and fecal output are monitored. Any negative effect of opioids on gastrointestinal motility usually resolves once the administration is discontinued following the postoperative period (eg, 2 to 3 days), without the need for additional medical intervention. In addition, equipotent dosages of these opioids were not used so direct comparisons cannot be made between the mu-opioid and its effect on the gastrointestinal tract of rabbits. Differences in the results may be due to the fact that higher dosages of morphine[37] than methadone[38] were used.

Another adverse effect of opioids is respiratory depression. Morphine administered at 4 mg/kg IV in conscious rabbits resulted in a reduction in respiratory rate, heart rate, blood pH, and PaO_2.[15] Fentanyl at high doses has been shown to induce chest wall rigidity in anesthetized rabbits.[39] In combination with medetomidine and midazolam, fentanyl produced transient apnea in rabbits that required intubation.[40] Buprenorphine as well has been shown to reduce respiratory rate, increase arterial carbon dioxide tension, produce mild hypoxemia, and reduce arterial oxygen tension when administered to healthy awake rabbits at 0.03 or 0.06 mg/kg IM or SC.[41,42] Although these adverse effects were tolerated in these studies, the effect on clinically ill rabbits should be considered.

In addition, 3 mg/kg of IV morphine can induce hypertension and hyperglycemia in conscious rabbits.[43] This is suspected to be secondary to increased sympathoadrenal activity and secretion of adrenaline.[43] Following administration of 0.24 mg/kg high concentration buprenorphine SC, two rabbits developed neurologic signs including depression, nystagmus, and ataxia.[29] One of those rabbits seizured and was euthanized due to the severity of neurologic signs. Necrosis of the hippocampus was observed on necropsy, which was presumably caused by hypoxia likely secondary to the seizure; although the etiology of the seizure was undetermined.[29] Sedation can occur following opioid administration, it may be marked at higher doses and in already depressed rabbits.[12] In addition, this sedative effect may be more profound if combined with other drugs such as benzodiazepines.[42]

TRAMADOL

The analgesic action of tramadol can be explained by its dual mechanism of action. It acts centrally as a mu-opioid receptor agonist and also inhibits the reuptake of serotonin and norepinephrine.[44] Tramadol is converted by P450 in the liver to the active metabolite, O-desmethyltramadol (M1) which has a higher affinity for mu receptors than the parent compound itself.[45,46] Studies evaluating tramadol in rabbits have produced conflicting evidence as to the drug's efficacy as an analgesic. Despite that, tramadol is often clinically used to treat mild to moderate pain.

In a study evaluating midazolam and ketamine alone or in combination with tramadol, neither group produced a change in response to toe pinch.[47] Following oral administration of 11 mg/kg of tramadol, plasma concentrations of tramadol considered analgesic in other species were not reached.[46] The M1 metabolite reached plasma concentrations therapeutic in other species for only 45 min in 2/6 rabbits in this study. Rabbits that received 10 or 20 mg/kg tramadol SC twice a day during and following gastrotomy had lower glucose, decreased cortisol, and decreased heart rate compared with control rabbits suggestive of potential analgesia, although these are considered a nonsensitive parameter for pain assessment.[48] Tramadol at 4.4 mg/kg IV resulted in a statistically significant but clinically unimportant decrease in the MAC of isoflurane in rabbits, which may or may not be associated with analgesic effects.[49]

Potential adverse effects of tramadol include gastrointestinal motility reduction and sedation. Tramadol in vitro has been shown to decrease peristalsis in the rabbit small intestine in a dose-dependent manner.[50] In vivo however, a single dose of tramadol administered at 10 m/kg IM had no effect on gastrointestinal contractions or transit time in rabbits.[37] A study evaluating IM tramadol at 10 to 15 mg/kg in male rabbits found that creatinine, alanine aminotransferase(ALT), aspartate aminotransferase (AST), and alkaline phosphatase (ALP) were increased in the rabbits that received tramadol compared with the control group.[51] In addition on histopathology, cellular degeneration of the renal tubules and fatty degeneration of the liver were present in the tramadol treatment group as opposed to the control group.[51] It is not mentioned how many rabbits developed these changes or the severity of it. Thus, monitoring for renal and hepatic damage may be recommended with long-term treatment. It is important to note that the tablet and compounded formulation of tramadol are both bitter, and palatability may be a concern with clinical use.

NONSTEROIDAL ANTI-INFLAMMATORY DRUGS

NSAIDs are one of the most commonly prescribed analgesic medications in rabbits. In addition to their analgesic properties, they are also anti-inflammatory and anti-pyretic. NSAIDs inhibit cyclooxygenase (COX) enzymes and the formation of prostanoids.[52] There are at least two isoenzymes of COX with COX-1 expression mainly in tissues, and COX-2 by inflammatory cells. Both isoenzymes are important for normal physiologic function.[52] NSAIDs may be classified by the ratio of COX-1 to COX-2 inhibition. Meloxicam and carprofen are classified as COX-2 preferential and are the most used NSAIDs in rabbits. Nonselective NSAIDs such as ketoprofen have been uncommonly used in rabbits clinically, though the pharmacokinetics have been studied following transdermal application.[53]

Meloxicam has been evaluated in various pharmacokinetic and safety studies in rabbits. Rabbits that received 1 mg/kg of meloxicam orally once a day maintained plasma concentrations that have been shown to be effective in other species.[54] Another study showed minimal accumulation and no adverse effects were reported when the same dose for used for up to 29 days.[55] Lower dosages (0.2 to 0.3 mg/kg PO) have been evaluated and resulted in inadequate plasma concentrations.[56,57] A study comparing the analgesic effect of meloxicam at different dosages in rabbits following ovariohysterectomy showed that only the group that received meloxicam at 1 mg/kg orally once a day the first day followed by 0.5 mg/kg PO once a day showed some degree of pain control.[58] In this study, however, even with high meloxicam dosages, some behaviors indicative of pain were still displayed, suggesting the use of additional analgesics may be required for this procedure.

A metanalysis evaluating analgesic drugs used in rabbits after surgical procedures found that carprofen was the most common NSAID prescribed during the periods of time evaluated (2000 to 2001 and 2005 to 2006).[2] Despite its widespread use, carprofen has been studied in rabbits in a limited capacity. In rabbits, pharmacokinetic parameters after carprofen at 4 mg/kg IV are similar to other species,[59] and its bioavailability is high (>90%) following 2 mg/kg SC administration.[60] However, when carprofen was given intra-articular as nanoparticles, the bioavailability was only 51.4%. When carprofen (5 mg/kg SC every 24 h) was used in combination with buprenorphine (0.05 to 0.01 SC every 6 h) in rabbits following maxillary surgery, there was no difference in facial expression of pain or bone healing compared with saline treatment, implying it was not an adequate pain management protocol for this procedure.[61] However, this invasive surgical procedure may necessitate a different analgesic drug combination and/or dosaging to control pain. The same study showed no difference in levels of the acute phase protein SAA between treatment groups.[61] SAA is a nonspecific inflammatory marker and may have reflected the severity of the surgical procedure rather than the anti-inflammatory effects of carprofen.

In other species, gastrointestinal injury, kidney injury, hepatic damage, and coagulation abnormalities are possible side effects after NSAID administration. Rabbits that received 1.5 mg/kg of meloxicam once a day for 7 days developed mild hepatic and renal changes on histopathology, which were found to resolved on day 10 posttreatment.[62] Rabbits that received 3 mg/kg developed severe hepatic necrosis and glomerular damage that was persistent at day 10 posttreatment. There is a single case report of a rabbit that was diagnosed with gastric ulceration on necropsy and was receiving meloxicam (0.2 mg/kg PO every 12 h).[63] However, given that this is a subclinical dose of meloxicam, other causes of the gastrointestinal ulceration must be considered. These adverse effects have not been evaluated or reported with other NSAIDs in rabbits. Overall, adverse events following NSAID treatment are rare in rabbits when administered at the appropriate dosage, but monitoring of renal, hepatic, and gastrointestinal function is warranted.

Grapiprant (Galliprant) is a more recently developed anti-inflammatory drug. Grapiprant is an antagonist of the prostaglandin E2 receptor 4 receptor for prostaglandin E2,[64] which mediates pain and inflammation. Because grapiprant does not interfere with prostaglandins function like COX-inhibiting NSAIDs do, it is possible its use could be associated with less gastrointestinal and renal adverse effects as opposed to traditional NSAIDs. This theory however has not been validated in rabbits. A recent study compared grapiprant (2 mg/kg IV) to meloxicam (0.5 mg/kg SC) in an inflammatory pain model in rabbits.[64] Both grapiprant and meloxicam increased the thermal withdrawal latency compared with saline for up to 10 h and plasma concentrations of grapiprant were detectable for up to 10 h, indicating this may be an effective analgesic drug in rabbits for this duration of time.[64] Further studies evaluating oral pharmacokinetics are needed for accurate dosage recommendations of grapiprant, as the oral bioavailability and equivalent oral dose remain unknown.

GABAPENTIN

Gabapentin produces analgesia by blocking N-type voltage-dependent neuronal calcium channels, leading to a reduction of calcium influx into neurons, in turn reducing neuronal transmission. Gabapentin has been shown to be an effective analgesic in other species, especially for neuropathic pain. A meta-analysis in humans concluded that gabapentinoids did not produce significant analgesics effects for acute pain.[65] However, the effect on acute pain in rabbits is unknown. Rabbits that received 25 mg/kg of gabapentin SC reached plasma concentrations that are analgesic in humans.[66] Rabbits that received gabapentin following a spinal cord ischemic injury had lower tissue injury markers compared with control rabbits indicating it may have neuroprotective properties.[67,68] Clinical dosing is currently extrapolated from other species, and administration every 8 to 12 h is recommended. This may be challenging for some owners for outpatient care. Sedation is the most common side effect of gabapentin, and mild sedation was observed in rabbits after oral administration of 25 and 50 mg/kg for up to 3 h.[69]

ALPHA-2 ADRENERGIC AGONIST

Alpha-2 adrenergic agonists can provide sedation, analgesia, and muscle relaxation. In addition, these drugs are reversible. Most of the studies about this class of drug in rabbits focused on evaluating their sedative properties with fewer studies assessing their analgesic efficacy. These drugs can produce negative cardiovascular effects by decreasing heart rate, altering blood pressure, and reducing cardiac output.[70] Myocardial necrosis and fibrosis has been seen following anesthesia of rabbits with xylazine and ketamine, most likely as a result of coronary vasoconstriction.[71] No statistical difference was seen in rabbits that received alpha-2 agonists compared with non-alpha-2 protocols in a retrospective study on perianesthetic mortality in rabbits.[72] However, careful patient selection is needed when selecting this drug.

KETAMINE

Ketamine is a dissociative anesthetic that mainly acts as an NMDA receptor antagonist, and interacts with opioid, monoaminergic, and muscarinic receptors. Subanesthetic dosages of ketamine can produce analgesia, especially effective for somatic pain in other species. In addition, preoperative administration may help decrease sensitization to pain in dogs.[73,74] Ketamine as a continuous rate infusion (40 μg/kg/min) has been shown to reduce the MAC of isoflurane in rabbits.[75] Clinically, ketamine has been used as a bolus and continuous rate of administration in rabbits as an anesthetic agent.[26,75,76] However, similar to alpha-2 agonists, most of the studies evaluating ketamine in rabbits focus on the sedative and anesthetic properties of the drug. Unfortunately, little to no research exists on the analgesic properties of ketamine in rabbits.

OTHER DRUGS

Maropitant is a selective neurokinin 1 (NK1)-receptor antagonist. It is approved for the use and treatment of emesis in dogs and cats. Although rabbits cannot vomit, it is unknown if they can experience nausea as a sensation. NK1-receptor antagonists may also play a role in visceral pain. NK-1 receptor antagonists have been shown to decrease the number of abdominal contractions in response to colorectal stimulation in rabbits.[77] Rabbits that received 1 mg/kg maropitant citrate IV and SC reached plasma concentrations that have been anti-emetic in other species, but overall had a lower C_{max} than in dogs.[78] Plasma concentrations in that study were lower than those that are associated with visceral analgesia in dogs.[79] When maropitant was administered at a higher dose in three rabbits (10 mg/kg SC), plasma concentrations were still present at 24 h. In both studies, a dermal reaction at the injection site occurred in several rabbits following SC administration.[78,80] The efficacy of maropitant as a visceral analgesic in rabbits has not yet been evaluated.

Cannabinoids have gained interested in veterinary medicine for the treatment of chronic pain. The pharmacokinetics of cannabidiol (CBD) and cannabidiolic acid (CBDA) in hemp oil has been evaluated in rabbits following a single 15 mg/kg of CBD with 16.4 mg/kg CBDA oral dose, with and without food. CBDA reached higher plasma concentrations and the administration of food slurry with the hemp oil resulted in lower CBD and CBDA (approximately 50%) plasma concentrations. No adverse effects were reported following a single dose administration at these doses.[81] However, the clinical significance of the plasma concentrations reached remains unknown as the analgesic effects of these cannabinoids and long-term adverse effects have not been yet investigated in rabbits.

LOCAL ANESTHETICS

Lidocaine is a sodium channel blocker, which inhibits action potential transmission along nerve fibers. Systemic administration may reduce the MAC of inhalant, provide visceral analgesia and improve gastrointestinal tract motility.[22,82,83] In addition, IV lidocaine has been shown to have anti-inflammatory properties in rabbit endotoxemia models.[84] A recent study compared lidocaine (2 mg/kg bolus followed by 100 μg/kg/min for 2 days) to buprenorphine (0.06 mg/kg IV every 8 h for 2 days) in rabbits that underwent an ovariohysterectomy.[22] Rabbits that received lidocaine had higher gastrointestinal motility, food intake and fecal output compared with those receiving buprenorphine.[85] Although pain scores did not differ between treatment groups, rabbits in the lidocaine group showed a higher number of normal behaviors compared with the buprenorphine group. Pain scores also did not greatly differ over time, which may mean this scoring system was not a reliable indicator of pain in this model. These results indicate that lidocaine administered as a continuous rate infusion may be a good alternative option for postoperative pain with minimal gastrointestinal adverse effects in rabbits.

LOCOREGIONAL TECHNIQUES

There are some general considerations when using locoregional techniques. The local block techniques should be performed after rigorous asepsis. The total dose (mg) of local anesthetic (LA) being used should be below the toxic doses reported or suggested for rabbits. Lidocaine and bupivacaine are the most often used LA. Although not well documented, doses of lidocaine and bupivacaine for infiltration or regional block of 4 and 2 mg/kg, respectively, should avoid toxicity.[86] Transient arrhythmias, indicative of cardiovascular toxicity, occurred after 2.2 to 2.8 mg/kg IV bupivacaine in both anesthetized paralyzed and awake rabbits.[87,88] Signs of central nervous system toxicity were not reported, but with more potent LA, cardiac toxicity has been found to arise concurrently with seizures or even precede them.[89]

The total volume administered when performing a local block plays a crucial role in the effectiveness of the nerve block. The LA of choice can be diluted with saline to the required total volume, if needed. The use of locoregional techniques has the potential to decrease the use of perioperative analgesic medications and inhaled anesthetic required to maintain general anesthesia and their associated dose-dependent adverse effects. Potential complications of locoregional techniques include neurologic signs, systemic toxicity, drug error, infection, and allergic reaction.[90] Although unknown in rabbits, these complications are in general rare. Three cardiac arrests (0.014%), one death (0.005%), 16 seizures (0.075%), four neurologic injuries (0.019%) and four radiculopathies (0.019%) were reported in humans after reviewing 21,278 peripheral nerve blocks.[90,91] Information about the clinical efficacy and safety of some of the blocks described below is unfortunately still limited in rabbits.

INFRAORBITAL NERVE BLOCK

The infraorbital nerve arises from the maxillary branch of the trigeminal nerve and provides sensory innervation to the upper incisor teeth, upper lip, and adjacent soft tissues.

The infraorbital nerve can be blocked by infusion of LA at the infraorbital foramen, where the nerve emerges from the skull. This can be palpated on the lateral aspect of the maxilla, midway and slightly rostral to an imaginary line connecting the lacrimal process to the facial tuberosity, and near the first maxillary cheek tooth.[92–95] A 27-gauge, 1.3 cm needle is inserted into the foramen to a depth of about 2 mm and, after negative aspiration, 0.05 mL of 1% to 2% lidocaine can be injected to desensitize the nerve.[92] Deposition of the LA outside the infraorbital foramen only desensitizes the skin of the muzzle and the upper lip (**Fig. 1**).[96]

Information on clinical efficacy and possible complications of this technique have not been published in rabbits. However, the infraorbital nerve occupies most of the infraorbital canal in New Zealand White rabbits,[97] and direct nerve damage is likely when LA is injected into the foramen itself.[97] Neuropraxia has been reported as a complication after infraorbital nerve block with 0.05 mL of lidocaine 1% in a

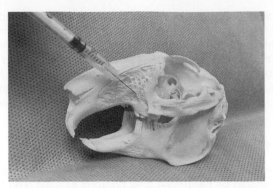

Fig. 1. Infraorbital nerve block at the infraorbital foramen in a rabbit skull.

companion rabbit (*O cuniculus*). Total recovery and normal use of both lips occurred within 10 days of the block.[92]

MAXILLARY NERVE BLOCK

The maxillary nerve provides sensory innervation to the hard and soft tissues of the ipsilateral maxilla, skin of the nose, cheek, upper lip, and possibly ipsilateral hard and soft palate (via the pterygopalatine nerve), and nasal mucosa (via the caudal nasal nerve). In large-breed rabbits, a maxillary nerve block using a "caudal infraorbital" strategy has been anecdotally described.[95] According to the author, a 27-gauge needle is advanced about 1 cm into the infraorbital canal, and LA is slowly injected after negative aspiration, whereas digital pressure is applied over the rostral end of the canal (**Fig. 2**).[95] The goal is to spread the LA into the infraorbital canal up to the maxillary nerve. Information on appropriate volume to use, clinical efficacy, and possible complications of this technique have not been published in rabbits. Because of its small size, it may not be possible to thread the needle into the canal in small rabbits, and we do not recommend this approach, as direct damage to the infraorbital nerve (which occupies most of the infraorbital canal in New Zealand White rabbits) is possible.[92,97]

A different technique in New Zealand White rabbits showed complete and effective staining of the maxillary nerve, and no complications were reported.[97] In this study,

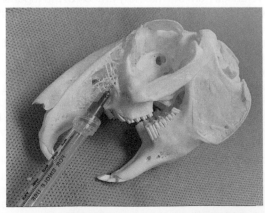

Fig. 2. Maxillary nerve block at the infraorbital foramen in a rabbit skull.

staining of the nerve occurred in 13/14 rabbits and algesiometer-applied force tolerance was significantly different between the treated and the control side of the rabbit. A 25-gauge, 16 mm needle is inserted below the zygomatic arch and caudal to the lateral canthus of the eye, and slowly advanced dorsally, medially, and caudally toward the pterygopalatine fossa until it contacts the bone. The needle is then withdrawn slightly and 0.25 to 0.5 mL of LA is injected after negative aspiration (**Fig. 3**).[97] A 12-MHz linear ultrasound probe can be placed on the upper lid to visualize the globe and pterygopalatine fossa, to confirm the spread of the LA.[98]

PALATINE NERVE BLOCK

According to Lichtenberger and Ko,[95] the anterior palatine nerve can be blocked as it exits the palatine foramen to desensitize the ipsilateral palate. The palatine foramen is located halfway between the palatal aspect of the third upper premolar tooth and the palatal midline (**Fig. 4**).[95] However, given the anatomy of the oral cavity of rabbits, visualization is limited, and information on appropriate volume to use, clinical efficacy, and possible complications of this technique have not been published in rabbits.

INFERIOR ALVEOLAR NERVE BLOCK

The inferior alveolar nerve is a branch of the mandibular nerve, and sensory innervation of the hard and soft tissues of the ipsilateral mandible, including any mandibular teeth, lower lip, and intermandibular tissues. This nerve can be blocked in rabbits as it enters the mandibular foramen on the medial surface of the mandible, using an extraoral approach. The mandibular foramen is located approximately midway between the distal aspect of the last molar and the ventral border of the mandible, caudal to the last molar and about 10 mm above the incisura vasorum facialium of the mandible in New Zealand White rabbits.[95,99]

A 25- to 27-gauge needle is inserted percutaneously at the incisura vasorum facialium of the mandible, at a 120°, and directed caudally and dorsally along the medial aspect of the mandible, toward the estimated location of the mandibular foramen (**Fig. 5**).[94,99,100] This technique was efficacious at limiting the response to surgical stimulation during mandibular surgery in a study in rabbits, when compared with a control group that received the same anesthetic protocol without the local block.[99] However, 5 mL of lidocaine 2% were used for this block in the above-mentioned study performed in New Zealand White rabbits weighting about 2 kg, which equals about

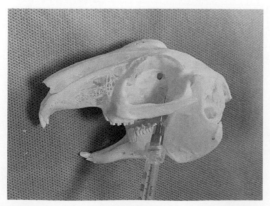

Fig. 3. Maxillary nerve block at the maxillary foramen in a rabbit skull.

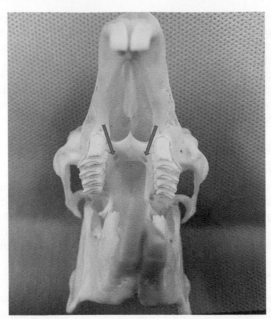

Fig. 4. Ventral view of a rabbit skull showing the palatine foramen (blue *arrows*).

50 mg/kg of lidocaine.[99] This lidocaine dose exceeds what is considered safe in any species, and it is not recommended for clinical use. Thus, the efficacy of this technique when a lower, and more appropriate, volume of LA is used remains unknown.

An additional approach to the mandibular nerve block has been reported in rabbits, but information on its clinical efficacy and possible complications has not been published. The needle is inserted percutaneously at the ventral border of the mandibular notch, and advanced cranially and dorsally along the medial aspect of the mandible, to the estimated location of the mandibular foramen (**Fig. 6**).[95,98] The volume of LA solution reported for this block in rabbits is about 0.5 to 1 mL total volume, assuming the toxic dose is not been exceeded.[95]

A nerve stimulator can be used to more precisely localize the mandibular nerve, but not the inferior alveolar nerve which only provides sensory innervation.[98] The insulated

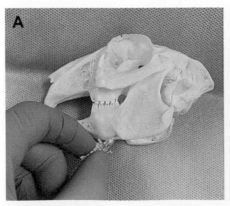
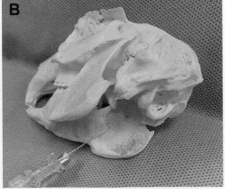

Fig. 5. Inferior alveolar nerve block in a rabbit skull: lateral (*A*) and medial (*B*) view.

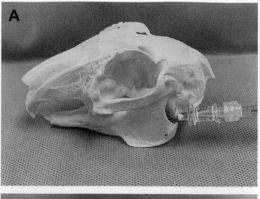

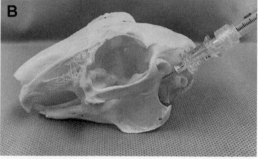

Fig. 6. Inferior alveolar nerve block with needle is inserted the ventral border of the mandibular notch in a rabbit skull (*A*). Inferior alveolar nerve block with needle is inserted the at the temporomandibular joint in rabbit skull (*B*).

needle connected to the nerve stimulator inserted in this case is at the level of the temporomandibular joint, and advanced rostromedially along the mandible until contraction of the masticatory muscle is observed, which indicates the proximity of the needle to the mandibular nerve.[98] Information on clinical efficacy and possible complications of this technique have not been published in rabbits. If LA is injected proximal to the mandibular foramen, this results in a mandibular nerve block—rather than an inferior alveolar nerve one—which also desensitizes the lingual nerve. The latter originates from the mandibular nerve, just rostral to the inferior alveolar nerve, and provides sensory innervation to the tongue, so when blocked self-inflicted chewing injuries are possible until normal sensation reappears.

The mandibular nerve was also accidently stained in 37.5% of rabbits while attempting an auriculotemporal nerve block with an angled approach in cadavers, due to the proximity of these nerves.[101]

MENTAL NERVE BLOCK

The mental nerve supplies sensory fibers to ipsilateral rostral lower lip, rostral intermandibular tissues, and lower incisor. It arises from the mandibular nerve as it extends into the mental foramen, and it can be blocked at this level. The mental foramen is located in the upper third of the lateral aspect of the body of the mandible, ventral and rostral to the first mandibular premolar tooth.[94,95] Deposition of the LA outside the mental foramen only desensitizes labial soft tissue rostral to it (**Fig. 7**).[95,98] The volume of LA solution reported for this block in rabbits is about 0.5 mL total volume,

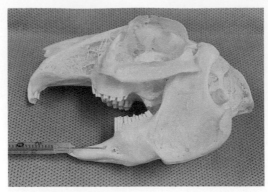

Fig. 7. Mental nerve block in a rabbit skull.

assuming the toxic dose is not been exceeded.[95] Information on clinical efficacy and possible complications of this technique have not been published in rabbits.

RETROBULBAR BLOCK

This block provides analgesia to the eye globe, and it is mainly used in veterinary medicine for enucleation procedures. Two techniques are described in New Zealand White rabbits.[102,103]

A 23-gauge, 25 mm hypodermic needle is inserted at the lateral aspect of the inferior orbital rim and advanced under ultrasonographic guidance (12-MHz linear probe) upward and medially in the retrobulbar area. The retrobulbar cone is visualized, and after confirming negative aspiration, 0.15 to 0.35 mL/kg (maximum volume 0.5 mL/kg) of LA is injected into the periconal space outside the muscular cone.[102] Alternatively, the needle can be further advanced inside the muscular cone to perform an intraconal injection.[93] A "pop sensation" is felt crossing the muscle cone where the needle is stopped.

A landmark-based only technique in rabbits uses a 20-gauge, 25 mm needle inserted at the lateral canthus of the eye, between the eyeball and the orbital bone. The needle is advanced toward the opposite mandible, until the medial orbital wall is being felt, and LA injected extraconaly. The efficacy of this block was assessed in a limited capacity in anesthetized New Zealand White rabbits, where 0.3 mL of lidocaine 4% provided adequate conditions for intraocular surgery, with no complications.[103] Care must be taken with all ophthalmic blocks to avoid the large retrobulbar venous plexus in rabbits.

GREATER AURICULAR AND AURICULOTEMPORAL NERVE BLOCKS

The greater auricular nerve is a superficial branch of the cervical plexus and provides sensory innervation of the pinna and vertical ear canal, alongside sensory branches of the facial nerve. The auriculotemporal branch of the mandibular nerve provides sensory innervation to the medial horizontal ear canal.[101]

To block the greater auricular nerve, a 23-gauge, 25 mm needle is inserted in the sternocephalicus muscle, caudal to the wings of the atlas. The needle is advanced rostrally over the transverse process of C1 toward the jugular groove, deep in the SC tissue of the neck. As the needle is slowly retracted the LA solution is injected.[98,101] A layer of adipose tissue lays over the greater auricular nerve in New Zealand White

rabbits, preventing nerve staining If the dye Is injected more superficially in the SC tissue as described in dogs.[101] This technique produced a reliable motor and sensory
blockade of the pinna when 0.3 mL/kg of bupivacaine 0.5% was used in a clinical
study in rabbits, although its duration varied between 30 and 184 min.[104] Animals
should be monitored for temporary loss of palpebral reflex, as accidental auriculopal-
pebral nerve block for up to 240 min was reported in the same study.[104]

The auriculotemporal nerve can be blocked by inserting a 23-gauge, 25 mm needle
between the external acoustic meatus and the caudal border of the ramus of the
mandible, either perpendicularly to the skin or with a 45° angle, and advanced about
0.5 to 1 cm depth where 0.075 mL/kg of LA solution is injected.[101] In rabbit cadavers,
inadvertent mandibular nerve staining was greater when the needle was inserted at a
45° angle.[101] Unfortunately, successful staining of the auriculotemporal nerve with this
technique was low in both rabbit cadavers and in a clinical study, even when the volume of the LA solution was increased to 0.3 mL/kg.[101,104]

To more precisely localize the auriculotemporal nerve, an insulated needle connected to a nerve stimulator can be used, and the needle advanced until caudal
displacement of the pinna is seen.[98] The efficacy of this technique has not been evaluated in a clinical study.

INTRATESTICULAR BLOCK

Intratesticular injections of LA are commonly performed for castration procedures. A
25-gauge, 16 mm needle is inserted through the testicle starting from the caudal
pole and aiming for the spermatic cord.[95,105] Volumes of LA 0.05 to 1 mL per testicle,
depending on the size of the animal, have been reported.[95,105] Upon LA injection, the
testicle becomes firmly turgid. At this point, the needle is withdrawn and the injection
repeated in the other testicle, and the remaining drug can be used for an incisional
block.[95]

BRACHIAL PLEXUS BLOCK

The brachial plexus of the rabbit is formed by the ventral rami of the spinal nerves C5-
T1.[106] It is located medial to the scapula in the axillary region,[106] and can be blocked to
desensitize the thoracic limb. Different techniques using ultrasound guidance and/or
electrolocation have been reported in rabbits, and result in a safe and effective
blockade of the nerves.[98,107] To perform the techniques described below, the rabbit
is positioned in lateral recumbency, with the leg to be blocked positioned uppermost.
Extension of the elbow is the expected motor response elicited upon electrical stimulation of the brachial plexus. A 12-MHz linear probe and a 22 to 23 gauge, 35 to
50 mm insulated needle, connected to a nerve stimulator, are used. The limb to be
blocked is extended and abducted, and the ultrasound probe placed on the axillary
region. The plexus is visualized as an area of hyperechoic structures, dorsal to the axillary artery and vein. The insulated needle is inserted longitudinally into the probe and
advanced until extension of the elbow is observed, and LA injected after negative aspiration.[107] After injection of 0.8 mL/kg of ropivacaine 0.4%, Fonseca and colleagues[107]
reported a sensory block lasting 319 ± 51 min, and motor blockade for 274 ± 14 min.

A subscalenic approach has been described in rabbits by Otero and Portela,[98] but
information on clinical efficacy and possible complications of this technique have not
been published. The upper limb and scapula are both displaced caudally, and the ultrasound probe is positioned parallel to the longitudinal axis of the scalenus muscle
and cranial to the first rib, above the costochondral joint. The brachial plexus is visualized below the scalenus muscle and in front of the first rib. If an ultrasound machine

is not available, this block can be performed under electrolocation only. In this case, with the upper limb and scapula displaced caudally, the first rib is palpated. The insulated needle connected to a nerve stimulator is inserted perpendicular to the skin, cranial to the first rib and above the costochondral joint, and advanced until the extension of the elbow is observed.[99]Alternatively, the insulated needle can be inserted cranial to the acromion and parallel to the longitudinal axis of the spine, with a 20 to 30° angle to the table, and advanced medially to the scapula and parallel to the rib cage until the extension of the elbow is observed.[98] The upper limb and scapula are not extended caudally in this case. Clinical efficacy and possible complications of this technique in rabbits have not been published.

RADIAL, ULNAR, MUSCULOCUTANEOUS, AND MEDIAN NERVE BLOCK

The radial, ulnar, musculocutaneous, and median nerves arise from the brachial plexus and provide motor and sensory innervation to the distal thoracic limb. Two nerve stimulator-assisted techniques, with or without an ultrasound machine, have been reported in rabbits to perform the radial, ulnar, musculocutaneous, and median (RUMM) block, but information on clinical efficacy and possible complications of these techniques have not been published.[98] Stimulation of the nerves produces characteristic motor responses: carpus extension (radial nerve), carpus flexion and digit protonation (ulnar and median nerves), and elbow flexion (musculocutaneous nerve).

One technique involves two injections performed at the caudal border of the humerus:

The first injection blocks the musculocutaneous, ulnar, and median nerves: the insulated needle connected to a nerve stimulator is inserted at the middle third of the humerus, on the medial aspect of the leg, cranial and caudal to the brachial artery, and advanced until characteristic motor responses are elicited.[98] The second injection blocks the radial nerve, and it is performed on the lateral aspect of the leg, between the middle and distal third of the humerus. As above, the needle is advanced until the characteristic motor response is seen.[98]

If ultrasound guidance is used, a 12-MHz linear probe is placed on the belly of the triceps muscle, at the proximal third of the humerus, perpendicular to the long axis of the leg. The radial, ulnar, musculocutaneous, and median nerves are visualized cranial and caudal to the brachial artery. The insulated needle connected to the nerve stimulator is introduced in plane with the ultrasound probe and advanced cranially until the characteristic motor responses are elicited.[98]

FEMORAL AND SCIATIC NERVES BLOCKS

The sciatic and the femoral nerves arise from the lumbosacral (LS) plexus, and innervate the stifle and the structures distal to it.[108] Nerve stimulator and ultrasound-guided sciatic and femoral nerve blocks have been described in rabbits.[98,109] The femoral nerve is blocked in the inguinal region. The rabbit is placed in lateral recumbency with the limb to be blocked uppermost, abducted at 90° angle, and extended caudally. The femoral artery is palpated, and a 22-gauge, 25-mm insulted needle connected to a nerve stimulator is inserted in the caudal portion of the sartorius muscle, cranial to the femoral artery, and perpendicular to the skin. The needle is advanced until stifle extension (produced by the femoral nerve stimulation) is observed.[98,109]

A similar technique can be performed under ultrasound guidance.[98] In this case, a 12-MHz linear probe is placed at the femoral triangle, at 90° angle to the long axis of the leg, to visualize the femoral artery and vein and the femoral nerve. The needle inserted in the cranial portion of the sartorius muscle, in-plane to the ultrasound probe, and directed caudally toward the femoral nerve.[98]

A pre-iliac approach technique to block the femoral nerve is reported in rabbits,[98] and results in blockade of the nerve proximal to the origin of its cutaneous branch, the saphenous nerve.[110] An insulated needle is inserted with a 30° to 45° angle to the skin, at the intersection between a line originating from the spinous process of L6 and perpendicular to the spine, and a second line originating from the cranial aspect of the iliac crest and parallel to the spine. Advance the needle caudomedially toward the greater trochanter of the femur, until stifle extension occurs.[98] If an ultrasound is used for the pre-iliac approach to the femoral nerve block, the rabbit is placed in dorsal recumbency, and a 12-MHz linear ultrasound probe is placed on the ventral aspect of the sublumbar musculature, at the level of L7, with a transverse orientation to the long axis of the spine. This allows direct visualization of the needle as it gets advanced caudomedially longitudinally to the probe.[98]

A separate injection is performed to block the sciatic nerve. The rabbit is placed in lateral recumbency with the limb to be blocked uppermost. The needle is inserted at approximately one-third the distance between the greater trochanter of the femur and the ischiatic tuberosity, closer to the greater trochanter, at 60° to 90° angle to the skin, and advanced until plantar extension and contraction of the caudal thigh muscles is seen.[98,109] The sciatic nerve can also be blocked under ultrasound guidance through a mediolateral approach.[98] A 12-MHz linear probe ultrasound probe is placed on the proximal third of the thigh, with the rabbit positioned in lateral recumbency and the sciatic nerve is visualized. A needle is inserted in the belly of the semitendinosus, in-plane to the ultrasound probe, and advance cranially toward the sciatic nerve.[98]

Only one clinical study is published investigating the efficacy and complications of a nerve stimulator–guided sciatic-femoral block in pet rabbits. In this case series, injection of 0.05 mL/kg of lidocaine 2% around the femoral and sciatic nerve produced effective blockade in rabbits anesthetized for orthopedic surgery distal to the knee, and no side effects were reported. Unfortunately, the overall duration of the block was not tested.[109]

EPIDURAL

Epidural injections are commonly performed at the LS junction to desensitize the pelvic limb and tissues caudal to it. Rabbits have 6 or 7 lumbar vertebra, 4 sacral vertebra, and the spinal cord terminates within the first, most commonly second, or third sacral vertebra.[108]

With the rabbit in sternal recumbency, the hind limbs are extended cranially, the LS junction is palpated as a depression on the midline at the level of the most prominent portion of the wings of the ileum. A 22 to 25g, 25 to 38 mm spinal or Touhy needle is introduced caudal to the last lumbar vertebra and advanced into the spinal canal until a "pop sensation," indicative of flavum ligament crossing, is felt. Correct needle placement can be also confirmed by lack of resistance (LOR) to air or saline introduced in the epidural space with a low-resistance syringe. Although the use of saline to perform the LOR technique can result in dilution of the LA solution, the use of air was associated with the reduced spread and uneven cranial distribution of contrast medium within the epidural space in research dogs, when compared with saline.[111] In the same study, air-induced compression of the spinal cord was seen with CT epidurography in some cases, but no neurologic complications were observed.[111]

If using the "hanging drop technique" to verify the correct positioning of the needle in the epidural space, the stylet of the needle is removed after being advanced through the skin and SC tissue, and the hub of the needle is filled with sterile saline. The needle is further advanced and once it crosses the flavum ligament the saline drop will aspirate in, due to negative pressure within the epidural space produced by the bulging of the flavum ligament during needle advancement. Because the dural sac of rabbits extends to the sacrum, there is a high chance of subdural injections while attempting epidural injections at the LS junction. Regardless of the technique used, always use a syringe to ensure negative aspiration and confirm the lack of both cerebrospinal fluid (CSF) and blood before injecting any solution. Presence of CSF indicates the needle is in the subdural space. Because of the small amount of CSF in rabbits, some authors report concerns whether the lack of CSF in the hub of the needle can be used as a confirmation of the needle tip being positioned in the epidural space, as presence of CSF in the hub of the needle is not always observed.[112] Moreover, with the "hanging drop technique," after the stylet is removed, a plug of tissue might clog the needle, preventing CSF from being seen. In other species, electrolocation is useful at discriminating whereas the needle is placed in the epidural or subarachnoid space, but the same is not true for rabbits.[112]

To reduce the chance of performing an accidental spinal injection, ultrasound and electrolocation have been used for sacrococcygeal epidural injections in rabbits.[98] The ultrasound allows to measure the distance between the skin and yellow ligament, which is then used to guide the insertion of the insulated needle connected to a nerve stimulator in the epidural space. The needle is advanced until it penetrates the yellow ligament, and contraction of the tail is seen. After negative aspiration, the solution is injected and its correct placement into the epidural space can be confirmed via ultrasound.[98]

Doses of 0.2 mL/kg of 2% lidocaine and 0.125% to 0.5% bupivacaine 0.1 to 0.4 mL/ kg have been used in rabbits to desensitize the hindlimbs and anything caudal to it without significant complications, in both clinical and experimental settings.[88,95,105,113,114] Epidural administration of 0.2 mL/kg of 2% lidocaine at the LS pace results in rapid-onset (1 to 3 min) of sensory and motor block to the hindquarters for 20 to 40 min in rabbits, without signs of toxicity.[113,114] Bupivacaine 0.3% injected epidurally at the LS space in New Zealand White rabbits produced, as expected, a longer lasting sensory and motor blockade compared with lidocaine.[88] In this study, rabbits weighing 2.5 to 2.7 kg received 3 mg or 6 mg of bupivacaine 0.3%. With the lower dose, motor blockade was rapid (5 ± 2 min) and lasted 113 ± 66 min; sensory blockade was achieved in 16 ± 4 min and lasted 75 ± 20.[88] Prolongation of both motor and sensory blockade was seen after 6 mg (176 ± 38 and 119 ± 36 min, respectively).[88] More significant hypotension occurred after 6 mg than after 3 mg epidural bupivacaine.[88] Morphine 0.1 mg/kg is commonly added to the LA mixture.[85,95,114] All drugs should be preservative free.

If CSF is detected while attending an LS epidural, a volume lower than that was originally intended for epidural injection is delivered, although clear indications are lacking in rabbits. In dogs, spinal injection of 0.05 mL/kg of bupivacaine 0.5% at the LS space will result in a block up to L3 dermatome. When morphine is added to the LA solution the suggested dose for spinal injection in dogs is 0.01 to 0.03 mg/kg.[115]

SUMMARY

Pain management is an essential component of veterinary care for rabbits for painful conditions and in the perioperative period. Although analgesic drugs and techniques are increasingly used in rabbits, they are likely still underutilized. Successful analgesic treatment necessitates knowledge of rabbit-specific anatomy, physiology, behavior, and metabolism. Although there are many similarities to pharmacologic drugs and techniques to dog and cat medicine, rabbit-specific knowledge of the current literature is essential for appropriate analgesic management. Ideally, an analgesic plan will include multimodal analgesia focusing on both pharmacologic intervention, non-pharmacologic intervention, and locoregional techniques.

CLINICS CARE POINTS

- Although studies have shown a negative effect of opioids on gastrointestinal motility in healthy rabbits, no studies have evaluated the gastrointestinal effect of these drugs in painful animals. Opioid analgesics are warranted in painful rabbits if appropriate nutritional support is provided, and patient monitoring is conducted.

- Multi-modal analgesia is likely underutilized in rabbit medicine and should be considered as a component of a complete analgesic plan.

- Locoregional analgesia may be a useful component of an analgesic plan. However, rabbit-specific anatomy must be considered as some of the techniques differ from those in other small animals.

- Most studies evaluating analgesia originate from healthy laboratory animal rabbits. Clinical response and translation of these dosages and protocols may therefore differ in clinically debilitated animals.

REFERENCES

1. Association AVM. AVMA pet ownership and demographics sourcebook. Veterinary Economics Division; 2018.
2. Coulter CA, Flecknell PA, Leach MC, et al. Reported analgesic administration to rabbits undergoing experimental surgical procedures. BMC Vet Res 2011;7:12.
3. Nunamaker EA, Stolarik DF, Ma J, et al. Clinical efficacy of sustained-release buprenorphine with meloxicam for postoperative analgesia in beagle dogs undergoing ovariohysterectomy. J Am Assoc Lab Anim Sci 2014;53:494–501.
4. Goldschlager GB, Gillespie VL, Palme R, et al. Effects of multimodal analgesia with LowDose buprenorphine and meloxicam on fecal glucocorticoid metabolites after surgery in New Zealand white rabbits (Oryctolagus cuniculus). J Am Assoc Lab Anim Sci 2013;52:571–6.
5. Woolf CJ, Chong M-S. Preemptive analgesia—treating postoperative pain by preventing the establishment of central sensitization. Anesth Analg 1993;77:362–79.
6. Shafford HL, Schadt JC. Effect of buprenorphine on the cardiovascular and respiratory response to visceral pain in conscious rabbits. Vet Anaesth Analg 2008;35:333–40.
7. Fleischer S, Sharkey M, Mealey K, et al. Pharmacogenetic and Metabolic Differences Between Dog Breeds: Their Impact on Canine Medicine and the Use of the Dog as a Preclinical Animal Model. AAPS J 2008;10:110–9.
8. KuKanich B, Wiese AJ. Opioids. Veterinary Anesthesia and Analgesia; 2015. p. 207–26.
9. Hayashida M, Fukunaga A, Fukuda K-i, et al. A rabbit model for evaluation of surgical anesthesia and analgesia: characterization and validation with isoflurane anesthesia and fentanyl analgesia. J Anesth 2004;18:282–91.

10. Barter LS, Hawkins MG, Pypendop BH. Effects of fentanyl on isoflurane minimum alveolar concentration in New Zealand White rabbits (Oryctolagus cuniculus). Am J Vet Res 2015;76:111–5.

11. Tearney CC, Barter LS, Pypendop BH. Cardiovascular effects of equipotent doses of isoflurane alone and isoflurane plus fentanyl in New Zealand White rabbits (Oryctolagus cuniculus). Am J Vet Res 2015;76:591–8.

12. Foley PL, Henderson AL, Bissonette EA, et al. Evaluation of fentanyl transdermal patches in rabbits: blood concentrations and physiologic response. Comp Med 2001;51:239–44.

13. Mirschberger V, von Deimling C, Heider A, et al. Fentanyl Plasma Concentrations after Application of a Transdermal Patch in Three Different Locations to Refine Postoperative Pain Management in Rabbits. Animals 2020;10:1778.

14. Weaver LA, Blaze CA, Linder DE, et al. A Model for Clinical Evaluation of Perioperative Analgesia in Rabbits (Oryctolagus cuniculus). J Am Assoc Lab Anim Sci : JAALAS 2010;49:845–51.

15. Weinstock M, Erez E, Roll D. Antagonism of the cardiovascular and respiratory depressant effects of morphine in the conscious rabbit by physostigmine. J Pharmacol Exp Ther 1981;218:504–8.

16. Hayashida M, Fukunaga A, Hanaoka K. Detection of acute tolerance to the analgesic and nonanalgesic effects of remifentanil infusion in a rabbit model. Anesth Analg 2003;97:1347–52.

17. Yu EH, Tran DH, Lam SW, et al. Remifentanil tolerance and hyperalgesia: short-term gain, long-term pain? Anaesthesia 2016;71:1347–62.

18. Chang S-F, Moore L, Chien YW. Pharmacokinetics and bioavailability of hydromorphone: effect of various routes of administration. Pharm Res 1988;5:718–21.

19. Roerig S, Fujimoto JM, Wang RI. Isolation of hydromorphone and dihydromorphine glucuronides from urine of the rabbit after hydromorphone administration. Proc Soc Exp Biol Med 1973;143:230–3.

20. Cone EJ, Darwin WD, Buchwald WF, et al. Oxymorphone metabolism and urinary excretion in human, rat, guinea pig, rabbit, and dog. Drug Metab Dispos 1983;11:446–50.

21. Guedes A, Papich M, Rude E, et al. Pharmacokinetics and physiological effects of intravenous hydromorphone in conscious dogs. J Vet Pharmacol Ther 2008; 31:334–43.

22. Schnellbacher RW, Divers SJ, Comolli JR, et al. Effects of intravenous administration of lidocaine and buprenorphine on gastrointestinal tract motility and signs of pain in New Zealand White rabbits after ovariohysterectomy. Am J Vet Res 2017;78:1359–71.

23. DiVincenti L, Meirelles LAD, Westcott RA. Safety and clinical effectiveness of a compounded sustained-release formulation of buprenorphine for postoperative analgesia in New Zealand White rabbits. J Am Vet Med Assoc 2016;248: 795–801.

24. Flecknell P, Liles J. Assessment of the analgesic action of opioid agonist-antagonists in the rabbit. J Assoc Vet Anaesthetists Great Britain Ireland 1990;17:24–9.

25. Robertson S, Taylor P, Lascelles B, et al. Changes in thermal threshold response in eight cats after administration of buprenorphine, butorphanol and morphine. Vet Rec 2003;153:462–5.

26. Murphy KL, Roughan JV, Baxter MG, et al. Anaesthesia with a combination of ketamine and medetomidine in the rabbit: effect of premedication with buprenorphine. Vet Anaesth Analg 2010;37:222–9.

27. DiVincenti L Jr, Meirelles LA, Westcott RA. Safety and clinical effectiveness of a compounded sustained-release formulation of buprenorphine for postoperative analgesia in New Zealand white rabbits. J Am Vet Med Assoc 2016;248: 795–801.

28. Askar R, Fredriksson E, Manell E, et al. Bioavailability of subcutaneous and intramuscular administrated buprenorphine in New Zealand White rabbits. BMC Vet Res 2020;16:1–10.

29. Andrews DD, Fajt VR, Baker KC, et al. A Comparison of Buprenorphine, Sustained release Buprenorphine, and High concentration Buprenorphine in Male New Zealand White Rabbits. J Am Assoc Lab Anim Sci 2020;59:546–56.

30. Freijs E. Comparison of plasma levels and analgesic effect between oral transmucosal and subcutaneous administration of buprenorphine in rabbits. Department of Clinical Science, Swedish University of Agricultural Sciences; 2016. p. 1–24.

31. Portnoy L, Hustead D. Pharmacokinetics of butorphanol tartrate in rabbits. Am J Vet Res 1992;53:541–3.

32. Nomura Y, Hayashi S. Pre- and Post-Synaptic Effects of Spiradoline and U-50488H, Selective Kappa Opioid Receptor Agonists, in Isolated Ileum. Scand J Gastroenterol 1992;27:295–302.

33. Cosola C, Albrizio M, Guaricci A, et al. OPIOID AGONIST/ANTAGONIST EFFECT OF NALOXONE IN. J Physiol Pharmacol 2006;57:439–49.

34. Deflers H, Gandar F, Bolen G, et al. Influence of a single dose of buprenorphine on rabbit (Oryctolagus cuniculus) gastrointestinal motility. Vet Anaesth analgesia 2018;45:510–9.

35. Martin-Flores M, Singh B, Walsh CA, et al. Effects of buprenorphine, methylnaltrexone, and their combination on gastrointestinal transit in healthy New Zealand white rabbits. J Am Assoc Lab Anim Sci 2017;56:155–9.

36. Feldman ER, Singh B, Mishkin NG, et al. Effects of Cisapride, Buprenorphine, and Their Combination on Gastrointestinal Transit in New Zealand White Rabbits. J Am Assoc Lab Anim Sci 2021;60(2).

37. Deflers H, Gandar F, Bolen G, et al. Effects of a Single Opioid Dose on Gastrointestinal Motility in Rabbits (Oryctolagus cuniculus): Comparisons among Morphine, Butorphanol, and Tramadol. Vet Sci 2022;9:28.

38. P D, Di Girolamo N RM. Effects of injectable analgesics on selected gastrointestinal physiologic parameters in rabbits. Proc ExoticsCon 2021;342–3.

39. Soares JHN, Brosnan RJ, Smith A, et al. Rabbit model of chest wall rigidity induced by fentanyl and the effects of apomorphine. Respir Physiol Neurobiol 2014;202:50–2.

40. Henke J, Astner S, Brill T, et al. Comparative study of three intramuscular anaesthetic combinations (medetomidine/ketamine, medetomidine/fentanyl/midazolam and xylazine/ketamine) in rabbits. Vet Anaesth Analg 2005;32:261–70.

41. Shafford HL, Schadt JC. Respiratory and cardiovascular effects of buprenorphine in conscious rabbits. Vet Anaesth Analg 2008;35:326–32.

42. Schroeder CA, Smith LJ. Respiratory rates and arterial blood gas tensions in healthy rabbits given buprenorphine, butorphanol, midazolam, or their combinations. J Am Assoc Lab Anim Sci 2011;50:205–11.

43. May CN, Ham IW, Heslop KE, et al. Intravenous morphine causes hypertension, hyperglycaemia and increases sympatho-adrenal outflow in conscious rabbits. Clin Sci 1988;75:71–7.

44. Raffa RB, Friderichs E, Reimann W, et al. Opioid and nonopioid components independently contribute to the mechanism of action of tramadol, an'atypical'opioid analgesic. J Pharmacol Exp Ther 1992;260:275–85.

45. Duvall A. Tramadol. J Exot Pet Med 2017;26:74–7.

46. Souza MJ, Greenacre CB, Cox SK. Pharmacokinetics of orally administered tramadol in domestic rabbits (Oryctolagus cuniculus). Am J Vet Res 2008;69:979–82.

47. Oguntoye CO, Oyewande OA, Afolabi OO. Evaluation of Tramadol-Midazolam-Ketamine Anaesthesia in Rabbits. Niger J Physiol Sci 2018;33:145–9.

48. Udegbunam RI, Onuba AC, Okorie-Kanu C, et al. Effects of two doses of tramadol on pain and some biochemical parameters in rabbits post-gastrotomy. Comp Clin Path 2015;24:783–90.

49. Egger CM, Souza MJ, Greenacre CB, et al. Effect of intravenous administration of tramadol hydrochloride on the minimum alveolar concentration of isoflurane in rabbits. Am J Vet Res 2009;70:945–9.

50. AL-Fathee MY, Taqa GA, AL- Jameel MY. The Effect of Tramadol on the Peristaltic Movement Small Intestine in Rabbit. Rafidain J Sci 2011;22:1–10.

51. Ali OK, Ahmed A, Mawlood A. Effects of tramadol on histopathological and biochemical parameters in male rabbits. Am J Biol Life Sci 2015;3:85–90.

52. Papich MG, Messenger K. Non-steroidal anti-inflammatory drugs. Veterinary Anesthesia and Analgesia; 2015. p. 227–43.

53. Audeval-Gerard C, Nivet C, El Amrani A-I, et al. Pharmacokinetics of ketoprofen in rabbit after a single topical application. Eur J Drug Metab Pharmacokinet 2000;25:227–30.

54. Fredholm DV, Carpenter JW, KuKanich B, et al. Pharmacokinetics of meloxicam in rabbits after oral administration of single and multiple doses. Am J Vet Res 2013;74:636–41.

55. Delk KW, Carpenter JW, KuKanich B, et al. Pharmacokinetics of meloxicam administered orally to rabbits (Oryctolagus cuniculus) for 29 days. Am J Vet Res 2014;75:195–9.

56. Turner PV, Chen CH, Taylor MW. Pharmacokinetics of meloxicam in rabbits after single and repeat oral dosing. Comp Med 2006;56:63–7.

57. Carpenter JW, Pollock CG, Koch DE, et al. Single and multiple-dose pharmacokinetics of meloxicam after oral administration to the rabbit (Oryctolagus cuniculus). J Zoo Wildl Med 2009;40:601–6.

58. Leach MC, Allweiler S, Richardson C, et al. Behavioural effects of ovariohysterectomy and oral administration of meloxicam in laboratory housed rabbits. Res Vet Sci 2009;87:336–47.

59. Parra-Coca A, Boix-Montañés A, Calpena-Campmany AC, et al. In vivo pharmacokinetic evaluation of carprofen delivery from intra-articular nanoparticles in rabbits: A population modelling approach. Res Vet Sci 2021;137:235–42.

60. Hawkins M, Taylor I, Craigmill A, et al. Enantioselective pharmacokinetics of racemic carprofen in New Zealand white rabbits. J Vet Pharmacol Ther 2008;31:423–30.

61. Hedenqvist P, Trbakovic A, Thor A, et al. Carprofen neither reduces postoperative facial expression scores in rabbits treated with buprenorphine nor alters long term bone formation after maxillary sinus grafting. Res Vet Sci 2016;107:123–31.

62. Ahmad A, Nawaz RS, Qureshi TA, et al. Histopathological effect of Meloxicam (Preferential COX-2 inhibitor NSAID) on liver and kidney of Rabbit. Int J Biosiences 2017;11(3):148–58.

63. Scarabelli S, Nardini G. Gastrointestinal vasculitis and necrosis In a rabbit under long-term meloxicam treatment. J Exot Pet Med 2020;34:26.

64. De Vito V, Salvadori M, Poapolathep A, et al. Pharmacokinetic/pharmacodynamic evaluation of grapiprant in a carrageenan-induced inflammatory pain model in the rabbit. J Vet Pharmacol Ther 2017;40:468–75.

65. Verret M, Lauzier F, Zarychanski R, et al. Perioperative Use of Gabapentinoids for the Management of Postoperative Acute Pain: A Systematic Review and Meta-analysis. Anesthesiology 2020;133:265–79.

66. Kozer E, Levichek Z, Hoshino N, et al. The Effect of Amitriptyline, Gabapentin, and Carbamazepine on Morphine-Induced Hypercarbia in Rabbits. Anesth Analg 2008;107.

67. Kale A, Börcek AÖ, Emmez H, et al. Neuroprotective effects of gabapentin on spinal cord ischemia-reperfusion injury in rabbits. J Neurosurg Spine 2011;15: 228–37.

68. Pang DSJ. Anesthetic and analgesic Adjunctive drugs. Veterinary Anesthesia and Analgesia; 2015. p. 244–59.

69. Burton M, Conway R, Mishkin N, et al. Pharmacokinetics of gabapentin after single, oral administration in domestic rabbits (Oryctolagus cuniculus). ICARE 2022;114.

70. Baumgartner C, Bollerhey M, Ebner J, et al. Effects of medetomidine-midazolam-fentanyl IV bolus injections and its reversal by specific antagonists on cardiovascular function in rabbits. Can J Vet Res 2010;74:286–98.

71. Marini RP, Li X, Harpster NK, et al. Cardiovascular pathology possibly associated with ketamine/xylazine anesthesia in Dutch belted rabbits. Lab Anim Sci 1999;49:153–60.

72. Lee HW, Machin H, Adami C. Peri-anaesthetic mortality and nonfatal gastrointestinal complications in pet rabbits: a retrospective study on 210 cases. Vet Anaesth Analg 2018;45:520–8.

73. Berry SH. Injectable Anesthetics. Veterinary Anesthesia and Analgesia; 2015. p. 277–96.

74. Slingsby LS, Waterman-Pearson AE. The post-operative analgesic effects of ketamine after canine ovariohysterectomy—a comparison between pre- or postoperative administration. Res Vet Sci 2000;69:147–52.

75. Gianotti G, Valverde A, Sinclair M, et al. Prior determination of baseline minimum alveolar concentration (MAC) of isoflurane does not influence the effect of ketamine on MAC in rabbits. Can J Vet Res = Revue canadienne de recherche veterinaire 2012;76:261–7.

76. Lipman NS, Marini RP, Erdman SE. A comparison of ketamine/xylazine and ketamine/xylazine/acepromazine anesthesia in the rabbit. Lab Anim Sci 1990;40: 395–8.

77. Okano S, Ikeura Y, Inatomi N. Effects of Tachykinin NK1 Receptor Antagonists on the Viscerosensory Response Caused by Colorectal Distention in Rabbits. J Pharmacol Exp Ther 2002;300:925–31.

78. Ozawa SM, Hawkins MG, Drazenovich TL, et al. Pharmacokinetics of maropitant citrate in New Zealand White rabbits (Oryctolagus cuniculus). Am J Vet Res 2019;80:963–8.

79. Boscan P, Monnet E, Mama K, et al. Effect of maropitant, a neurokinin 1 receptor antagonist, on anesthetic requirements during noxious visceral stimulation of the ovary in dogs. Am J Vet Res 2011;72:1576–9.

80. Sadar MJ, McGee WK, Au GG, et al. Pilot pharmacokinetics of a higher dose of subcutaneous maropitant administration in healthy domestic rabbits (Oryctolagus cuniculus). J Exot Pet Med 2022;41:1–2.

81. Rooney T, Carpenter JW, KuKanich B, et al. Pharmacokinetics of cannabidiol administered orally in the Rabbit (Oryctolagus cuniculus). ExoticsCon 2021;199.

82. Valverde A, Doherty TJ, Hernández J, et al. Effect of lidocaine on the minimum alveolar concentration of isoflurane in dogs. Vet Anaesth Analg 2004;31:264–71.

83. Schnellbacher RW, Carpenter JW, Mason DE, et al. Effects of lidocaine administration via continuous rate infusion on the minimum alveolar concentration of isoflurane in New Zealand White rabbits (Oryctolagus cuniculus). Am J Vet Res 2013;74:1377–84.

84. van der Wal SEI, van den Heuvel SAS, Radema SA, et al. The in vitro mechanisms and in vivo efficacy of intravenous lidocaine on the neuroinflammatory response in acute and chronic pain. Eur J Pain 2016;20:655–74.

85. Antończyk A, Liszka B, Skrzypczak P, et al. Comparison of analgesia provided by lidocaine or morphine delivered epidurally in rabbits undergoing hindlimb orthopedic surgery. Pol J Vet Sci 2019;22:31–5.

86. Barter LS. Rabbit analgesia. Vet Clin Exot Anim Pract 2011;14:93–104.

87. Bernards CM, Artru AA. Effect of intracerebroventricular picrotoxin and muscimol on intravenous bupivacaine toxicity. Evidence supporting central nervous system involvement in bupivacaine cardiovascular toxicity. Anesthesiology 1993;78:902–10.

88. Dollo G, Malinovsky J-M, Péron A, et al. Prolongation of epidural bupivacaine effects with hyaluronic acid in rabbits. Int J Pharm 2004;272:109–19.

89. Mahajan A, Derian A. Local anesthetic toxicity. Treasure Island (FL): StatPearls Publishing; 2021.

90. Campoy L, Read MR. Small animal regional anesthesia and analgesia. John Wiley & Sons; 2013.

91. Auroy Y, Narchi P, Messiah A, et al. Serious complications related to regional anesthesia: results of a prospective survey in France. J Am Soc Anesthesiologists 1997;87:479–86.

92. d'Ovidio D, Adami C. Neuropraxia after infraorbital nerve block in a pet rabbit (Oryctolagus cuniculus). Vet Anaesth Analg 2021;48:817–9.

93. d'Ovidio D, Adami C. Locoregional Anesthesia in Exotic Pets. Vet Clin North Am Exot Anim Pract 2019;22:301–14.

94. Böhmer E. Dentistry in rabbits and rodents. 1st edition. Chichester United Kingdom: Wiley Blackwell; 2015.

95. Lichtenberger M, Ko J. Anesthesia and analgesia for small mammals and birds. Vet Clin North Am Exot Anim Pract 2007;10:293–315.

96. Woodward TM. Pain management and regional anesthesia for the dental patient. Top Companion Anim Med 2008;23:106–14.

97. Peña T, Campoy L, de Matos R. Investigation of a maxillary nerve block technique in healthy New Zealand White rabbits (Oryctolagus cuniculus). Am J Vet Res 2020;81:843–8.

98. Otero PE, Portela DA. Manual of small animal regional anesthesia: Illustrated anatomy for nerve stimulation and ultrasound-guided nerve blocks. 5M Publishing; 2019.

99. Yong-Di L, Zheng-Long T, Jian-Qin T, et al. Anatomy of the Inferior Alveolar Nerve in Rabbits and its Block Anesthesia. Int J Oral Dent Health 2018;4:051.

100. Lennox AM. Clinical technique: small exotic companion mammal dentistry—anesthetic considerations. J Exot Pet Med 2008;17:102–6.

101. de Miguel Garcia C, Radkey DI, Hetzel S, et al. Injection techniques for auricular nerve blocks in the rabbit cadaver. Vet Anaesth Analg 2020;47:274–9.
102. Najman IE, Ferreira JZ, Abimussi CJ, et al. Ultrasound-assisted periconal ocular blockade in rabbits. Vet Anaesth Analg 2015;42:433–41.
103. Hazra S, Palui H, Biswas B, et al. Anesthesia for intraocular surgery in rabbits. Scand J Lab Anim Sci 2011;38:81–7.
104. de Miguel Garcia C, Doss G, Travis ML, et al. Efficacy of greater auricular and auriculotemporal nerve blocks performed in rabbits. Vet Anaesth Analg 2020; 47:567–73.
105. Hawkins M, Pascoe P. Anesthesia, Analgesia and Sedation of Small Mammals. In: Quezenberry K, Christoph M, Orcutt C, et al, editors. Ferrets, rabbits and Rodents: clinical medicine and surgery. Philadelphia: Saunders; 2020.
106. Osofsky A, LeCouteur RA, Vernau KM. Functional neuroanatomy of the domestic rabbit (Oryctolagus cuniculus). Vet Clin North Am Exot Anim Pract 2007;10: 713–30.
107. Fonseca C, Server A, Esteves M, et al. An ultrasound-guided technique for axillary brachial plexus nerve block in rabbits. Lab Animal 2015;44:179–84.
108. Greenaway J, Partlow G, Gonsholt NL, et al. Anatomy of the lumbosacral spinal cord in rabbits. J Am Anim Hosp Assoc 2001;37:27–34.
109. d'Ovidio D, Rota S, Noviello E, et al. Nerve stimulator–guided sciatic-femoral block in pet rabbits (Oryctolagus cuniculus) undergoing hind limb surgery: a case series. J Exot pet Med 2014;23:91–5.
110. Portela DA, Otero PE, Briganti A, et al. Femoral nerve block: a novel psoas compartment lateral pre-iliac approach in dogs. Vet Anaesth Analg 2013;40: 194–204.
111. Iseri T, Nishimura R, Nagahama S, et al. Epidural spread of iohexol following the use of air or saline in the 'loss of resistance'test. Vet Anaesth Analg 2010;37: 526–30.
112. Otero PE, Portela DA, Brinkyer JA, et al. Use of electrical stimulation to monitor lumbosacral epidural and intrathecal needle placement in rabbits. Am J Vet Res 2012;73:1137–41.
113. Doherty MM, Hughes PJ, Korszniak NV, et al. Prolongation of lidocaine-induced epidural anesthesia by medium molecular weight hyaluronic acid formulations: pharmacodynamic and pharmacokinetic studies in the rabbit. Anesth Analg 1995;80:740–6.
114. Gusak V, Turkovic V, Nesek-Adam V, et al. Lidocaine serum concentration after epidural administration in combination with morphine and fentanyl in rabbit–A preliminary study. Res Vet Sci 2013;94:651–5.
115. Novello L, Corletto F, Rabozzi R, et al. Sparing effect of a low dose of intrathecal morphine on fentanyl requirements during spinal surgery: a preliminary clinical investigation in dogs. Vet Surg 2008;37:153–60.
116. Hedenqvist P, Orr HE, Roughan JV, et al. Anaesthesia with ketamine/medetomidine in the rabbit: influence of route of administration and the effect of combination with butorphanol. Vet Anaesth Analg 2002;29:14–9.
117. Fisher P, Graham J. Rabbits. Exotic animal formulary. St. Louis, MO: Elsevier; 2018. p. 494–531.

Pain Recognition in Ferrets

Yvonne van Zeeland, DVM, MVR, PhD, Dip ECZM (Avian, Small mammal), CPBC,
Nico Schoemaker, DVM, PhD, Dip ECZM (Small mammal, Avian)*

KEYWORDS

- Ferret • *Mustela putorius furo* • Pain recognition • Grimace scale • Behavior

KEY POINTS

- Recognition of pain in ferrets can be challenging.
- Pain assessment requires a combined evaluation of physiologic and behavioral parameters, as most of these on their own are nonspecific.
- Similar to other animals, a grimace scale seems to be a useful tool to recognize pain in ferrets.

INTRODUCTION

Over the past decades, increasing attention has been paid to animal welfare, which involves the minimizing of suffering, pain, and discomfort. To minimize pain and deliver effective pain management, an understanding of the pathophysiology of pain and knowledge of the pharmacologic and pharmacodynamic effects of analgesics is required. In addition, it is equally important for veterinarians (and caregivers) to have the knowledge and skills to accurately assess whether an animal is suffering from pain or whether the administered analgesia is sufficient to provide effective pain relief. However, the recognition and accurate assessment of the severity of pain can be challenging as animals are unable to verbally communicate, and often tend to hide their pain.[1] Signs may also be subtle, hence being easily overlooked by the inexperienced observer that is not familiar with the normal physiology and behavior of the species involved.[2] Pain assessment in animals heavily relies on the assessment of behavioral, physiologic, and other clinical parameters that serve as indirect indicators of pain, and is therefore subject to some degree of variability among observers. While the basic principles of pain recognition apply to all species, there are also signs that are more species-specific. Hence, a sound understanding of the species-specific behaviors and pain signs is required. This review will focus on pain and pain recognition in ferrets.

Division of Zoological Medicine, Department of Clinical Sciences, Faculty of Veterinary Medicine, Utrecht University, Yalelaan 108, Utrecht 3584 CM, the Netherlands
* Corresponding author.
E-mail address: N.J.Schoemaker@uu.nl

Vet Clin Exot Anim 26 (2023) 229–243
https://doi.org/10.1016/j.cvex.2022.07.011

Pain in Ferrets – Definition, Causes, and Pathophysiology

Like other animals, ferrets can experience pain for numerous reasons, including acute or chronic inflammatory diseases, neoplasia, trauma, surgery, and/or diagnostic procedures. Pain may either originate from the triggering of nociceptive nerve fibers by inflammation, chemical, or physical damage (*nociceptive pain*), or from a lesion or disease within the nervous system itself (*neuropathic pain*).[3,4] Two types of nociceptive pain can be distinguished, that is, *somatic pain*, which results from injuries to musculoskeletal tissues such as the skin, muscles, bones, joints, or connective tissue, and *visceral pain*, which arises from distension or inflammation of internal organs. Somatic pain is often well localized and described as intense, dull, throbbing, or sore, while visceral pain can present as gnawing, squeezing, or cramping, and is usually more diffuse and difficult to localize.[5,6] Visceral pain has also been associated with autonomic changes (eg, nausea, gastrointestinal disturbances, changes in body temperature, blood pressure, and heart rate), and may be referred to other parts of the body due to convergence on pathways within the spinal cord that also convey somatosensory information.[5,7,8] Neuropathic pain in humans can involve burning, shooting, stabbing, or tingling/electric-like sensations that can either be diffuse or follow a specific nerve path.[5] It is important to identify what type of pain is experienced, as effective pain management differs across the various types of pain. For example, non-steroidal anti-inflammatory drugs such as meloxicam are often effective in alleviating somatic pain, whereas neuropathic pain can respond favorably to gabapentin, a gamma-aminobutyric acid (GABA) analog.

Unfortunately, when assessing the patient, difficulties often arise when trying to assess whether the animal is in pain, let alone identify the type of pain involved. Challenges may also arise in relation to the recognition of chronic pain. Acute pain is often readily identified due to its immediate association with surgery, trauma, or disease of sudden onset, such as the pain associated with a trichobezoar or foreign body leading to ileus and distension of the gastrointestinal tract, or pain resulting from a bite sustained by another ferret or trauma resulting in a leg fracture. In contrast, chronic disease conditions such as neoplasia, dental disease, or arthritis, and their associated pain, often generate more subtle signs which are harder to recognize and assess. Moreover, pain can last well beyond the expected healing time for an injured tissue,[9] making it more difficult to identify whether an observed behavior or other sign is indicative of (chronic) pain or not.[10] Nevertheless, if a specific disease condition is identified, based on the analogy principle inferences can be made from knowledge obtained from human patients to help determine whether and to what extent pain is experienced. In addition, it can be taken into account that the various body tissues and organs have different sensitivities to painful stimuli. Examples of tissues that are considered very sensitive to pain include the mucous membranes, cornea, and dental pulp, whereas parenchymatous organs are often found to respond less to pain.[11] These principles and guidelines can help veterinarians to make decisions on whether and from which analgesic regimen and additional recommendations regarding husbandry and/or diet (eg, provision of soft bedding for ferrets suffering from chronic arthritis, or offering soft, liquid foods to animals with periodontal disease) the patient may benefit. Additionally, certain physiologic, biochemical, and behavioral parameters can be assessed, which can provide additional information regarding the need for and efficacy of an analgetic regimen in the individual patient.

Physiologic Parameters

One way to assess pain is by the evaluation of physiologic parameters that change in response to a painful stimulus. Nociception leads to the activation of the sympathetic nervous system, which in turn leads to catecholamine release (epinephrine, norepi-nephrine) which induces a series of cardiovascular, respiratory, and other physiologic changes as part of the fight-or-flight response. Some typical effects include an increase in body temperature, heart and respiratory rate, blood pressure, peripheral vasoconstriction, sweating, and pupillary dilation.[12] While many of these parameters can be measured in ferrets (**Table 1** for reference ranges), the handling and restraint needed to record them can influence the recorded values. For example, heart/pulse rate, body temperature, and respiratory frequency may easily and quickly rise following agitation (**Fig. 1**). A study evaluating the use of respiratory and heart rate in dogs indicated limited value of these parameters when assessing pain in hospital-ized animals.[13] While no studies have been performed to evaluate the value of clinical parameters for pain assessment in ferrets, findings are likely to be similar. Hence, the weight attributed to these clinical parameters remains questionable.

Evaluating blood pressure is generally more difficult to perform in awake ferrets due to their activity level and liveliness. In a study evaluating noninvasive blood pressure measurement in healthy animals, attempts were made to measure blood pressure in conscious animals by scruffing the loose skin on the back of the neck. Using this tech-nique, the authors were unable to obtain reliable measurements, hence rendering sedation with butorphanol and midazolam (0.2 mg/kg IM each) as the sole method to successfully obtain reliable measurements.[14] However, as butorphanol and mida-zolam can provide some analgesia, and lead to altered mentation, the usefulness of blood pressure measurements in relation to pain assessment remains questionable. In preliminary studies, the authors have attempted to measure blood pressure in conscious ferrets by offering liquid food (Convalescence support, Royal Canin). How-ever, as nearly all ferrets started trembling while eating, collecting measurements were not possible.

Another parameter that has been suggested to be helpful as an indicator of pain in animals is body weight as weight loss may indicate reduced food intake which can result from pain. Similarly, checking the quality and quantity of feces could be helpful to assess digestive function, which could be altered due to pain. However, for all pa-rameters, it should be noted that changes may also result from other pathology and that these are not necessarily caused by pain.[15] In addition, it is important to realize that ferrets display obvious sexual dimorphism (males being twice the size of females) and may undergo seasonal body weight changes, which can include a weight gain of 30% to 40% in autumn and winter.[16]

In human medicine, the value of physiologic parameters has been extensively stud-ied as these may provide helpful clues to identify pain in people that are unable to

Table 1 Physiologic indicators of discomfort	
Parameter	Reference Value
Respiratory rate[17,18]	33–36/min
Heart rate[16,17]	200–250 bpm
Blood pressure (diastole/systole)[14,16]	51–87/95–155 mm Hg
Temperature[17,18]	37.8–40 °C 98.6–104 °F
Body weight[18]	Female (jill): 600–950 g Male (hob): 1–2 kg
Cortisol[18,19]	6.6 (0.0–101.5) nmol/L

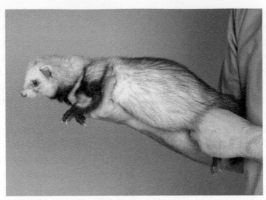

Fig. 1. The pulse frequency will increase under influence of pain, but is also influenced by agitation. When the ferret is rested on the lower arm the femoral pulse can easily be counted, minimally influenced by stress.

verbally communicate or self-report their pain, for example, those with severe or profound intellectual disability. Such studies have included more or less invasive technologies, such as electrocardiography (ECG) or photoplethysmography for the measurement of heart rate variability, pulse oximetry to measure changes in respiratory pattern, electromyography (EMG) to measure muscle tension, pupillometry to measure changes in pupillary diameter, skin conductance tests to measure changes in electrodermal activity related to sweating, and electroencephalography (EEG) or neuroimaging techniques (eg, [functional] magnetic resonance imaging, (f)MRI; positron emission tomography, PET) to record brain activity.[20–22] Of these, respiratory pattern analysis, muscle tension, and pupillometry have been shown to reliably indicate the presence of acute pain, whereas (f)MRI can assess changes in the brain as a result of both acute and long-term, chronic pain.[22] Of these, only PET and fMRI have been evaluated for assessing pain in animal models.[23,24] While these studies have shown similar changes in the brain as in humans following chronic pain and pharmacologic intervention, these techniques remain impractical from a clinical perspective because of their invasiveness, limited availability, and associated expenses. Electroencephalography has been more commonly used to study pain in animals. While these studies have mostly involved laboratory (eg, rabbits,[25] rats,[26,27] mice,[28]) and production animals (eg, sheep,[29,30] deer,[31] cattle,[32,33] pigs,[34] poultry[35]), some studies have evaluated its usefulness to assess pain in companion animals (eg, dogs,[36] horses,[37,38]). In ferrets, EEGs have also been performed.[39–41] However, their application is mostly limited to studies on sleep and brain dysfunction, rather than the study of pain. In addition, EEG has its practical limitations as locating pain centers in the brain and separating pain responses from other emotional states such as fear and anxiety may be difficult. Moreover, EEG interpretation may be hindered by movement artifacts.[42]

Biochemical Parameters

Aside from the activation of the sympathetic system, nociception will also lead to the activation of the hypothalamic–pituitary–adrenal axis. Corticotrophin-releasing hormone (CRH) produced by the hypothalamus will stimulate the release of adrenocorticotropic hormone (ACTH) by the anterior pituitary gland which leads to the production and release of glucocorticosteroids from the adrenal cortex. Of these, cortisol is the main glucocorticoid hormone in mammals, and its release will lead to a plethora of changes, including increased gluconeogenesis (which can eventually lead to weight loss), and suppression of the immune system (which can increase susceptibility to infections).[9,43] In animal models and patients with conditions associated with chronic pain (eg, fibromyalgia, irritable bowel syndrome, rheumatoid arthritis), marked HPA axis abnormalities have been noted, indicating a relationship between chronic pain and stress.[44–46] In many of these patients, abnormal cortisol levels can be observed.[47–49] As such, assessing the activity of the HPA system can be considered to assess pain or distress and has mostly involved the measurement of cortisol in plasma, saliva, urine, or feces of animals undergoing painful procedures such as abdominal surgery,[50] electroimmobilization,[51] and castration.[52] Sladky and colleagues (2000) evaluated fecal cortisol concentrations in laboratory ferrets (n = 12) undergoing ovariohysterectomy and bilateral anal sacculectomy following epidural anesthesia with morphine (0.1 mg/kg) or saline (0.1 mL/ferret).[53] While fecal cortisol concentrations were higher in all animals during the first 24h after surgery, increases were statistically significant only in the ferrets receiving the saline epidural, suggesting that morphine helps to attenuate the physiologic responses to surgically induced pain, and indicating that fecal cortisol can be used to assess pain in ferrets.[53] However, it is important to realize that—similar to physiologic parameters—values may be affected by other events which might not necessarily be associated with pain, such as stress induced by handling and restraint.[54,55] In addition, plasma concentrations, in particular, can periodically fluctuate and depend on circadian rhythms,[56–58] rendering serial measurements before and after treatment a necessity to properly evaluate the changes.[9]

Other biochemical parameters that have been measured in other animal species in relation to pain include plasma (nor)epinephrine, ACTH, glucose, and lactate.[59–62] Plasma epinephrine has been shown to increase rapidly but briefly after painful procedures such as tail docking and castration in lambs, castration in pigs, dehorning in calves, and ovariohysterectomy in dogs.[63–65] Plasma norepinephrine changes were found to show a similar pattern, though increases generally occurred later and lasted longer compared with epinephrine.[63] As such, these hormones may be useful to consider as a parameter to evaluate acute pain, but as these hormone measurements are not routinely conducted in practice, evaluation of pain by the measurement of these hormones is not routinely conducted. Prunier and colleagues (2005) evaluated the effects of painful procedures (eg, castration, tail docking) on cortisol, ACTH, glucose, and lactate in piglets, and found lactate to increase following castration, most likely as a result of (adrenalin-induced) catabolism of muscular glycogen.[59] Alternatively, increased lactate levels may have resulted from the increased muscular activity and anaerobic glycogenolysis associated with defensive movements made on experiencing acute pain.[62] In addition to lactate, glucose and free fatty acids are expected to increase following the release of catecholamines and/or cortisol. In horses and rabbits, glucose values have been found to significantly rise in animals suffering from highly painful, life-threatening diseases such as colic, gastrointestinal ileus, or liver lobe torsion.[66,67] However, in horses with chemically induced synovitis, no significant differences were found in glucose values following treatment with epidural analgesia and/or phenylbutazone, compared with a placebo.[68] Hence, the value of glucose as a sensitive and specific marker for pain remains questionable. Similarly, attempts were made to connect pain related to castration in male pigs with fluctuations in plasma concentrations of various other substances, including tumor necrosis factor-alpha, interleukin-1 beta, C-reactive protein, serum amyloid A and haptoglobin, have been unsuccessful.[69]

Behavioral Parameters

Already in 1985, Morton and Griffiths suggested that changes in behavior patterns could be useful to assess whether an animal is in pain, thereby emphasizing that behavior analysis should constitute a substantial part of pain assessment.[12] Behavior data also avoid the induction of stress or pain that can result from the collection of biochemical or physiologic parameters. However, a solid understanding of the normal behavior of a given species is essential to be able to correctly identify and interpret painful behavior. This is particularly true for the prey species that hide and disguise pain and display a "conservation-withdrawal" reflex rather than a "fight-or-flight" response that is commonly exhibited by the domesticated and predatory species.[2] Despite ferrets being predatory and domesticated species, pain can be seemingly difficult to recognize in this species. Some factors that might explain why ferrets might display less pain behaviors are the innate solitary lifestyle of its ancestor, limiting the need for obvious pain display, and their overall higher tolerance for pain.

Behavioral changes that are commonly observed in animals with pain include:

- Reduced (general) activity, including diminished play behavior and exploration of novel items or new environments.
- Restlessness.
- Changes in temperament, for example, sudden onset of aggression in animals that are otherwise friendly, or apathy/lethargy in animals that are otherwise fierce.
- Isolation and withdrawal behavior, for example, hiding in the back of the cage.
- Altered posture and/or gait, for example, lameness, increased muscle tension/rigidity, or loss of the normal hunched posture of ferrets.
- Lack of or reduced grooming behavior, resulting in a ruffled, unkempt appearance of the hair coat, or excessive biting licking.
- Piloerection, twitching/shivering (despite normal body temperature).
- Hypersensitivity to touch, sound, and/or temperature change.
- Diminished food and water intake.
- Bruxism (teeth grinding).
- Vocalizations differing in pitch and pattern from normal vocalizations.[1,2,12,55,70,71,72]

Many of the aforementioned parameters are nonspecific and may be affected by many other conditions or disorders. Moreover, behaviors may not uniformly manifest across species and can be subtle. For example, a study evaluating behavioral responses to tooth pulp inflammation in ferrets demonstrated ipsilateral tongue protrusions (ie, tongue protrusions aimed toward the affected side) to be the single most significant behavior change indicative of pain, whereas other behaviors, including face-wash strokes, headshakes, fore limb flairs, paw-licks, ear grasps and chin rubs, seemed less specific.[73] These findings emphasize the importance of familiarizing oneself with the normal behavior of the species as well as the individual to obtain proper baseline measurements for comparison.[12,70,74] In addition, sufficient time and close monitoring of the behavior are required to enable the detection of subtle behavior changes. In practice, this task is therefore usually performed by the owner or veterinary technician, who can be instructed to evaluate the animal's behavior and look for subtle changes therein. These behavior observations should normally take place without disturbing the animal at a time when it is awake and active. In ferrets, this poses an additional challenge as they may spend up to 70% of their time sleeping, with relatively short episodes of activity in between.[40,75]

Specific behaviors that have been reported as indicators of pain in ferrets include general malaise, anorexia/decreased appetite, lethargy, depression, inactivity/immobility, staying rolled up into a ball,[76,77] or reluctance to curl into this sleeping position (which is normal for a ferret).[78,79] Respirations may be more frequent and deeper, and the ferret may show a strained facial expression, squinting (**Fig. 2**), focal muscle fasciculations, or focal muscle bristling of the tail fur (**Fig. 3**).[2,76,77] Rather than walking with a normal, hunched posture, the ferret may have a stiff gait, and walk lame or with its head elevated and extended forward.[76,78,79,80] Additionally, ferrets may show aggression, biting, and/or teeth-bearing when disturbed.[76] Ferrets in pain may also stop grooming, hide themselves, grind their teeth, produce high-pitched vocalizations (eg, screeching, whining, crying), or grunt (particularly when handled).[76,77] However, the value of most of these parameters is primarily based on expert opinion with no studies performed to establish their clinical validity as indicators of pain.

When evaluating pain behavior in an animal it is also important to take into account that different forms of pain might induce different types of pain-related behaviors. For example, excessive biting or licking a particular body area or aversive responses to external palpation will often indicate localized pain in this area. Dental pain will commonly result in teeth grinding and reduced water and food intake, while ferrets with otitis media are more likely to show head shaking, ear scratching, dysphagia, and reluctance to open their mouth. Abdominal or visceral pain, which may result from for example, gastric ulceration, foreign body, trichobezoar, *Helicobacter* gastritis, or epizootic catarrhal enteritis (ED), is more likely to result in a stiff, stilted gait, or walking hunched with an arched back, immobility, reduced appetite or teeth grinding, especially when presented with food.[80]

Postoperative and traumatic pain usually manifests as a reluctance to move and an overall tensed facial expression with dull, half-open, noninquisitive eyes.[79] In addition, shivering or trembling despite normal body temperature may be seen, which disappears following the administration of an appropriate dose of analgesics. Sladky and colleagues (2000) reported specific behavioral changes in female ferrets that underwent ovariohysterectomy and anal sacculotomy and received epidural morphine for postoperative analgesia.[53] Compared with the treatment group, control animals displayed restricted/labored breathing patterns, trembling, and attenuation of movement on rubbing the site of incision over the edge of the nest box when climbing it, suggesting these behaviors to indicate pain. The latter in particular, has been shown to be a robust pain indicator in dogs and cats as well.[81–83] Other behavioral parameters, such as licking the incision site, drowsiness, and depression did not differ between

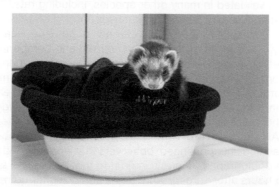

Fig. 2. A 5.5-year-old female, hospitalized in the clinic for acute liver failure. Notice the squinting of the eyes indicating a form of discomfort in this ferret.

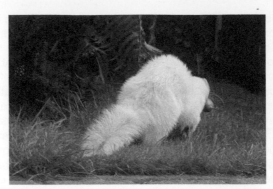

Fig. 3. This ferret is demonstrating the bristling of the hairs on the tail. This behavior can be seen either during excitement but can also be a sign of pain/discomfort (photo credit: B. van der Laan).

the control and treatment groups, suggesting these are less reliable as indicators for pain.

Facial Expressions

Pain can give rise to changes in facial expression as a result of activation of the sympathetic nervous system, which results in pupillary dilatation and muscle tension leading to ocular squinting, sunken eyes, and flattened ears.[12,70] Such facial changes may help to minimize sensory input,[84] but are also hypothesized to serve a function in soliciting for social support from conspecifics that can potentially help to diminish the experienced discomfort.[85]

Kinematic analysis of facial movements following a short-lasting, painful stimulus (IV catheter placement) using an infrared motion capture system and reflective markers on the eyelids, nostrils, facial crest, and midline, indicated consistent changes in facial expression on the delivery of the painful stimulus.[86] As changes are often subtle, these can be difficult to recognize for the inexperienced observer. Nevertheless, systematic evaluations of specific facial features have been shown effective to allow the recognition of these subtle changes. These features, which include changes in the eyes, cheek, nose, whiskers, and ears, are summarized in a so-called facial grimace scale (FGS). Facial grimace scales have initially been developed for mice,[87] and have since been adjusted and validated in many other species, including rats,[88] rabbits,[89] horses,[90,91] cats,[92] cattle,[93] sheep,[94] pigs,[95] and sheep.[96]

Reijgwart and colleagues, (2017) developed a grimace scale for ferrets.[97] Following a study of the facial musculature of ferrets and comparing lateral photographs of 19 ferret faces at six-time points before and after intraperitoneal telemetry probe implantation, they identified five Action Units (AUs) as potential indicators of pain in ferrets: orbital tightening, nose bulging, cheek bulging, ear changes and whisker retraction (**Fig. 4**). To evaluate whether these AUs could reliably assess pain related to the procedure, photographs taken before and after the procedure were scored 0 (AU not present), 1 (moderately present), or 2 (obviously present) by 11 (experienced and unexperienced) observers that were blinded to the treatment and timing of the photographs. Analysis indicated that AU-scores assigned to photographs taken 5 hours after surgery were significantly higher compared with time-matched baseline scores, suggesting that an FGS can be helpful to recognize pain in ferrets as well. In particular, orbital tightening had a high sensitivity, specificity,

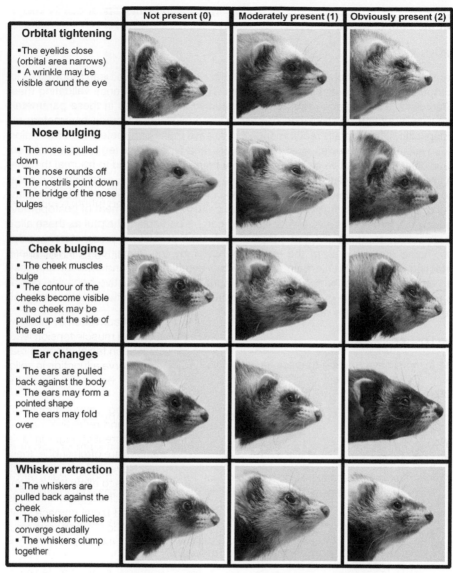

	Not present (0)	Moderately present (1)	Obviously present (2)
Orbital tightening • The eyelids close (orbital area narrows) • A wrinkle may be visible around the eye			
Nose bulging • The nose is pulled down • The nose rounds off • The nostrils point down • The bridge of the nose bulges			
Cheek bulging • The cheek muscles bulge • The contour of the cheeks become visible • the cheek may be pulled up at the side of the ear			
Ear changes • The ears are pulled back against the body • The ears may form a pointed shape • The ears may fold over			
Whisker retraction • The whiskers are pulled back against the cheek • The whisker follicles converge caudally • The whiskers clump together			

Fig. 4. The ferret grimace scale. Photographs visualizing the normal appearance and changes (0 = not present, 1 = moderately present, 2 = obviously present) of the 5 Action Units that are used in the Ferret Grimace Scale. Reprinted with permission.[93]

and accuracy, while other facial features (nose and cheek bulging and ear flattening) had little to no extra value in making this distinction. In fact, whisker retraction was attributed to a negative weight, resulting in lower accuracy, indicating this should be left out of the FGS altogether in its current form. However, as no analgesia was provided, postanesthetic effects on facial expression could not completely be ruled out, warranting further studies to validate the use of this FGS in ferrets. Additionally, the value of frontal images (as used in other species), as opposed to photographs taken laterally, could be compared, although this method was attempted in a pilot study but had a high failure rate as the ferrets' agility resulted in many poor quality images that were out of focus.

SUMMARY

Many physiologic, biochemical, and behavioral parameters have been reported as indicators of pain in ferrets and other animals. The scientific evidence validating these parameters is limited and requires further studies into changes in these parameters following induction or alleviation of pain using analgesia. As many parameters are nonspecific, it is generally recommended to assess these parameters in combination, taking into account species-specific behaviors, and type of pain (eg, visceral pain, somatic pain, postoperative pain, inflammatory pain, or pain related to trauma) that may be involved, as their clinical presentation may differ. In addition, establishing a baseline for the individual ferret is important to be able to quickly and reliably detect behavioral or physiologic changes associated with pain. In the assessment of postoperative pain, pain score sheets and grimace scales can be particularly helpful as these allow for objective, standardized and effective evaluation of relevant parameters. In addition, home assessments of the ferret's behavior by the owner can be valuable in detecting signs of chronic pain, whereby the behavior with and without analgesia can be compared. In these situations, a return to normal attentive behavior, curling up under a towel to sleep, and adequate appetite are all suggestive that the analgesia provided to the ferret is adequate.

DISCLOSURE

The authors have nothing to disclose.

REFERENCES

1. Short CE. Fundamentals of pain perception in animals. Appl Anim Behav Sci 1998;59:125–33.
2. Mayer J. Use of behavior analysis to recognize pain in small mammals. Lab Anim 2007;36(6):43–8.
3. International Association for the Study of Pain. IASP Taxonomy. Pain terms. Neuropathic pain. 2017. Available at: www.iaspain.org/Taxonomy#Neuropathicpain.
4. Murnion BP. Neuropathic pain: current definition and review of drug treatment. Aust Prescr 2018;41(3):60.
5. McCaffrey M, Pasero C. Pain: clinical manual. 2nd edition. St Louis (MO): CV Mosby; 1999.
6. Roberston SA. Pain management in laboratory animals-are we meeting the challenge? J Am Vet Med Assoc 2002;221(2):205–8.
7. Giamberardino MA, Vecchiet L. Pathophysiology of visceral pain. Curr Pain Headache Rep 1997;1(1):23.
8. Paine P, Kishor J, Worthen SF, et al. Exploring relationships for visceral and somatic pain with autonomic control and personality. Pain 2009;144(3):236–44.
9. Molony V, Kent J. Assessment of acute pain in farm animals using behavioral and physiological measurements. J Anim Sci 1997;75(1):266–72.
10. Mogil JS, Crager SE. What should we be measuring in behavioral studies of chronic pain in animals? Pain 2004;112(1–2):12–5.
11. Henke J, Erhardt W. Schmerzmanagement bei Klein- und Heimtieren. Stuttgart, Germany: Enke Verlag; 2001.

12. Morton DB, Griffiths PHM. Guidelines on the recognition of pain, distress and discomfort in experimental animals and hypothesis for assessment. Vet Rec 1985;116(16):431–6.

13. Holton LL, Scott EM, Nolan AM, et al. Relationship between physiological factors and clinical pain in dogs scored using a numerical rating scale. J Small Anim Pract 1998;39(10):469–74.

14. van Zeeland YRA, Wilde A, Bosman IH, et al. Non-invasive blood pressure measurement in ferrets (Mustela putorius furo) using high definition oscillometry. Vet J 2017;228:53–62.

15. Sanford J. Guidelines for detection and assessment of pain and distress in experimental animals. In: Short CE, Poznak von A, editors. Animal pain. New York (NY): Churchil Livingstone; 1992. p. 518–24.

16. Wolfensohn S, Lloyd M. Carnivores. In: Wolfensohn S, Lloyd M, editors. Handbook of laboratory animal management and welfare. 3rd edition. Oxford, UK: Blackwell Publishing Ltd; 2008. p. 281–303.

17. Schoemaker NJ. Ferrets, Skunks and Otters. In: Meredith A, Johnson-Delaney C, editors. BSAVA manual of exotic pets. 5th edition. Gloucestershire, British Small Animal Veterinary Association; 2010. p. 127–38.

18. Fox JG. Normal clinical and biologic parameters. In: Fox JG, Marini RP, editors. Biology and diseases of the ferret. 3rd edition. Baltimore (MD): Williams & Wilkins; 2014. p. 157–87.

19. Hein J, Spreyer F, Sauter-Louis C, et al. Reference ranges for laboratory parameters in ferrets. Vet Rec 2012;171(9):218. https://doi.org/10.1136/vr.100628.

20. Cowen R, Stasiowska MK, Laycock H, et al. Assessing pain objectively: the use of physiological markers. Anaesthesia 2015;70(7):828–47.

21. Jiang M, Mieronkoski R, Syrjälä E, et al. Acute pain intensity monitoring with the classification of multiple physiological parameters. J Clin Monit Comput 2019; 33(3):493–507.

22. Korving H, Sterkenburg PS, Barakova EI, et al. Physiological measures of acute and chronic pain within different subject groups: a systematic review. Pain Res Manag 2020. https://doi.org/10.1155/2020/9249465.

23. Borsook D, Becerra L. CNS animal fMRI in pain and analgesia. Neurosci Biobehav Rev 2011;35(5):1125–43.

24. Thompson SJ, Bushnell MC. Rodent functional and anatomical imaging of pain. Neurosci Lett 2012;520(2):131–9.

25. Zattoni J, Giunta F, Corssen G. Effects of phentanyl on spontaneous EEG activity, on EEG reactivity to pain, and on primary cortical potentials resulting from electrical stimulation of the trigeminal nerve in the rabbit. Surv Anesthesiol 1966; 10(5):428.

26. Murrell JC, Johnson CB. Neurophysiological techniques to assess pain in animals. J Vet Pharmacol Ther 2006;29(5):325–35.

27. Diesch TJ, Mellor DJ, Johnson CB, et al. Electroencephalographic responses to tail clamping in anaesthetized rat pups. Lab Anim 2009;43(3):224–31.

28. Li YD, Ge J, Luo YJ, et al. High cortical delta power correlates with aggravated allodynia by activating anterior cingulate cortex GABAergic neurons in neuropathic pain mice. Pain 2020;161(2):288–99.

29. Ong RM, Morris JP, O'dwyer JK, et al. Behavioural and EEG changes in sheep in response to painful acute electrical stimuli. Aust Vet J 1997;75(3):189–93.

30. Johnson CB, Sylvester SP, Stafford KJ, et al. Effects of age on the electroencephalographic response to castration in lambs anaesthetized with halothane in oxygen from birth to 6 weeks old. Vet Anaesth Analg 2009;36(3):273–9.

31. Johnson CB, Wilson PR, Woodbury MR, et al. Comparison of analgesic techniques for antler removal in halothane-anaesthetized red deer (Cervus elaphus): electroencephalographic responses. Vet Anaesth Analg 2005;32(2):61–71.
32. Gibson TJ, Johnson CB, Murrell JC, et al. Components of electroencephalographic responses to slaughter in halothane-anaesthetised calves: Effects of cutting neck tissues compared with major blood vessels. N Z Vet J 2009;57(2):84–9.
33. Drnec K. Electroencephalography (EEG) and measures of nociception in domestic cattle (Doctoral dissertation. College Park): University of Maryland; 2013.
34. Kells NJ, Beausoleil NJ, Sutherland MA, et al. Electroencephalographic assessment of oral meloxicam, topical anaesthetic cream and cautery iron for mitigating acute pain in pigs (Sus scrofa) undergoing tail docking. Vet Anaesth Analg 2017; 44(5):1166–74.
35. McIlhone AE, Beausoleil NJ, Kells NJ, et al. Effects of noxious stimuli on the electroencephalogram of anaesthetised chickens (Gallus gallus domesticus). PLoS one 2018;13(4):e0196454.
36. Kongara K, Chambers JP, Johnson CB. Effects of tramadol, morphine or their combination in dogs undergoing ovariohysterectomy on peri-operative electroencephalographic responses and post-operative pain. N Z Vet J 2012;60(2): 129–35.
37. Murrell JC, Johnson CB, White KL, et al. Changes in the EEG during castration in horses and ponies anaesthetized with halothane. Vet Anaesth Analg 2003;30(3): 138–46.
38. Stomp M, D'ingeo S, Henry S, et al. EEG individual power profiles correlate with tension along spine in horses. PLoS one 2020;15(12):e0243970.
39. Majkowski J, Lee MH, Kozlowski PB, et al. EEG and seizure threshold in normal and lissencephalic ferrets. Brain Res 1984;307(1–2):29–38.
40. Jha SK, Coleman T, Frank MG. Sleep and sleep regulation in the ferret (Mustela putorius furo). Behav Brain Res 2006;172(1):106–13.
41. Hsu N, Jha SK, Coleman T, et al. Paradoxical effects of the hypnotic Zolpidem in the neonatal ferret. Behav Brain Res 2009;201(1):233–6.
42. Barnett JL. Measuring pain in animals. Aust Vet J 1997;12:878–9.
43. Thau L, Gandhi J, Sharma S. Physiology, cortisol. StatPearls; 2021 [Internet].
44. Clauw DJ, Chrousos GP. Chronic pain and fatigue syndromes: overlapping clinical and neuroendocrine features and potential pathogenic mechanisms. Neuroimmunomodulation 1997;4(3):134–53.
45. Bomholt SF, Harbuz MS, Blackburn-Munro G, et al. Involvement and role of the hypothalamo-pituitary-adrenal (HPA) stress axis in animal models of chronic pain and inflammation. Stress 2004;7(1):1–14.
46. Ulrich-Lai YM, Xie W, Meij JT, et al. Limbic and HPA axis function in an animal model of chronic neuropathic pain. Physiol Behav 2006;88(1–2):67–76.
47. Griep EN, Boersma JW, Lentjes EG, et al. Function of the hypothalamic–pituitary–adrenal axis in patients with fibromyalgia and low back pain. J Rheumatol 1998; 25(7):1374–81.
48. Korszun A, Young EA, Singer K, et al. Basal circadian cortisol secretion in women with temporomandibular disorders. J Dent Res 2002;81(4):279–83.
49. Tennant F, Hermann L. Normalization of serum cortisol concentration with opioid treatment of severe chronic pain. Pain Med 2002;3(2):132–4.
50. Pearson RA, Mellor DJ. Some physiological changes in pregnant sheep and goats before, during and after surgical insertion of uterine catheters. Res Vet Sci 1975;19(1):102–4.

51. Jephcott EH, McMillen IC, Rushen J, et al. A comparison of electro-immobilisation and, or, shearing procedures on the ovine plasma concentrations of beta-endorphin/beta-lipotrophin. Res Vet Sci 1987;43(1):97–100.

52. Mellor DJ, Murray L. Changes in the cortisol responses of lambs to tail docking, castration and ACTH injection during the first 7 days after birth. Res Vet Sci 1989; 46(3):392–5.

53. Sladky KK, Horne WA, Goodrowe KL, et al. Evaluation of epidural morphine for postoperative analgesia in ferrets (Mustela putorius furo). J Am Assoc Lab Anim Sci 2000;39(6):33–8.

54. Colborn DR, Thompson D Jr, Roth T, et al. Responses of cortisol and prolactin to sexual excitement and stress in stallions and geldings. Sci J Anim 1991;69(6): 2556–62.

55. Weary DM, Niel L, Flower FC, et al. Identifying and preventing pain in animals. Appl Anim Behav Sci 2006;100(1–2):64–76.

56. McNatty KP, Cashmore M, Young A. Diurnal variation in plasma cortisol levels in sheep. J Endocrinol 1972;54(2):361–2.

57. Tapp WN, Holaday JW, Natelson BH. Ultradian glucocorticoid rhythms in monkeys and rats continue during stress. Am J Physiol 1984;247(5 Pt 2):866–71.

58. Gardy-Godillot M, Durand D, Dalle M, et al. Diurnal pattern of plasma cortisol in preruminant calves fasted or fed different milk proteins. J Dairy Sci 1989;72(7): 1842–6.

59. Prunier A, Mounier AM, Hay M. Effects of castration, tooth resection, or tail docking on plasma metabolites and stress hormones in young pigs. J Anim Sci 2005; 83(1):216–22.

60. Mormede P, Andanson S, Auperin B, et al. Exploration of the hypothalamic-pituitary-adrenal function as a tool to evaluate animal welfare. Physiol Behav 2007;92(3):317–39.

61. Merlot E, Mounier AM, Prunier A. Endocrine response of gilts to various common stressors: a comparison of indicators and methods of analysis. Physiol Behav 2011;102(3–4):259–65.

62. Landa L. Pain in domestic animals and how to assess it: a review. Vet Med 2012; 57(4):185–92.

63. Prunier A, Bonneau M, Von Borell EH, et al. A review of the welfare consequences of surgical castration in piglets and the evaluation of non-surgical methods. Anim Welf 2006;15(3):277–89.

64. Mellor DJ, Stafford KJ, Todd SE, et al. A comparison of catecholamine and cortisol responses of young lambs and calves to painful husbandry procedures. Aust Vet J 2002;80(4):228–33.

65. Mastrocinque S, Fantoni DT. A comparison of preoperative tramadol and morphine for the control of early postoperative pain in canine ovariohysterectomy. Vet Anaesth Analg 2003;30(4):220–8.

66. Parry BW. Use of clinical pathology in evaluation of horses with colic. Vet Clin North Am Equine Pract 1987;3(3):529–42.

67. Harcourt-Brown FM, Harcourt-Brown SF. Clinical value of blood glucose measurement in pet rabbits. Vet Rec 2012;170(26):674. https://doi.org/10.1136/vr.100321.

68. Bussières G, Jacques C, Lainay O, et al. Development of a composite orthopaedic pain scale in horses. Res Vet Sci 2008;85(2):294–306.

69. Moya SL, Boyle LA, Lynch PB, et al. Effect of surgical castration on the behavioural and acute phase responses of 5-day-old piglets. Appl Anim Behav Sci 2008; 111(1–2):133–45.

70. Stasiak KL, Maul D, French E, et al. Species-specific assessment of pain in laboratory animals. Contemp Top Lab Anim Sci 2003;42(4):13–20.
71. Gregory NG. Pain. In: Gregory NG, editor. Physiology and behaviour of animal suffering. Hoboken (NJ: John Wiley & Sons; 2008. p. 94–130.
72. van Oostrom H, Schoemaker NJ, Uilenreef JJ. Pain management in ferrets. Vet Clin North Am Exot Anim Pract 2011;14(1):105–16.
73. Chattipakorn SC, Sigurdsson A, Light AR, et al. Trigeminal c-Fos expression and behavioral responses to pulpal inflammation in ferrets. Pain 2002;99(1–2):61–9.
74. Flecknell PA. Analgesia in small mammals. Semin Avian Exot Pet Med 1998; 7(1):41–7.
75. Thurber A, Jha SK, Coleman T, et al. A preliminary study of sleep ontogenesis in the ferret (Mustela putorius furo). Behav Brain Res 2008;189(1):41–51.
76. Johnston MS. Clinical approaches to analgesia in ferrets and rabbits. Semin Avian Exot Pet Med 2005;14(4):229–35.
77. Lichtenberger M, Ko J. Anesthesia and analgesia for small mammals and birds. Vet Clin North Am Exot Anim Pract 2007;10(2):293–315. https://doi.org/10.1016/j. cvex.2006.12.002.
78. Brown SA. Clinical techniques in domestic ferrets. Semin Avian Exot Pet Med 1997;6(2):75–85.
79. Pollock C. Emergency medicine of the ferret. Vet Clin North Am Exot Anim Pract 2007;10(2):463–500.
80. Fisher PG. Ferret behavior. In: Bradley Bays T, Lightfoot T, Mayer J, editors. Exotic pet behavior. Cambridge (MA): Elsevier; 2006. p. 163–205.
81. Hardie EM, Hansen BD, Carroll GS. Behavior after ovariohysterectomy in the dog: what's normal? Appl Anim Behav Sci 1997;51:111–28.
82. Firth AM, Haldane SL. Development of a scale to evaluate postoperative pain in dogs. J Am Vet Med Assoc 1999;214(5):651–9.
83. Murrell JC, Psatha EP, Scott EM, et al. Application of a modified form of the Glasgow pain scale in a veterinary teaching centre in the Netherlands. Vet Rec 2008; 162(13):403–8.
84. Susskind JM, Lee DH, Cusi A, et al. Expressing fear enhances sensory acquisition. Nat Neurosci 2008;11(7):843–50. https://doi.org/10.1038/nn.2138.
85. Langford DJ, Tuttle AH, Brown K, et al. Social approach to pain in laboratory mice. Soc Neurosci 2010;5(2):163–70. https://doi.org/10.1080/17470910903216609.
86. Love EJ, Gillespie L, Colborne GR. Facial expression of pain in horses. Vet Anaesth Analg 2011;38(1):4–7.
87. Langford DJ, Bailey AL, Chanda ML, et al. Coding of facial expressions of pain in the laboratory mouse. Nat Methods 2010;7(6):447–9. https://doi.org/10.1038/ nmeth.1455.
88. Sotocinal SG, Sorge RE, Zaloum A, et al. The Rat Grimace Scale: a partially automated method for quantifying pain in the laboratory rat via facial expressions. Mol Pain 2011;7:55. https://doi.org/10.1186/1744-8069-7-55.
89. Keating SC, Thomas AA, Flecknell PA, et al. Evaluation of EMLA cream for preventing pain during tattooing of rabbits: changes in physiological, behavioural and facial expression responses. PLoS One 2012;7:e44437. https://doi.org/10. 1371/journal.pone.0044437.
90. Dalla Costa E, Minero M, Lebelt D, et al. Development of the Horse Grimace Scale (HGS) as a pain assessment tool in horses undergoing routine castration. PLoS One 2014;9:e92281. https://doi.org/10.1371/journal.pone.0092281.
91. Gleerup KB, Forkman B, Lindegaard C, et al. An equine pain face. Vet Anaesth Analg 2015;42(1):103–14. https://doi.org/10.1111/vaa.12212.

92. Holden E, Calvo G, Collins M, et al. Evaluation of facial expression in acute pain in cats. J Small Anim Pract 2014;55(12):615–21. https://doi.org/10.1111/jsap.12283.

93. Gleerup KB, Andersen PH, Munksgaard L, et al. Pain evaluation in dairy cattle. Appl Anim Behav Sci 2015;171:25–32. https://doi.org/10.1016/j.applanim.2015.08.023.

94. McLennan KM, Rebelo CJ, Corke MJ, et al. Development of a facial expression scale using footrot and mastitis as models of pain in sheep. Appl Anim Behav Sci 2016;176:19–26.

95. Di Giminiani P, Brierley VL, Scollo A, et al. The assessment of facial expressions in piglets undergoing tail docking and castration: toward the development of the piglet grimace scale. Front Vet Sci 2016;14(3):100. https://doi.org/10.3389/fvets.2016.00100.

96. Guesgen MJ, Beausoleil NJ, Leach M, et al. Coding and quantification of a facial expression for pain in lambs. Behav Process. 2016;132:49–56. https://doi.org/10.1016/j.beproc.2016.09.010.

97. Reijgwart ML, Schoemaker NJ, Pascuzzo R, et al. The composition and initial evaluation of a grimace scale in ferrets after surgical implantation of a telemetry probe. PloS one 2017;12(11):e0187986.

Treatment of Pain in Ferrets

Olivia A. Petritz, DVM, DACZM[a],*,
Ricardo de Matos, LMV, MSc, DABVP(Avian), DECZM[b]

KEYWORDS

• Analgesia • Ferret • Non-steroidal anti-inflammatory drugs • Opioids

KEY POINTS

• A recent pharmacokinetic study found a single subcutaneous dose of meloxicam (0.2 mg/kg) resulted in plasma concentrations considered to provide analgesia in horses, but there were significant differences in pharmacokinetic parameters between male and female ferrets.

• A previous pharmacokinetic study of a single dose of hydromorphone (0.1 mg/kg SC) to ferrets found no appreciable negative adverse effects at that dose but it had a short duration of plasma concentration above the therapeutic concentration in other species (<2 hours).

• Transmucosal detomidine gel (2 and 4 mg/m²) was previously evaluated in ferrets and both doses tested resulted in a reversible, rapid, safe, and effective sedation for physical exam and venipuncture.

• Constant rate infusions (CRIs) result in a sustained analgesic effect in ferrets and other species, and several drugs (butorphanol, ketamine, fentanyl) have been used solely or in combination via this delivery system to provide intraoperative and postoperative analgesia.

• Gabapentin, a GABA (gamma-aminobutyric acid) analog, has been used with increasing frequency in domestic mammals for the treatment of neuropathic pain; however, there are no current pharmacokinetic nor pharmacodynamic studies of its use in ferrets, only published case reports.

INTRODUCTION

Domestic ferrets (*Mustela putorius furo*) are commonly kept as companion animals and used in biomedical research worldwide. When presented for veterinary care, ferrets like many other domestic and nondomestic species, often require pain management as part of a comprehensive treatment plan. Recognition and ideally quantification of pain, such as a ferret grimace scale,[1] are important first steps before

[a] Department of Clinical Sciences, North Carolina State University, College of Veterinary Medicine, 1060 William Moore Drive, Raleigh, NC 27607, USA; [b] Section of Zoological Medicine, Department of Clinical Sciences, Cornell University College of Veterinary Medicine, S2-208 Veterinary Center, Ithaca, NY 14853, USA
* Corresponding author. NCSU, 1060 William Moore Dr, Raleigh, NC 27607.
E-mail address: oapetrit@ncsu.edu

Vet Clin Exot Anim 26 (2023) 245–255
https://doi.org/10.1016/j.cvex.2022.07.012
1094-9194/23/© 2022 Elsevier Inc. All rights reserved.
vetexotic.theclinics.com

an appropriate analgesic plan can be developed. Please refer to the article "Pain recognition in ferrets" in this same issue for additional information on pain recognition in ferrets. To select an appropriate analgesic, quantification of pain, as well as additional logistics, should be considered, such as outpatient vs inpatient, owner/caretaker compliance, and availability of intravenous access. A multimodal approach to pain management is preferred, which includes combining analgesic drugs of multiple classes and/or techniques to have a positive impact on several different points of the pain pathway.[2] When combined appropriately, these analgesic drugs often work synergistically and lead to individual drug dosage reduction, which in turn can reduce potential negative side effects. This article reviews the current published literature on analgesics in domestic ferrets, and a list of the drugs, doses, dosing intervals, and routes of administration discussed herein is provided in **Table 1**.

Non-steroidal Anti-inflammatory Drugs

Non-steroidal anti-inflammatory drugs (NSAIDs) inhibit the action of cyclooxygenase 1 and 2 (COX-1 and COX-2). Both enzymes produce prostaglandins, which are responsible for pain and pyrexia that accompanies generalized inflammation. Some prostaglandins produced by the COX-1 enzymes activate platelets and provide protection for the gastrointestinal mucosal barrier—beneficial processes to maintain homeostasis. Therefore, newer NSAIDs inhibit COX-2 exclusively, to reduce negative side effects that can occur by blocking beneficial COX-1 prostaglandin production. Meloxicam and carprofen, both COX-2 inhibitors, are anecdotally the most commonly used NSAIDs in ferrets.

The pharmacokinetics of a single subcutaneous dose of meloxicam has recently been evaluated in ferrets.[3] To date, this is the only pharmacokinetic study on any NSAID published in this species, and there are no pharmacodynamic studies of any NSAID in ferrets. In that study, 0.2 mg/kg of meloxicam was administered subcutaneously to 9 male and 9 female ferrets, and a population pharmacokinetic modeling approach was used due to sample volume limitations of the individual ferrets. This dose was sufficient to result in plasma concentrations considered to provide analgesia in horses (0.73 µg/mL)[4] for male but not female ferrets; however, the analgesic efficacy was not assessed in this study. Interestingly, there was a significant difference between the pharmacokinetics in male and female ferrets—females exhibited a higher volume of distribution, faster drug elimination, ad lower plasma concentrations, compared with males. The females were significantly smaller in body weight than the males; however, the meloxicam dose was normalized for body weight, per kg. The authors of that study hypothesized that bioavailability, which was not evaluated, could have accounted for the gender differences in addition to possible differences in metabolism and/or body composition. No adverse effects were noted after the single subcutaneous dose of meloxicam, but repeated dosing was not assessed.

No pharmacokinetic studies on carprofen in ferrets have been performed to date. However, it has been used in clinical reports for postoperative analgesia[5] and it is included in several textbooks, review articles, and formularies as an analgesic in this species.[6–8] Dosage ranges are variable, but the most commonly reported is 1–5 mg/kg PO or SC every 12 to 24 hours.[6–9] Due to the concerns for potential side effects of gastrointestinal ulceration of this NSAID, some authors have recommended giving concurrently with an H2 receptor antagonist, such as famotidine.[6]

Ibuprofen is a commonly used NSAID in human medicine for its analgesic, anti-inflammatory, and antipyretic effects. Ibuprofen nonselectively inhibits cyclooxygenase enzymes by blocking the conversion of arachidonic acid into various prostaglandins that mediate pain and inflammation. Despite its positive therapeutic

Table 1
Ferret analgesia drugs, dose intervals, and routes of administration

Drug	Dose (mg/kg)	Route	Interval (h)	References
Opioids				
Buprenorphine	0.01–0.05	SC, IV, IM	6–12	van Zeeland[8] 2021
	0.04–0.06	Transmucosal	6–8	Ko[15] 2014
	0.012	Epidural	4–6	Hawkins[17] 2016, Hawkins[28] 2021
	0.04	SC, IV, IM		Katzenbach etal[13] 2018
Butorphanol	0.05–0.5	SC, IV, IM	2–4	van Zeeland[8] 2021, Hawkins[28] 2021
	0.3	SC		Katzenbach etal[13] 2018
	Loading dose, 0.05–0.2; intraoperative rate, 0.1–0.4 mg/kg/h	IV		Hawkins[28] 2021
Fentanyl	Loading dose, 2–5 µg/kg; intraoperative rate, 5–10 µg/kg/h; postoperative rate, 0.5–2 µg/kg/h	IV		Hawkins[28] 2021
	Loading dose, 5–10 µg/kg; intraoperative rate, 10–30 µg/kg/h; postoperative rate, 1.25–5 µg/kg/h	IV		Johnson-Delaney[6] 2016, Hawkins[17] 2016
Hydromorphone	0.1	SC	< 2	Katzenbach etal[13] 2018
	0.1–0.2	SC, IV, IM	6–8	van Zeeland[8] 2021
	0.05–0.3	SC, IM		Hawkins[28] 2021
Morphine	0.05–5	SC, IM	2–6	van Zeeland[8] 2021
	0.05–1	SC, IM	2–4	Hawkins[28] 2021
	0.1	Epidural[a]		Hawkins[17] 2016, Sladky et al[35] 2000
Oxymorphone	0.05–0.2	SC, IV, IM	6–8	van Zeeland[8] 2021, Pollock[18] 2002
	0.02–0.05	SC, IM	6–8	Hawkins[28] 2021
Tramadol	10 mg/kg	PO	24	van Zeeland[8] 2021, Lichtenberger[29] 2007

(continued on next page)

Table 1
(continued)

Drug	Dose (mg/kg)	Route	Interval (h)	References
NSAIDs				
Carprofen	1–4	PO, SC	12–24	van Zeeland [8] 2021
	1–5	PO	12–24	Johnson-Delaney [6] 2016, Hawkins [9] 2015
Meloxicam	0.2	SC	24	Chinnadurai et al [3] 2014
Local analgesics				
Bupivacaine (0.125%)	1	SC – line or ring block		Ko [15] 2014
	1	Epidural		Hawkins [17] 2016
Lidocaine	1	SC – line or ring block		Ko [15] 2014
Other drugs				
Detomidine gel	2–4 mg/m²	Topically		Phillips [30] 2015
Gabapentin	10 mg/kg	PO	8–12	Dias et al [47] 2019, Paushter et al [48], 2021, Morera et al [49] 2011
Ketamine	Loading dose, 2–5 mg/kg; perioperative rate, 1–2 mg/kg/h; Postoperative rate, 0.25–1 mg/kg/h	IV		Hawkins [28] 2021

[a] Preservative-free morphine solution should be used for epidural administration.

effects on people, its use is not recommended in certain species, such as domestic dogs and cats, due to its narrow safety margin. Ferrets are especially sensitive to the toxic effects of ibuprofen. In a retrospective study of 43 cases of ibuprofen toxicity reported to the ASPCA, 93% of ferrets developed neurologic signs, 55% developed gastrointestinal signs such as vomiting, anorexia, diarrhea, and melena, and 13% developed renal dysfunction as evidenced by polyuria, polydipsia, and dysuria.[10] In that study, the minimum lethal dose was 220 mg/kg, which means even a single 200 mg tablet can result in a toxic dose of 100 to 400 mg/kg in a ferret. There are several formularies that list therapeutic doses for ibuprofen in ferrets[6,7]; however, based on the reported narrow safety range, the authors do not recommend the use of this NSAID in this species.

Opioids

Opioids provide analgesia either through an agonist effect (buprenorphine, hydromorphone, fentanyl, morphine) or an agonist-antagonist effect (butorphanol) in the different types of opioid receptors (μ, κ, δ, and nociceptin). They are used either for perioperative analgesia or combined with a sedative as a neuroleptic-analgesic.[11] Although the clinical effects of opioids in ferrets appear to be similar to other more common species, there are limited pharmacokinetic and pharmacodynamic studies of this group of drugs in ferrets.

Buprenorphine, historically characterized as a partial μ-opioid receptor agonist, is considered a full agonist as its analgesic effects in humans does not have the ceiling effect that characterizes a partial μ agonist. There is, however, a ceiling effect for respiratory depression, which reduces the potential of this adverse effect.[12] Buprenorphine is frequently used to provide analgesia in ferrets, at a dose of 0.01 to 0.05 mg/kg IV, IM or SC. A pharmacokinetics study of buprenorphine given at a dose of 0.04 mg/kg intramuscularly to ferrets demonstrated a quick decrease in the blood concentration of buprenorphine. Since the minimal analgesic blood concentration of buprenorphine in ferrets has not been determined, it is not possible to elucidate how often the medication must be given to be effective based on blood concentrations alone.[13] The analgesia time seems to last between 4 and 6 hours, which supports is frequent use.[13] Studies in cats have shown that buprenorphine is absorbed following oral transmucosal administration.[14] As absorption is depended on the saliva's pH and with ferrets' saliva pH being similar to that of cats, oral transmucosal administration of buprenorphine at a dose of 0.04 to 0.06 mg/kg every 6 to 8 hours has been proposed for providing long-lasting analgesia in ferrets.[15] Other formulations of buprenorphine (transdermal hydrogel, sustained-release formulation, high concentration formulation) may be viable options to consider in ferrets. Additional studies are required to assess the efficacy and safety of these formulations in ferrets.

Butorphanol, a mixed agonist-antagonist with a preference for the κ-opioid receptor, is also used frequently in ferrets at a dose of 0.05 to 0.5 mg/kg IM or SC. The pharmacokinetic properties of butorphanol were recently investigated in ferrets.[13] A single dose of butorphanol 0.3 mg/kg given subcutaneously was well tolerated. The mean maximum concentration was 48.6 ng/mL which was reached at 13 minutes. This is slightly above the determined effective analgesic blood concentration of butorphanol in cats (40 ng/mL). When comparing the blood concentrations of butorphanol in ferrets with the effective analgesic concentration for dogs and humans, they remained above the dog analgesic dose (6 ng/mL) for 200 minutes, and above the human analgesic dose (1.5 ng/mL) for 360 minutes. As for buprenorphine, since the minimal effective analgesic dose is not known for this species it is difficult to translate the results of the study into dosing frequency recommendations.[13] The authors of this study suggest a dosing interval of 2 to 4 hours.

Other opioids that have been used in ferrets include the μ-opioid receptor agonists morphine, hydromorphone, oxymorphone, and fentanyl, and the atypical opioid tramadol.[16] The doses, mode, and frequency of administration are listed in **Table 1**. Morphine, hydromorphone and oxymorphone have similar analgesia properties and duration, with all drugs potentially causing severe sedation in ferrets.[17] Morphine can cause dose-dependent respiratory depression, nausea and vomiting in ferrets.[13,18–20] Agitation has also been reported in ferrets given morphine at a dose of 1 mg/kg subcutaneously.[13] Antiemetic drugs such as metoclopramide, maropitant or ondansetron can be given before morphine administration to reduce the occurrence of vomiting.[21] A pharmacokinetic study of a single dose of hydromorphone 0.1 mg/kg given subcutaneously to ferrets suggested that the drug is safe and has a short duration of analgesia (less than 2 hours) at that dose in this species.[13] Hydromorphone analgesia can be extended and its sedative effects be reduced with administering as a CRI, as a single drug or when administered with ketamine.[22] Methadone is a long-acting synthetic opioid analgesic with potent μ-opioid agonist and some affinity for the κ and δ opioid receptors. In addition, it inhibits serotonin and norepinephrine reuptake in the central nervous system and antagonizes the NMDA receptor. For these reasons, it reduces hyperalgesia and opioid tolerance in addition to its analgesic effects.[23] Although its use has not been reported in ferrets, it may be a useful option in this species, especially considering its reduced gastrointestinal side effects reported in dogs.[23]

Fentanyl, a short-acting opioid with effects similar to morphine, is most frequently used in ferrets as constant rate infusion (CRI) for intra and postoperative analgesia, or for analgesia in trauma patients. Due to its potency, ferrets receiving this medication should be reassessed periodically to determine the effectiveness of the analgesia and the development of bradycardia and/or respiratory depression.[11,16] Remifentanil may be an alternative to fentanyl for CRI use. This ultrashort-acting μ-opioid receptor agonist is metabolized differently (via esterase hydrolysis in the blood and tissues instead of in the liver and kidneys) preventing drug accumulation and prolonged respiratory and cardiovascular depression when the medication is discontinued. Animals receiving the medication may develop tolerance, requiring an increase in dose to maintain the same level of analgesia.[24,25]

Tramadol is a weak μ-opioid receptor agonist, with inhibitory effects on serotonin and norepinephrine reuptake. Its analgesic properties vary between species due to variation in its metabolism and the relative levels of the parent drug (stronger serotonin and norepinephrine reuptake inhibitor) and the active M1 metabolite (more potent μ-opioid receptor agonist). The proposed doses for ferrets have been extrapolated from other mammals, with limited information on their efficacy and safety. In one study with a relatively small sample size, tramadol given intramuscularly at 5 and 10 mg/kg resulted in agitation and self-biting presumed to be secondary to irritation at the injection site. This was more pronounced for the 10 mg/kg dose.[26] The use of tapentadol, also an atypical opioid medication, has not been reported or evaluated in ferrets. Although tapentadol has a similar mechanism of action to tramadol, it is 2 to 3 times more potent than tramadol. In addition, it is active in its original form, with no active metabolites as for tramadol, and the effect of cytochrome p450 enzymes in its metabolism is not significant.[27] This has the potential to reduce the interspecies analgesic response to tapentadol, as it occurs for tramadol.

Close monitoring of ferrets receiving opioids is recommended, as they are reported to be more sensitive to the sedative and respiratory depressant effects of these medications.[20] The dose should be adjusted as needed. Opioids can be reversed with pure (naloxone and naltrexone) or partial antagonists (nalbuphine and butorphanol). Pure antagonists are more likely to reverse all effects of the opioid given, including its analgesic effects, and this should be considered clinically before their use.[16,28]

Alpha-2 Adrenoreceptor Agonists

This group of drugs includes xylazine, detomidine, medetomidine, and dexmedetomidine. They provide analgesia, sedation, and muscle relaxation. Medetomidine can be used either in the perioperative setting as a sedative, or in an intensive care setting as an analgesic and/or sedative administered as a CRI. Lower doses are recommended in ferrets due to the significant cardiovascular depressant effects associated with higher doses in this species.[29] A dose of 0.02 mg/kg given intramuscularly to ferrets provided approximately 15 minutes of analgesia (loss of toe pinching reflex) and 74 minutes of anesthesia (lateral recumbency).[26] Medetomidine is no longer commercially available, and there are currently no pharmacokinetic nor pharmacodynamic studies of dexmedetomidine in ferrets. A commercially available formulation of detomidine gel was evaluated in ferrets for sedation for clinical procedures.[30] Both doses tested (2 and 4 mg/m^2) resulted in a reversible, rapid, safe, and effective sedation for physical exam and venipuncture. The drug caused decreased heart rate and rectal temperature, piloerection of the tail and, in some ferrets, muscle twitching. Alpha 2 agonists can be reversed effectively with yohimbine, atipamezole, and tolazoline.

N-Methyl-D-Aspartate-Receptor Antagonists

Ketamine is a widely used N-methyl-D-aspartate (NMDA) receptor antagonist in veterinary medicine. In addition to being a dissociative anesthetic, there are numerous studies and systematic reviews in human medicine which describe this drug as a powerful analgesic, particularly in subanesthetic intravenous doses.[31] Ketamine does not cause hyperalgesia or nausea, like what is commonly seen with opioid analgesics. Intravenous constant-rate infusions (CRIs) of low or "microdoses" of ketamine have been described for use in perioperative and postoperative analgesia in several small mammal species, including ferrets[6,17,28] These low doses typically do not cause dysphoric effects, which can be seen with higher doses, such as those used for heavy sedation or anesthetic induction. Ketamine CRIs can be titrated to effect and reduce other anesthetic drugs as part of a multi-modal anesthetic approach in addition to providing intraoperative analgesia. Loading, intraoperative, and postoperative dosages for a ketamine CRI in ferrets can be found in **Table 1**.

Local and Regional Anesthesia

Local anesthetic agents can be used in ferrets for preemptive analgesia and as part of a multimodal approach to pain management. Their main advantages are the potential to provide analgesia with minimal or no systemic effects and to reduce the concentration of gas anesthetic used during a surgical procedure. Possible techniques include incisional line blocks, ring blocks, splash blocks, topical application, nerve blocks, and epidural injections.[18,29] The reader is referred to other publications for additional details on the indications and techniques for different nerve blocks in ferrets.[32,33] The most commonly used drugs are lidocaine and bupivacaine. They provide a short onset of analgesia, with a duration of effect depends on the drug (shorter for lidocaine) and mode of administration. Bupivacaine absorbed to porcine small intestine submucosa (SIS) was effective in providing analgesia in ferrets undergoing surgically created and SIS repaired abdominal hernia defect. The effects lasted for 2 to 4 days and there were no clinical side effects reported.[34] Other formulations and drugs approved for use in dogs that may be of benefit to ferrets include the long-lasting (up to 72 hours) liposome-encapsulated formulation of bupivacaine, mepivacaine and ropivacaine approved.

The toxic doses and effects of lidocaine and bupivacaine in ferrets are similar to what is described in dogs and cats, with signs of toxicity including vomiting, arrhythmias, hypotension, depression, muscle tremors, ataxia, and nystagmus.[28] Opioids such as buprenorphine, oxymorphone or morphine can also be used, especially for epidural injections. These medications take longer to reach their peak effect and last longer when compared with lidocaine and bupivacaine. Combining these with an opioid will result in a short onset of analgesia, increased duration of effects, and reduced adverse effects since lower doses of each medication can be used.[17,18,29]

Epidural injections are usually performed at the lumbosacral space since it is relatively larger and because the dural sac in ferrets does not extend beyond L7. The procedure is in general similar to what is described for dogs and cats.[29] The main difference in this technique in ferrets is the frequent absence of the distinct "popping" sensation when the intervertebral ligaments are penetrated.[35,36] When cerebrospinal fluid is noted in the hub of the needle being used, the drug(s) dosage(s) should be reduced in half to prevent excessive diffusion of the drug cranially in the subarachnoid space and its associated effects.[36] The total volume of administration for an epidural injection should be less than 0.33 mL/kg, and preservative free saline used for drug dilution if needed.

Topical analgesia of the skin can be obtained with the use of eutectic mixture of local anesthetics (EMLA) cream, which contains 2.5% lidocaine and 2.5% prilocaine. This can facilitate the placement of intravenous catheters or venipuncture, with analgesia reported 30 to 60 minutes after clipping the fur, applying the product, and covering the area with a bandage. Toxicity can occur with prolonged contact time and application to a large or traumatized skin area.[17]

Miscellaneous Analgesics

Gabapentin

Gabapentin is a GABA (gamma-aminobutyric acid) analog, which was originally used for its anticonvulsant properties in humans and domestic animals. More recently, gabapentin has been used to treat neuropathic pain, and there is evidence in human medicine that shows this medication reduces opioid requirements and pain levels after soft tissue surgical procedures.[37–40] Interestingly, it does not bind directly to the GABA receptors, and the exact mechanism for gabapentin's anticonvulsant and analgesic effects has yet to be definitively elucidated.[41]

Due to the short terminal half-life of gabapentin in dogs and cats (~3–4 hours), dosing every 8 hours (10–20 mg/kg) is required to maintain minimum target concentrations which are efficacious in humans (2 μg/mL).[42] Pharmacodynamic studies in dogs and cats are limited, and there are several which failed to show analgesic efficacy of gabapentin—one in an experimental thermal antinociceptive model in cats[43] and 2 postoperative studies in dogs.[44,45] However, extrapolations from these studies for clinical use in these species should be conducted with caution due to the dosing interval used (every 12 hours, rather than the recommended 8 hours) and the fact that gabapentin is not thought to be efficacious for the treatment/prevention of acute pain. Recently, oral gabapentin (20 mg/kg) was shown to have a minimum alveolar concentration (MAC)-sparing effect of isoflurane when administered 2 hours before anesthesia in 6 dogs.[46]

To date, no pharmacokinetic nor pharmacodynamic studies of gabapentin have been performed in ferrets; however, there are several published case reports describing its use. In 2 reports,[47,48] gabapentin (10 mg/kg PO q8-12 hours) was proscribed in combination with meloxicam and in one case[49] with prednisone and tramadol for additional analgesia. No discussion of the perceived efficacy of this drug was mentioned by the authors, nor was it prescribed without an additional analgesic medication. Therefore, the efficacy and safety of this medication cannot be definitively determined from these published case reports, and clinical extrapolation should be conducted with caution.

CLINICS CARE POINTS

- Hydromorphone has a shorter duration of action, less than 2 hours, in ferrets than in other species and this should be considered clinically when this drug is used in this species.

- Unlike other exotic small mammals such as rabbits and rodents, the dose of meloxicam for a ferret is much lower and thus more similar to a domestic dog or cat based on published pharmacokinetic studies in this species.

DISCLOSURE

The authors have nothing to disclose.

REFERENCES

1. Reijgwart ML, Schoemaker NJ, Pascuzzo R, et al. The composition and initial evaluation of a grimace scale in ferrets after surgical implantation of a telemetry probe. PloS one 2017;12:e0187986.
2. Lamont LA. Multimodal pain management in veterinary medicine: the physiologic basis of pharmacologic therapies. Vet Clin North Am Small Anim Pract 2008;38: 1173–86.
3. Chinnadurai S, Messenger K, Papich M, et al. Meloxicam pharmacokinetics using nonlinear mixed-effects modeling in ferrets after single subcutaneous administration. J Vet Pharmacol Ther 2014;37:382–7.
4. Toutain P-L, Reymond N, Laroute V, et al. Pharmacokinetics of meloxicam in plasma and urine of horses. Am J Vet Res 2004;65:1542–7.
5. van Zeeland Y, Lennox A, Quinton J-F, et al. Prepuce and partial penile amputation for treatment of preputial gland neoplasia in two ferrets. J Small Anim Pract 2014;55:593–6.
6. Johnson-Delaney CA. Analgesia and anaesthesia. Ferret Medicine and surgery. Boca Raton, FL: CRC Press; 2016. p. 407–18.
7. Morrisey J, Johnston MS. Ferrets. In: Carpenter JW, editor. Exotic animal formulary. 5th edition. St. Louis, MO: Elsevier; 2018. p. 532–57.
8. van Zeeland YR, Schoemaker NJ. Analgesia, Anesthesia, and Monitoring. In: Graham JE, Doss GA, Beaufrère H, editors. Exotic Animal Emergency and Critical Care Medicine. Hoboken, NJ: Wiley Blackwell; 2021.
9. Hawkins MG. Advances in exotic mammal clinical therapeutics. Vet Clin Exot Anim Pract 2015;18:323–37.
10. Richardson JA, Balabuszko RA. Ibuprofen ingestion in ferrets: 43 cases January 1995–March 2000. J Vet Emerg Crit Care 2001;11:53–8.
11. Ko J, Marini RP. Anesthesia and analgesia in ferrets. Anesthesia and analgesia in laboratory animals. London, UK: Elsevier, Academic Press; 2008. p. 443–56.

12. Pergolizzi J, Aloisi AM, Dahan A, et al. Current knowledge of buprenorphine and its unique pharmacological profile. Pain Pract 2010;10:428–50.

13. Katzenbach JE, Wittenburg LA, Allweiler SI, et al. Pharmacokinetics of single-dose buprenorphine, butorphanol, and hydromorphone in the domestic ferret (Mustela putorius furo). J Exot Pet Med 2018;27:95–102.

14. Robertson S, Taylor P, Sear J. Systemic uptake of buprenorphine by cats after oral mucosal administration. Vet Rec 2003;152:675–8.

15. Ko J, Marini R. Anesthesia. In: Fox J, Marini R, editors. Biology and diseases of the ferret. Ames, IA: Wiley Blackwell; 2014. p. 259–83.

16. van Oostrom H, Schoemaker NJ, Uilenreef JJ. Pain management in ferrets. Vet Clin Exot Anim Pract 2011;14:105–16.

17. Hawkins MG. Advances in exotic mammal clinical therapeutics. J Exot Pet Med 2014;23:39–49.

18. Pollock C. Postoperative management of the exotic animal patient. Vet Clin Exot Anim Pract 2002;5:183–212.

19. Shiokawa M, Narita M, Nakamura A, et al. Usefulness of the dopamine system-stabilizer aripiprazole for reducing morphine-induced emesis. Eur J Pharmacol 2007;570:108–10.

20. Johnston M. Rabbit-and Ferret-Specific Considerations. Handbook of veterinary pain management. St. Louis, MO: Elsevier; 2015. p. 517–35.

21. Kapaldo N, Eshar D. Ferret Sedation and Anesthesia. Vet Clin Exot Anim Pract 2022;25:273–96.

22. Schnellbacher, Rodney, Comolli J. Constant rate infusions in exotic animals. J Exot Pet Med 2020;35:50–7.

23. Kreutzwiser D, Tawfic QA. Methadone for pain management: a pharmacotherapeutic review. CNS drugs 2020;34:827–39.

24. Criado AB, De Segura IAG. Reduction of isoflurane MAC by fentanyl or remifentanil in rats. Vet Anaesth analgesia 2003;30:250–6.

25. Hayashida M, Fukunaga A, Hanaoka K. Detection of acute tolerance to the analgesic and nonanalgesic effects of remifentanil infusion in a rabbit model. Anesth Analg 2003;97:1347–52.

26. Giral M, García-Olmo D, Gómez-Juárez M, et al. Anaesthetic effects in the ferret of alfaxalone alone and in combination with medetomidine or tramadol: a pilot study. Lab Anim 2014;48:313–20.

27. Roulet L, Rollason V, Desmeules J, et al. Tapentadol versus tramadol: a narrative and comparative review of their pharmacological, efficacy and safety profiles in adult patients. Drugs 2021;81:1257–72.

28. Hawkins M, Pascoe P. Anesthesia, analgesia, and sedation of small mammals. In: Quesenberry K, Orcutt CJ, Mans C, et al, editors. Ferrets, rabbits, and rodents: clinical medicine and surgery. 4th edition. St. Louis, MO: Elsevier; 2021. p. 536–58.

29. Lichtenberger M, Ko J. Anesthesia and analgesia for small mammals and birds. Veterinary Clin North Am Exot Anim Pract 2007;10:293–315.

30. Phillips BE, Harms CA, Messenger KM. Oral transmucosal detomidine gel for the sedation of the domestic ferret (Mustela putorius furo). J Exot pet Med 2015;24:446–54.

31. Vadivelu N, Schermer E, Kodumudi V, et al. Role of ketamine for analgesia in adults and children. J anaesthesiology, Clin Pharmacol 2016;32:298.

32. DiGeronimo PM, da Cunha AF. Local and Regional Anesthesia in Zoological Companion Animal Practice. Vet Clin Exot Anim Pract 2022;25:321–36.

33. Comolli J, d'Ovidio D, Adami C, et al. Technological advances in exotic pet anesthesia and analgesia. Vet Clin Exot Anim Pract 2019;22:419–39.
34. Johnson BM, Ko JC, Hall PJ, et al. Analgesic effect of bupivacaine eluting porcine small intestinal submucosa (SIS) in ferrets undergoing acute abdominal hernia defect surgery. J Surg Res 2011;167:e403–12.
35. Sladky KK, Horne WA, Goodrowe KL, et al. Evaluation of epidural morphine for postoperative analgesia in ferrets (Mustela putorius furo). J Am Assoc Lab Anim Sci 2000;39:33–8.
36. Eshar D, Wilson J. Epidural anesthesia and analgesia in ferrets. Lab Animal 2010;39:339–40.
37. Mathiesen O, Møiniche S, Dahl JB. Gabapentin and postoperative pain: a qualitative and quantitative systematic review, with focus on procedure. BMC Anesthesiol 2007;7:6.
38. Dirks J, Fredensborg BB, Christensen D, et al. A randomized study of the effects of single-dose gabapentin versus placebo on postoperative pain and morphine consumption after mastectomy. J Am Soc Anesthesiologists 2002;97:560–4.
39. Pandey CK, Singhal V, Kumar M, et al. Gabapentin provides effective postoperative analgesia whether administered pre-emptively or post-incision. Can J Anesth 2005;52:827–31.
40. Grover V, Mathew P, Yaddanapudi S, et al. A single dose of preoperative gabapentin for pain reduction and requirement of morphine after total mastectomy and axillary dissection: randomized placebo-controlled double-blind trial. J Postgrad Med 2009;55:257.
41. Sills GJ. The mechanisms of action of gabapentin and pregabalin. Curr Opin Pharmacol 2006;6:108–13.
42. KuKanich B. Outpatient oral analgesics in dogs and cats beyond nonsteroidal antiinflammatory drugs: an evidence-based approach. Vet Clin Small Anim Pract 2013;43:1109–25.
43. Pypendop BH, Siao KT, Ilkiw JE. Thermal antinociceptive effect of orally administered gabapentin in healthy cats. Am Vet Med Assoc 2010;71(9):1027–32.
44. Aghighi SA, Tipold A, Piechotta M, et al. Assessment of the effects of adjunctive gabapentin on postoperative pain after intervertebral disc surgery in dogs. Vet Anaesth analgesia 2012;39:636–46.
45. Wagner AE, Mich PM, Uhrig SR, et al. Clinical evaluation of perioperative administration of gabapentin as an adjunct for postoperative analgesia in dogs undergoing amputation of a forelimb. J Am Vet Med Assoc 2010;236:751–6.
46. Johnson BA, Aarnes TK, Wanstrath AW, et al. Effect of oral administration of gabapentin on the minimum alveolar concentration of isoflurane in dogs. Am J Vet Res 2019;80:1007–9.
47. Dias S, Fernández-Flores F, Pumarola M, et al. Multifocal embryonal tumor in the central nervous system of a ferret (mustela putorius furo). J Exot Pet Med 2019;28:185–92.
48. Paushter A, Early P, Perkins T, et al. Surgical resection of a parietal osteoma in a domestic ferret using advanced neurosurgical techniques. J Am Anim Hosp Assoc 2021;57:91–5.
49. Morera N, Juan-Sallés C, Torres JM, et al. Cryptococcus gattii infection in a Spanish pet ferret (Mustela putorius furo) and asymptomatic carriage in ferrets and humans from its environment. Med Mycol 2011;49:779–84.

Acupuncture in Zoological Companion Animals

Ronald B. Koh, DVM, MS, Dipl. ACVSMR, CVA, CCRP, CVMMP, CVCH, CVFT[a],*,
Tara M. Harrison, DVM, MPVM, Dipl. ACZM, Dipl. ACVPM, Dipl. ECZM (Zoo Health Management), CVA[b]

KEYWORDS

- Zoologic companion animals • Acupuncture • Pain • Analgesia
- Multimodal pain management

KEY POINTS

- Acupuncture is one of the most common integrative modalities in veterinary medicine for pain relief.
- A large and expanding body of scientific evidence supporting the use of acupuncture in the management of acute and chronic pain.
- Acupuncture blocks pain by activating a variety of bioactive chemicals through peripheral, spinal, and supraspinal (brain) mechanisms.
- Acupuncture is safe, has minimal side effects, and is well tolerated by most zoologic companion animals, including but not limited to rabbits, rodents, birds, and reptiles.
- Acupuncture is easy to implement clinically and can be used as an adjunct modality or as a nonmedication option in multimodal pain management to improve pain and functional recovery.

INTRODUCTION

Over the past years, the concept of pain management in veterinary medicine has evolved and led to the establishment of a new concept of multimodal approach to pain management, as the current standard of care.[1] The use of multimodal analgesia combining pharmacologic and nonpharmacologic techniques not only help optimize the quality and efficacy of analgesia but also may prevent the development of chronic or persistent pain. During the past decade, acupuncture has become more popular and evolved into one of the most used forms of integrative medicine interventions and nonpharmacologic therapeutic options for pain management in humans and animals in North America and Europe. There is ample evidence from basic and clinical

[a] Integrative Medicine Service, UC Davis Veterinary Medical Teaching Hospital, University of California, Davis, 1 Garrod Road, Davis, CA 95616, USA; [b] Exotic Animal Medicine Service, North Carolina State University, College of Veterinary Medicine, 1060 William Moore Drive, Raleigh, NC 27607, USA
* Corresponding author.
E-mail address: rbkoh@ucdavis.edu

Vet Clin Exot Anim 26 (2023) 257–280
https://doi.org/10.1016/j.cvex.2022.07.008
1094-9194/23/© 2022 Elsevier Inc. All rights reserved.

research for acupuncture is effective in the treatment of acute and chronic pain by influencing neural networks of the nervous system. While in the modern days' veterinary acupuncture has been predominantly used in horses and dogs, its popularity in zoologic companion animals (ZCA) has increased in recent years as an adjunct therapy for treating musculoskeletal, neurologic, and gastrointestinal disorders due to its minimal invasiveness and low risk of adverse events.[2] The integrative use of acupuncture has become even more important with the increasingly limited use of opiates in veterinary medicine due to the opiate crisis. The purpose of this article aims to provide guidance for using acupuncture for pain management in ZCA in clinical practice, based on available information and recommendations from experienced veterinary acupuncturists (RK and TH).

HISTORY

Acupuncture, an essential part of Traditional Chinese medicine (TCM) and Traditional Chinese Veterinary Medicine (TCVM), is an ancient medical technique that involves the practice of inserting fine needles into specific points through the skin for the treatment of disease, relieving pain, and improving general health.[3,4] The earliest known reference to acupuncture is found in the book *Huangdi Neijing* (*The Yellow Emperor's Inner Classic of Medicine*), from approximately the period 475 BC to 225 BC.[4] Like human acupuncture, the practice of veterinary acupuncture can be traced back thousands of years.[4] *Bo Le Zhen* Jing (Bole's Canon of Veterinary Acupuncture) is believed earliest veterinary acupuncture book written by Dr Bo Le during the *Qin-mu-gong* period (659 B.C. to 621 B.C.).[5] Since that time, acupuncture in animals has evolved to include food animals, dogs, cats, zoo animals, and ZCA. It has grown tremendously during the past decades with increasing numbers of research studies being performed to better understand its mechanism of action and clinical benefits for a variety of conditions, such as pain, osteoarthritis, nerve damage, vomiting, and calming or behavioral effects. In recent years, veterinary medicine programs in academic institutions have created an integrative medicine curriculum that included acupuncture as an integral part of patient care in disease management.[6]

TCVM emphasizes individualized treatment by using a unique theory and terminology to diagnose and treat a wide range of health problems in animals. Two concepts that are unique and fundamental to TCVM are *Qi* (usually translated as "vital energy") and Yin and Yang.[7] *Qi* flows through the body to maintain the proper functioning of body systems toward health and wellbeing. Yin and Yang are the harmonies of all the opposite and complementary forces that make up all aspects and phenomena of life, and when they are in balance, the body is in a harmonious and healthy state. Disharmony or imbalance of *Qi* and/or Yin and Yang causes disease and illness. Additionally, the Wu Xing or Five Elements is another unique theory that is central to the practice of TCVM. It describes stages of the constantly moving cycle between Yin and Yang in nature and is used to explain the body's physiology.[7] The Five Elements include wood, fire, earth, metal, and water. Each Element is associated with a number of characteristics, such as certain body organs, a color, a taste, an emotion, a constitution, and a season of the year (**Table 1**).[7] Before treatment, a TCVM practitioner will complete a detailed assessment based on the 4 diagnostic methods to evaluate the patient's condition, including observing (tongue, mental attitude, appearance and color of feces and urine), hearing/smelling (vocal, odor of body, feces, and urine), asking (history, diet, and environmental interaction), and touching/palpating (pulse, integument, nails, muscle, meridians, and acupoints).[7] The practitioner will then determine

Table 1
Each of the five elements has several characteristics

	Wood	Fire	Earth	Metal	Water
Season	Spring	Summer	Late Summer	Fall	Winter
Organs	Liver (LIV) Gallbladder (GB)	Heart (HT) Pericardium (PC) Small Intestine (SI) Triple Heater (TH)	Spleen (SP) Stomach (ST)	Lung (LU) Large Intestine (LI)	Kidney (KID) Bladder (BL)
Constitution	Competitive, confident, dominant, aggressive	Lively, playful, affectionate, sensitive	Friendly, relaxed, laid back, slow response to a stimulus	Aloof, quiet, independent, obey the rules	Careful, timid, fearful, self-contained

a TCVM pattern diagnosis based on examination findings, followed by the formulation of an individualized treatment plan that may include acupuncture, herbal therapy, food therapy, and Tui-na.

MECHANISM OF ACTION

The mechanism behind acupuncture involves the stimulation of specific anatomic points, known as acupuncture points or acupoints, in the body to achieve a therapeutic effect. There are an estimated 365 acupoints distributed along 14 theorized meridians that run on the body surface of an animal.[3] Additionally, different species may also have "Classical" acupoints which are extraacupoints that are without any meridian associations and have been used since the earliest recordings of acupuncture use in this species.[3] For an example, *Jiang-ya* in a classical acupoint at the nostril of horses that is known to relieve colic in that species.[3] The components of acupoints involve nerve fibers, low-threshold mechanoreceptors, mast cells, and microcirculatory complexes recognized through electron microscopy, which is referred to as the neural acupuncture unit (NAU).[8] Following acupuncture needle insertion, activation of the NAU has been shown to stimulate the release of various inflammatory mediators such as endorphins, enkephalins, and corticosteroids through modulating neurotransmitters within the nervous system.[8] Increasing evidence shows that acupuncture effectively alleviates pain in animal models by activating a variety of bioactive chemicals through peripheral, spinal, and supraspinal mechanisms.[9]

The peripheral analgesic effect of acupuncture takes place at the area of needle insertion and is mediated by the release of adenosine, a neuromodulator with antinociceptive properties. Adenosine inhibits nearby adenosine A1 receptors in nociceptive afferent nerve endings and thus suppresses pain locally.[10] Increase of endogenous cannabinoid CB2 receptors (CB2R) to upregulate peripheral opioids, as well as the inhibition of prostaglandin E2 (PGE2) synthesis and cyclooxygenase-2 (COX-2) expression in inflamed tissue, are also involved in local analgesia by acupuncture.[11,12] In addition, studies have shown that the needling of acupoints creates a microtraumatic environment which led a variety of local immunobiological reactions, such as decreasing proinflammatory cytokines (eg, IL-1β, TNF-α, and IL-6), recruiting mast cells, macrophages, and other local cells to release certain biomolecules (eg, histamine, serotonin, and so forth).[13] These elements may not only reduce inflammation and minimize pain and, but also eliminate edema and promote tissue healing throughout the recovery process. The local microtrauma caused by acupuncture is repaired quickly after needles are removed, but the series of immunobiological reactions induced by it may continue for a longer period.

Spinal mechanisms underpinning acupuncture analgesia have been extensively investigated. Acupuncture has shown to induce several spinal neurotransmitters, including opioids, serotonin, norepinephrine, and acetylcholine which work interactively in the spinal cord to alleviate pain. Furthermore, acupuncture also impedes the transmission of noxious inputs at the spinal level with the involvement of inhibiting cytokines, glutamate, glial cell, substance P, and N-methyl-D-aspartate (NMDA) receptors in the spinal cord.[9,14,15]

The supraspinal or brain mechanism of acupuncture on pain is less studied due to the complex neural regulatory events of pain pathway and perception within the brain. Nonetheless, numerous studies report that acupuncture inhibits pain within the brain through[9,14–17] (1) modulating the somatosensory cortex to affect pain sensory signals; (2) activating the hypothalamus to release β-endorphin into CSF and bloodstream; (3) activating the descending inhibitory system in the brainstem; (4) deactivating the limbic system to mediate analgesic and sedative effects.

ROLE OF ACUPUNCTURE IN PAIN MANAGEMENT

Pain management in ZCA can be challenging due to limited evidence and data on clinical efficacy, pharmacokinetics, and pharmacodynamics of analgesic drugs in some species. Nevertheless, once pain is recognized or suspected, pain management with all treatment options should be considered for better pain relief, minimizing unwanted side effects of treatments, and optimizing the quality of life in patients. Because pain perception involves various complex processes in the nervous system, a single analgesic drug or a sole therapeutic modality is often insufficient for complete alleviation of pain; thus, multimodal analgesic approach involving pharmacologic and nonpharmacologic interventions is frequently recommended.[1] This is especially true for chronic, neuropathic, or persistent pain because of its complex and multidimensional mechanisms. While pharmacologic options remain the mainstays, nonpharmacologic interventions are an important part of a comprehensive pain management plan. Acupuncture offers a safe and effective nonpharmacologic intervention with minimal adverse effects that most animals tolerate well.[2,3,17] It has become more accepted for pain relief in veterinary medicine and can be used independently or integrated into conventional analgesia protocols. In humans, positive results for pain relief in low back pain, neck pain, osteoarthritis, cancer-related pain, and postoperative pain by acupuncture are reported in several systematic reviews and meta-analyses.[18–21] Although clinical research in veterinary medicine is limited, several studies have demonstrated analgesia effect of acupuncture on pain related to osteoarthritis, hip dysplasia, postoperation, back pain, and laminitis.[22–33] Moreover, the pain management guidelines published by the American Animal Hospital Association, American Association of Feline Practitioners, and World Small Animal Veterinary Association endorse acupuncture as a safe adjunct treatment of pain management in dogs and cats that should be strongly considered as a part of multimodal pain management regimen.[1,34] Therefore, it seems to be a reasonable option for ZCA for the treatment of pain.

METHODS OF STIMULATION

Acupuncture needles vary by needle length (8–60 mm or 0.25–2.5 inches), needle gauge (thickness; 28- to 40-gauge (ga) or 0.16 to 0.35 mm (mm) in diameter), and handle style (metal or plastic) (**Fig. 1, Table 2**). What size of needle to choose to depend on the size of the animal, area of the body to be treated, as well as the behavior and temperament of the animal species. Acupoints can be stimulated by dry needle, electroacupuncture, aqua-acupuncture, laser acupuncture, acupressure, moxibustion, and material implantation.[3,17] Dry needle (DN) involves the insertion of fine, sterile needles into acupoints. The needles are typically left in place for a few seconds up to 20 minutes per treatment of ZCA. Unique local propagating bodily sensations, termed *de-Qi* (arrival of *Qi*), may be elicited when acupuncture needles are inserted into acupoints.[3,35] Inducing the *de-Qi* response regulates the movement of *Qi* along meridians.[3] It informs the acupuncturist of correct acupoint location and is believed to be closely related to the treatment efficacy of acupuncture analgesia.[3,35] In humans, the needle sensations may feel like heaviness, tingling, numbness, soreness, distension, and warmth.[35] In animals, observation of muscle twitching, flinching, or attempts to bite may indicate *de-Qi* with the stimulation of the needles.[3] In electroacupuncture (EA), acupoints are stimulated by applying low-level electrical current through needles for up to 20 minutes per treatment with the goal of a more vigorous stimulation of the acupoints. EA has more profound and prolonged analgesic effects than other techniques.[9] It is useful for neuralgia, nervous system injury, and persistent pain.[9] Low-frequency EA (2–10 Hz) produces longer-lasting alleviation of pain and inhibits nerve injury-related allodynia/hyperalgesia more potently than do higher

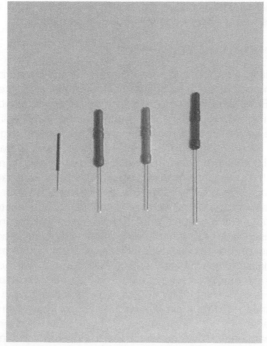

Fig. 1. A variety of needles size that is commonly used in ZCA. Sizes are left to right: 42, 36, 34, 32 gauge.

Table 2									
Common acupuncture needle thicknesses and lengths use in ZCA									
Needle Thickness	Gauge Number (ga)	32	34	36	38	40	42	44	46
	Diameter (mm)	0.24	0.22	0.20	0.18	0.16	0.14	0.12	0.10
Needle Length	Inches	0.12	0.16	0.25	0.5				
	Millimeters (mm)	3	4	7	13				

frequencies (100 Hz).[9] Generally ZCA may tolerate only a few minutes of EA stimulation but some rabbits or patients with paraparesis or paralysis are able to tolerate longer EA treatment. With aqua-acupuncture (AQ), a small amount of sterile fluid (eg, normal saline, vitamin $B_{12,}$ or 50:50 mixture of normal saline and vitamin B_{12}) is injected into acupoints for stimulation. It is commonly used after DN or EA to prolong the effect of acupoint stimulation.[3] Acupressure is a type of manual therapy technique that is performed using hands and fingers gradually pressing onto acupoints to simulate acupoints for pain relief and muscle relaxation.[3] Laser acupuncture (LA), also called acupuncture photobiomodulation therapy, is the use of nonthermal, low-intensity laser irradiation with red and infrared wavelengths (625–1000 nm) to stimulate acupoints and has been shown providing antiinflammatory and antinociceptive effects.[36] The advantages of this technique over traditional acupuncture include minimal sensation, short duration of treatment, and minimal risks of infection, trauma, and bleeding complications. Lastly, moxibustion involves using the heat of burning dried mugwort herb to stimulate acupoints or specific surficial regions to treat a wide variety of conditions.[3] For animal patients that are fractious, untouchable, or intolerance to needle insertion, acupressure, laser acupuncture and moxibustion offer advantage over other methods because they are noninvasive, painless, safer, and easy to control. For smoke-sensitive species or those that are more sensitive to a variety of smells, such as avian patients, moxibustion should be used with caution.

CLINICAL USE AND INTEGRATION INTO PRACTICE

Licensed veterinarians are advised to receive formal training in veterinary acupuncture before incorporating acupuncture into his or her conventional or integrative medicine practice settings. Basic or advanced certification veterinary acupuncture courses are offered at several institutions in the United States, Europe, and Asia (Box 1). Before acupuncture, underlying pain or medical conditions are always diagnosed as part of conventional care. Once standard treatment measures are underway, acupuncture can be used as an integrative modality to reduce acute or chronic pain. For outpatients, it can be offered at the clinic, once or twice a week. For inpatients, it can be performed in the hospital, once a day before discharge. Practices that do not offer acupuncture can refer patients to veterinarians with CVA (certified veterinary acupuncturist) credentials.

Veterinarians who perform acupuncture must obtain informed consent from clients beforehand. The discussion of acupuncture in the context of multimodal pain management must focus not only on the analgesic efficacy of acupuncture but also on expectations and potential adverse effects. A multimodal approach with acupuncture offers better pain control and may allow for a reduction in the dose of conventional analgesic agents; therefore, a decrease in their adverse effects. For patients resistant to pain medications or cannot tolerate their side effects, acupuncture can be a reasonable alternative treatment.

Acupuncture treatments should be tailored to the needs of the individual. In ZCA, the selection of appropriate needle size, stimulation method, treatment time, and frequency for acupuncture greatly depends on the specific species and their natural

Box 1
Acupuncture resources

a. University and institutes that offer veterinary acupuncture (canine or equine) training or certification programs in North America, South America, Europe, Asia, and Australia:
1. Chi University: chiu.edu
2. International Veterinary Acupuncture Society (IVAS): ivas.org
3. College of Integrative Veterinary Therapies (CIVT): civtedu.org
4. CuraCore: curacore.org
5. Canine Rehabilitation Institute (CRI): caninerehabinstitute.com

bNon-profit organizations that promote the art and science of veterinary acupuncture:
1. American Academy of Veterinary Acupuncture (AAVA): aava.org
2. World Association of Traditional Chinese Veterinary Medicine (AATCVM): watcvm.org
3. American Holistic Veterinary Medical Association (AHVMA): ahvma.org

behavior and temperament, diseases or conditions to be treated, the size of the animal, area of the body to be treated, as well as the balance between potential benefits and risks. For example, easily aroused, frightened, or stressed species are best treated with dry needle acupuncture with fewer acupoint selection (eg, 2–5 acupoints). Instead of leaving needles in the skin for a longer period, each needle is gently manipulated for only a few seconds (eg, 5–15 seconds) and then removed. For most species, however, sessions are typically tolerated for 3 to 5 minutes. Alternatively, aquapuncture can be considered for those patients that will not tolerate leaving needles in for a session as it requires less treatment time. Aquapuncture is typically performed using a combination of vitamin B_{12} (1000 mcg/mL) and normal saline in a 50:50 mixture. Volume injected at each acupoint depends on the size of the animal but can range from 0.02 mL to 0.5 mL. Providing food or treats can be helpful to keep the patient distracted, safe, and relaxed throughout their treatment. For those patients that do not tolerate needles at all, laser acupuncture is an ideal therapy and can be conducted by just touching the animal with the unit for sessions 3 to 10 minutes in length depending on the tolerance of the animal.

As with any therapy, not every patient responds to acupuncture; therefore, realistic expectations need to be set for clients. The authors often require clients to commit to sessions once or twice a week for at least 4 to 6 treatments, especially for chronic conditions. Although many patients may not need 4 treatments to experience benefits, shorter durations and lower intensities of treatment may result in suboptimal outcomes. Acupuncture has both immediate and cumulative analgesic effects following repeated treatments.[18]

SAFETY AND CONTRAINDICATIONS

Acupuncture is generally a safe and minimal invasive procedure with a low risk of adverse events when performed correctly by licensed veterinarians certified in veterinary acupuncture.[17] Common minor adverse effects after acupuncture include tiredness, increased water intake, soreness, muscle spasm, and minor bleeding, which typically resolve quickly.[3,] Other rare complications include local infection, dermatitis, and broken needle fragments.[3] To avoid direct needle injury to articular cartilage, local nerves or vessels, attention should be paid to anatomic landmarks and depth of needle insertion, especially in small species. Deep needle insertion should be avoided into acupoints around joint spaces (eg, TH-4 at the carpal joint space, ST-35a and ST-35b at the stifle joint space), around major vessels or nerves (eg, axillary artery and brachial plexus at HT-1, sciatic nerve at GB-30, spinal nerves at Bai-hui), and around the lung fields (eg, SP-21, GB-24, BL-12 to BL-19). Acupuncture on the face or around the eyes is generally not tolerated by ZCA and the acupuncturist should be extremely cautious when using acupoints around these areas. Acupuncture should also be used cautiously in patients who are severely debilitated or have clotting abnormalities.[37] Acupuncture needles should not be placed on infected or inflamed skin, open wounds, sites of tumor and fractures, around the abdomen of a pregnant animal, or in specific points that may contribute to premature parturition (ie, ST-36, SP-6, BL-40, BL-60, and BL-67).[3,37] Do not apply EA across the thoracic area (heart position) in animals with heart disease, or seizure disorders.[3,37]

CLINICAL APPLICATION IN ZOOLOGIC COMPANION ANIMALS
Rabbits

Rabbits are common pets in the United States. They are commonly brought to veterinary practices and owners expect similar treatments to domestic animals. These animals are prey animals and tend to be fearful when brought in for treatment. Research on the use of acupuncture has been conducted in laboratory animal rabbits primarily to evaluate the use of acupuncture for humans.[38–44] That said, there are approximate acupuncture meridians and transposition of points that have been published.[45] Treating rabbits with acupuncture requires modifications. Specifically, in creating a TCVM diagnosis, tongue color and pulse are used, these diagnoses, however, cannot be routinely conducted, or not conducted without stressing the animal out, which may change the color of the tongue and make the TCVM diagnosis inaccurate. Femoral pulses can be obtained and are less stressful to the animal than obtaining the tongue color. The practitioner should determine what level of stress is appropriate for the animal to obtain the femoral pulse. Frequently a TCVM diagnosis can be made for this species without using tongue color and pulse and through other diagnostic methods such as physical examination, radiographs, or bloodwork. When treating these animals, it is easiest to use 34 ga or 36 ga in 7 to 13 mm length (0.25–0.5 inches) length colored handled needles. The color-handled needles are especially helpful in longer-haired rabbits to keep track of whereby the needles were placed. Treatment times vary depending on the constitution of the animal. Most rabbits are the water element constitution, but there are some rabbits that are Wood element constitution and do not tolerate needle placement well. Typically, an initial treatment time of needles in the animal is 3 to 5 minutes long. Generally, if these animals tolerate dry needling, they will also tolerate EA and tend to calm down after EA starts. When using AQ along with DN and/or EA, use AQ at the end of the other treatments. Medial acupoints are challenging and stressful for the animal to access and generally are avoided. See **Figs. 2–4**.

The most common conditions treated with acupuncture in rabbits are musculoskeletal and gastrointestinal. For musculoskeletal conditions, rabbits are prone to spinal injuries, which can be treated with acupuncture points cranial and caudal to the lesion. Rabbits also develop osteoarthritis, typically in the caudal spine and pelvic regions. The most common gastrointestinal condition that rabbits develop is gastrointestinal stasis. This condition is multifactorial and can be caused by many conditions. This condition is typically treated similarly to colic in horses; however, if there is no response to treatment, one of the authors (TMH) has found that it tends to be a surgical cause for the stasis and additional diagnostics should be pursed. Pododermatitis can also be managed as a multimodal therapy in rabbits typically involving photobiomodulation along with acupuncture therapy.[46] **Table 3** and **Fig. 4** list acupoints that are commonly used in rabbits.

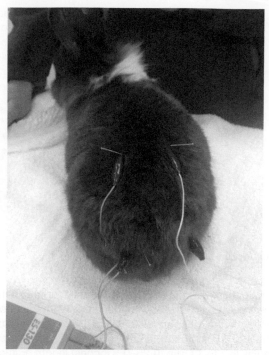

Fig. 2. A rabbit receiving acupuncture with dry needles and electroacupuncture for hindlimb osteoarthritis.

Rodents

There are many different rodent species, but perhaps the 2 most commonly seen in veterinary practice are rats and guinea pigs. Both of these species are prey species and as such tend to be Water element species. These animals are substantially more tolerant of acupuncture along the spine than on the limbs. The more distal the limb points, the more these animals tend to not tolerate them. In developing a TCVM diagnosis, these animals tend to be challenging to get an accurate tongue color

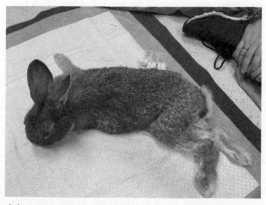

Fig. 3. A rabbit receiving acupuncture with dry needles for spinal cord injury resulting in paraparesis.

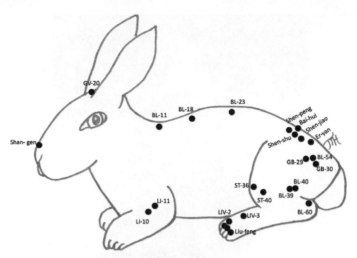

Fig. 4. Common acupuncture points used in a rabbit.

and femoral pulse palpation. It tends to be less stressful for the animal to not attempt to get tongue color or pulse palpation and to make the TCVM diagnosis through other methods as mentioned in the other species above. Rats tend to accept acupuncture therapies for about 3 to 5 minutes in length. Needles used tend to be the colored handled 36 ga needles in 7 to 13 mm (0.25–0.5 inches) length or 42 ga hand needles. Electroacupuncture tends to not be as tolerated in rats. Photobiomodulation (cold laser) therapy can be used in addition to or in place of acupuncture in these animals. Rats are prone to developing pododermatitis[46] and osteoarthritis. Both of these conditions tend to be chronic, long-term conditions as well as require chronic, long-term therapies. **Table 4** lists acupoints that are commonly used in rodents. See **Figs. 5–7**.

Guinea pigs are very common companion animals as well. These animals are also very challenging to evaluate tongue color as well as to get a femoral pulse in a minimally stressful way. These animals tend to be either Earth or Water Element personalities and are more tolerant of acupuncture. Determining the acupoints to use is typically based on other diagnostic methods as mentioned in the other species above. These animals tend to accept acupuncture and electroacupuncture for 3 to 5 minutes, but some will tolerate longer time periods for their therapy. It is not unusual to be able to acupuncture a guinea pig while providing food for distraction/as a reward. Guinea

Table 3	
Common acupoints for the treatment of medical conditions in rabbits	
Rabbit Medical Condition	**Acupoints to Include in Treatment**
Spinal injuries	Acupoints cranial and caudal to the lesion, as well as BL-11, BL-23, BL-40, BL-60, KID-3, ST-36, GV-20, Bai-hui, Shen-shu, Shen-peng, Shen-jiao, Er-yan, Liu-feng
Osteoarthritis – caudal spine/pelvic	BL-54, GB-29, GB-30, BL-40, BL-39, ST-36, KID-10
Gastrointestinal stasis	GV-20, LI-10, LI-11, ST-36, ST-40, ST-45, SP-6, Bai-hui, Shan-gen
Pododermatitis	LIV-2, LIV-3, BL-18, BL-40, BL-60, KID-3, Bai-hui

Table 4	
Common acupoints for the treatment of medical conditions in rodents	
Rodent Medical Condition	Acupoints to Include in Treatment
Osteoarthritis	BL-11, BL-23, BL-40, ST-36, GB-34, KID-3, Bai-hui, Er-yan, Shen-shu, Shen-peng, Shen-jiao
Pododermatitis	LIV-2, LIV-3, BL-18, BL-40, BL-60, KID-3, Bai-hui

pigs will frequently allow acupuncture while eating products such as romaine lettuce or other green vegetables. Needles used tend to be the colored handled 36 ga needles. See **Fig. 8**. Conditions that guinea pigs develop include osteoarthritis as a chronic condition, but they also can develop gastrointestinal stasis as an acute condition. Gastrointestinal stasis in guinea pigs is even more of a critical condition than rabbits and should be treated in a multimodal approach. Osteoarthritis or other traumatic conditions do respond well to acupuncture and photobiomodulation. Treatments should be at minimum weekly for at least 4 treatments to evaluate response to therapy. **Table 5** lists acupoints that are commonly used in guinea pigs. **Fig. 9** shows common acupuncture points used in guinea pigs.

Ferrets

Ferrets have been studied through laboratory animal medicine as to their response to acupuncture, particularly emesis.[47] Ferrets, similar to treating feline patients and it is possible to diagnose and similarly treat them by using tongue color and pulse to make

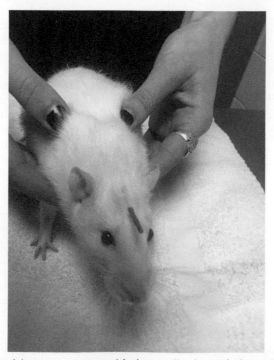

Fig. 5. A pet rat receiving acupuncture with dry needles for pododermatitis. Pictured is the acupuncture point GV-20 for calming.

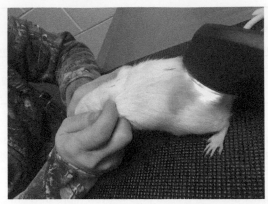

Fig. 6. A rat with pododermatitis receiving acupuncture and photobiomodulation (cold laser therapy) for the treatment of hind-end pain and pododermatitis.

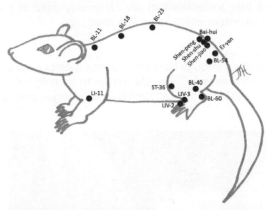

Fig. 7. Common acupuncture points used in a rat.

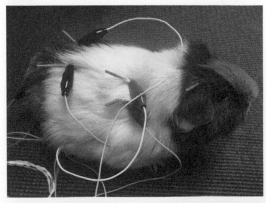

Fig. 8. A guinea pig receiving acupuncture with electroacupuncture for the treatment of hind end paresis due to being dropped by an owner. After three treatments this animal was able to ambulate normally.

Table 5	
Common acupoints for the treatment of medical conditions in guinea pigs	
Guinea Pig Medical Condition	**Acupoints to Include in Treatment**
Gastrointestinal stasis	LI-10, LI-11, ST-36,ST-40, ST-45, Shan-gen
Osteoarthritis	BL-11, BL-23, Bai-hui, Er-yan, Shen-shu, Shen-peng, Shen-jiao, BL-40, BL-60, KID-3

a TCVM diagnosis. Actually placing needles in a ferret can be very challenging; however, as most ferrets will not tolerate holding still or accepting needles to be placed and to stay in. Aquapuncture with a 50:50 mixture of vitamin B_{12} and normal saline with injections of 0.1 mL per acupoint or LA (photobiomodulation) are far easier methods to use when treating ferrets (**Fig. 10**). Conditions that can be treated with acupuncture as a multimodal approach involve pain relief for traumatic conditions or appetite stimulation. Ferrets can also be treated as an adjunct for *Helicobacter mustelae* infection-induced nausea or as an adjunct therapy for nausea from chemotherapy use. **Tables 6** list acupoints that are commonly used in ferrets. **Fig. 11** shows the location of common acupuncture points used in ferrets.

Reptiles

Acupuncture has not been commonly documented as being used in reptiles for treating medical conditions. Acupuncture has been documented in two studies, however, regarding recovery from anesthesia and was found to significantly improve recovery time from anesthesia.[48,49] In general, it has been found by the authors, that reptiles respond quite well to acupuncture and EA. If there is a reptile where needle placement cannot occur, then LA (photobiomodulation) could occur for those animals. Transpositional points and a generalized evaluation of points exist in a boa constrictor, and box turtle but otherwise do not exist in a published format.[50] Placement of acupuncture needles should occur between the scales, and not through the scales. This type of needle placement substantially improves the method of placement and also does not damage the scales that could contribute to dysecdysis at a later time point. In small to medium patients, the 42 ga in 4 to 7 mm (0.16–0.25 inches) length Japanese hand needles are easiest to place between the scales. Other animals larger, stiffer gauge needles, such as 32 ga needles may be easiest to place in the region between the scales. Certain reptiles do not have all points accessible, such as snakes (no limb points) and turtles or tortoises (no spinal bladder meridian points). Reptiles typically respond the most when needles are placed, but afterward are calm and may even

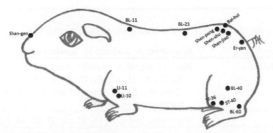

Fig. 9. Common acupuncture points used in a guinea pig. The open circle represents a point located in the center of the popliteal crease.

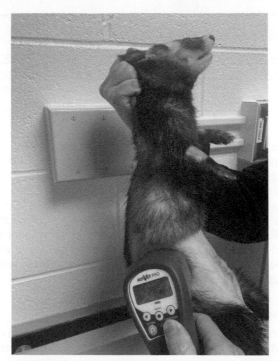

Fig. 10. A ferret receiving photobiomodulation for the treatment of a thermal burn.

Table 6	
Common acupoints for the treatment of medical conditions in ferrets	
Ferret Medical Condition	**Acupoints to Include in Treatment**
Appetite Stimulation	Shan-gen, Jian-wei, LI-10, ST-36, ST-40, ST-45
Nausea	ST-36, ST-37, ST-44, BL-20, BL-21

Table 7	
Common acupoints for the treatment of medical conditions in reptiles	
Reptile Medical Condition	**Acupoints to Include in Treatment**
Spondylosis/Spondylitis	Bladder meridian cranial and caudal to the affected area, BL-11, BL-23, BL, BL-40, BL-60, KID-3, ST-36, Bai-hui, Shen-Shu (note, most of these are not accessible in turtles/tortoises)
Anorexia	Shan-gen, LI-10, LI-11, ST-36, ST-40, BL-20, BL-21, BL-25
Arthritis/Nutritional Secondary Hyperparathyroidism	BL-11, BL-23, BL-54, GB-29, GB-30, BL-40, BL-60, KID-3, ST-36, Bai-hui, Er-yan, Shen-shu, Shen-peng, Shen-jiao

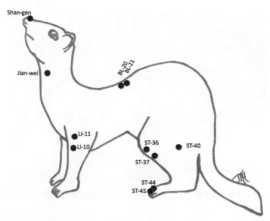

Fig. 11. Common acupuncture points used in a ferret.

fall asleep when EA is started. Sessions can range from seconds to 15 or 20 minutes depending on the tolerance of the animal. See **Figs. 12–16**. Amphibians can also be acupunctured, although it is less common. When acupuncture is used on amphibians, powder-free gloves should be worn and 42 ga Japanese hand needles should be used (**Fig. 17**).

Conditions that commonly occur and benefit from acupuncture include spondylosis or spondylitis which is a common condition that presents in snakes and other animals

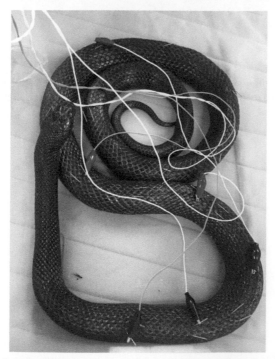

Fig. 12. A black rat snake receiving acupuncture with dry needles and electroacupuncture for the treatment of spinal spondylosis and osteoarthritis.

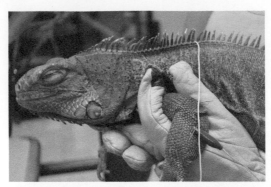

Fig. 13. A green iguana receiving acupuncture with electroacupuncture for the treatment of spinal problem.

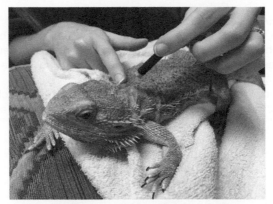

Fig. 14. A bearded dragon receiving acupuncture with dry needle and moxibustion as an adjunct treatment to manage pain and improve mobility caused by metabolic bone disease.

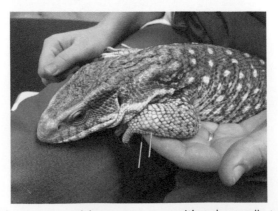

Fig. 15. A savannah monitor receiving acupuncture with a dry needle to relieve pain and improve left thoracic limb mobility caused by metabolic bone disease.

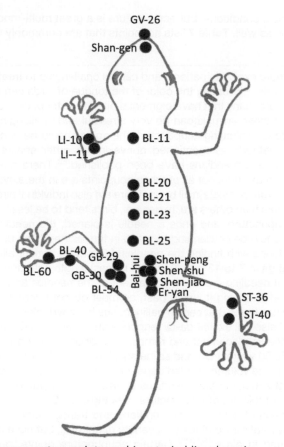

Fig. 16. Common acupuncture points used in a typical lizard species.

affected with nutritional secondary hyperparathyroidism. Arthritis can also be common in snakes as well as those animals affected with nutritional secondary hyperparathyroidism and several cases have been managed by the author (TMH) and others to a great benefit.[51] Anorexia is also a common condition that occurs in reptiles typically

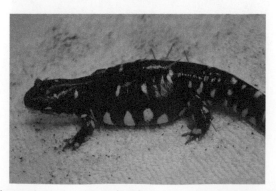

Fig. 17. A tiger salamander being treated with Japanese hand needles for acupuncture for the treatment of egg stasis.

due to other medical conditions, but acupuncture is a great multi-modal approach to treat this condition as well. **Table 7** lists acupoints that are commonly used in reptiles.

Aves

Birds tend to be more excitable patients and can be challenging to treat with traditional acupuncture methods. Evaluating the color of the tongue of birds can also be complicated in that there are many that have pigmentation of their tongues. Additionally, evaluating the pulse of these animals can be very stressful and challenging and likely not diagnostic, therefore, evaluating acupuncture therapies should be conducted through other diagnostic methods as mentioned above in the other species. Approximate acupuncture points and meridians have been published.[52] There are many different species of birds and as such, not all of these acupoints are in the exact same location and not all therapies are possible in all birds. There are also individual birds that are more tolerant of treatments than others are. In general, birds tend to be less tolerant of needle placement for acupuncture, and once a needle is placed, the needle can feel like a feather shaft and could be challenging to refind in the feathers. The use of the colored handled needles helps with finding the needles if the avian patient allows placement. Typically 34 or 36 ga in 7 to 13 mm (0.25–0.5 inches) length acupuncture needles are used. In general, if needling a patient, placement of the needles and stimulating it for a few seconds and removing it works best, as most do not tolerate longer sessions. The author (TMH) has found that certain gallinaceous birds will tolerate longer acupuncture sessions and also will exhibit *de-Qi* response and yawn with EA. For birds that do not tolerate the needle placement and removal, aquapuncture and the use of vitamin B_{12} and inject a 50:50 vitamin B_{12} and saline solution of 0.02 to 0.1 mL solution at acupoints instead, with the volume injected dependent on the size of the patient. Photobiomodulation (LA) at acupoints and meridians is also a successful form of treatment of patients that are not tolerant of acupuncture. See **Figs. 18–21**.

The approximation of acupuncture meridians and transpositional points has been documented in several publications on a variety of animals, but have been more thoroughly documented in birds.[45,50,52] Certain acupuncture points, particularly those along the spine can be challenging to use for the beginner avian veterinarian practitioner and should be used with caution. Acupuncture has been used as an adjunct therapy for arthritis, appetite stimulation, and pododermatitis. In a case report, dry needle acupuncture at ST-36, LI-4, BL-40, BL-60, GB-34, and *Ba-Feng* once per

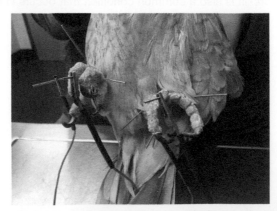

Fig. 18. An Amazon parrot receiving aquapuncture with dry needles and electroacupuncture for managing pain and mobility issues caused by gout.

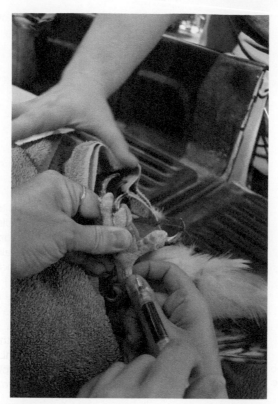

Fig. 19. A red-tailed hawk receiving aquapuncture with aquapuncture for the treatment of osteoarthritis. A small amount of diluted 50:50 vitamin B_{12} and saline solution was injected into acupoints.

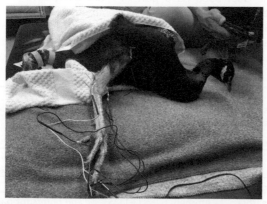

Fig. 20. A peacock receiving acupuncture with dry needles and electroacupuncture for osteoarthritis and weakness of the right limb caused by overcompensation. After the amputation of the left limb, a prosthetic device was fitted for his right limb to support activity.

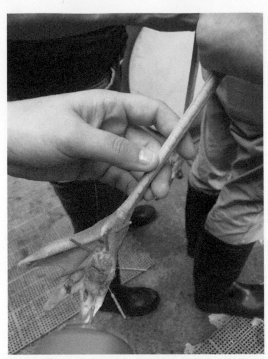

Fig. 21. A flamingo receiving acupuncture for the treatment of pododermatitis. "Circle the dragon" technique is shown in this photograph.

week for 2 months and biweekly for another 2 months had shown a significant clinical improvement in a bald eagle with persistent severe lameness due to chronic degenerative joint disease in the right stifle despite being treated with antiinflammatory or analgesic drugs.[53] Other severe clinical signs including reluctance to movement, inappetence, vocalization, depression, and pododermatitis were also clinically improved after eighth acupuncture treatment.[53] In addition, acupuncture has also been used for behavioral modification such as in the condition of feather destructive behaviors, but it is best used as a part of more integrative medicine or holistic approach to evaluate the cause of the feather destructive behavior through a thorough physical examination and diagnostic testing. If the destructive behavior is determined to be behavioral, acupuncture as well as other treatments and modifications such as potential diet change, enrichment, herbal medications, behavioral medications,

Table 8	
Common acupoints for the treatment of medical conditions in birds, those labeled (+/−) may not be readily accessible in all species of birds	
Avian Medical Condition	**Acupoints to Include in Treatment**
Arthritis	LI-10, LI-11, HT-3 (+/−), SI-4 (+/−), BL-11 (advanced avian skill), BL-23 (advanced avian skill), BL-40, BL-60, KID-3, ST-36
Appetite Stimulation	ST-36, ST-40, ST-45, Shan-gen
Feather Plucking/Feather Destructive Behavior	An-shen, HT-7, LI-11, ST-36, and points for pain near where picking
Pododermatitis	LIV-8 (+/−), GB-34, circle the dragon

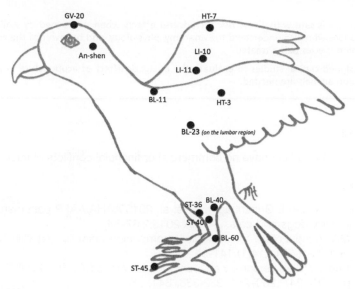

Fig. 22. Common acuspuncture points used in birds.

lighting changes, and so forth can be conducted as a more global approach to the condition. **Table 8** lists acupoints that are commonly used in birds. **Fig. 22** illustrates common acupuncture points used in birds.

SUMMARY

Multimodal pain management among ZCA is an important aspect of providing quality care and achieving optimal clinical outcomes. There is substantial evidence for acupuncture is safe and effective in the treatment of acute and chronic pain and can play an important role as part of multimodal-based therapeutic strategies for effective pain. With proper training, acupuncture can be easily implemented in a clinical setting and can be incorporated into conventional analgesia protocols for better pain control and faster recovery whether the patient is managed medically or surgically. Nonetheless, randomized controlled trials are needed to verify its therapeutic efficacy for pain relief in ZCA species. Although there are growing numbers of studies to support acupuncture for the management of pain in humans, dogs, cats, and horses, additional research involving well-designed clinical studies is needed to expand the knowledge and effect of acupuncture in these unique patients.

CLINICS CARE POINTS

- Acupuncture involves the insertion of very thin needles through the skin at acupuncture points on the body (referred to as a "neural acupuncture unit") that consists of nerve fibers, mechanoreceptors, mast cells, and microcirculatory complexes.

- The mechanisms of acupuncture analgesia are complex and generally associate with the local stimulus responses and functions of the peripheral and central nervous system to block pain perception, reduce inflammation, and promote tissue healing.

- Acupuncture provides a useful adjunct or occasionally alternative to multimodal pain management for better pain control and faster recovery, whether the patient is managed medically or surgically.

- Acupuncture is safe with a low risk for adverse effects when performed by well-trained veterinarians who also understand the anatomy, physiology, and behavior of the zoologic companion species being treated.
- Well-designed clinical studies to evaluate the analgesic effect of acupuncture in zoologic companion animals are needed.

DISCLOSURE

The authors of this article have no commercial or financial conflicts of interest.

REFERENCES

1. Epstein M, Rodan I, Griffenhagen G, et al. 2015 AAHA/AAFP pain management guidelines for dogs and cats. JAAHA 2015;2:67–84.
2. Koski MA. Acupuncture for zoological companion animals. Vet Clin North Am Exot Anim Pract 2011;14(1):141–54.
3. Xie H, Priest V. Xie's veterinary acupuncture. xii. Ames (IA): Blackwell Publishing; 2007. p. 3–15, 247, 260–261, 332-336, 341.
4. Xie H, Chrisman C. Equine acupuncture: from ancient art to modern validation. Am J Trad Chin Vet Med 2009;4(2):1–4.
5. Song D, Xie H. Annotated Yuan Heng's classical collection on the treatment of equine diseases. Beijing (China): China Agriculture Press; 2012. p. 5–6.
6. Memon MA, Shmalberg JW, Xie H. Survey of Integrative Veterinary Medicine Training in AVMA-Accredited Veterinary Colleges. J Vet Med Educ 2021;48(3): 289–94.
7. Xie H, Preast V. Traditional Chinese veterinary medicine: fundamental principles. 2nd edition. Reddick, FL: Jing Tang; 2013. p. 1–43, 249-302.
8. Wright BD. Acupuncture for the treatment of animal pain. Vet Clin North Am Small Anim Pract 2019;49(6):1029–39.
9. Zhang R, Lao L, Ren K, et al. Mechanisms of acupuncture-electroacupuncture on persistent pain. Anesthesiology 2014;120(2):482–503.
10. Goldman N, Chen M, Fujita T, et al. Adenosine A1 receptors mediate local antinociceptive effects of acupuncture. Nat Neurosci 2010;13(7):883–8.
11. Su TF, Zhang LH, Peng M, et al. Cannabinoid CB2 receptors contribute to upregulation of beta-endorphin in inflamed skin tissues by electroacupuncture. Mol Pain 2011;7:98.
12. Lee J, Jang K, Lee Y, et al. Electroacupuncture inhibits inflammatory edema and hyperalgesia through regulation of cyclooxygenase synthesis in both peripheral and central nociceptive sites. Am J Chin Med 2006;34:981–8.
13. Cui J, Song W, Jin Y, et al. Research progress on the mechanism of the acupuncture regulating neuro-endocrine-immune network system. Vet Sci 2021;8(8):149.
14. Tahir AH, Li JJ, Tang Y. Peripheral and spinal mechanisms involved in electroacupuncture therapy for visceral hypersensitivity. Front Neurosci 2021;15: 696843.
15. Dewey CW, Xie H. The scientific basis of acupuncture for veterinary pain management: A review based on relevant literature from the last two decades. Open Vet J 2021;11(2):203–9.
16. Kong JT, Schnyer RN, Johnson KA, et al. Understanding central mechanisms of acupuncture analgesia using dynamic quantitative sensory testing: a review. Evid Based Complement Alternat Med 2013;2013:187182.

17. Fry LM, Neary SM, Sharrock J, et al. Acupuncture for analgesia in veterinary medicine. Top Companion Anim Med 2014;29(2):35–42.
18. Xiang A, Cheng K, Shen X, et al. The immediate analgesic effect of acupuncture for pain: a systematic review and meta-analysis. Evid Based Complement Alternat Med 2017;2017:3837194.
19. Ko HF, Chen CH, Dong KR, et al. Effects of acupuncture on postoperative pain after total knee replacement: systematic literature review and meta-analysis. Pain Med 2021;22(9):2117–27.
20. Wu B, Yang L, Fu C, et al. Efficacy and safety of acupuncture in treating acute low back pain: a systematic review and bayesian network meta-analysis. Ann Palliat Med 2021;10(6):6156–67.
21. Yang J, Wahner-Roedler DL, Zhou X, et al. Acupuncture for palliative cancer pain management: systematic review. BMJ Support Palliat Care 2021;11(3):264–70.
22. Silva NEOF, Luna SPL, Joaquim JGF, et al. Effect of acupuncture on pain and quality of life in canine neurological and musculoskeletal diseases. Can Vet J 2017;58(9):941–51.
23. Lane DM, Hill SA. Effectiveness of combined acupuncture and manual therapy relative to no treatment for canine musculoskeletal pain. Can Vet J 2016;57(4): 407–14.
24. Jaeger GT, Larsen S, Søli N, et al. Double-blind, placebo-controlled trial of the pain-relieving effects of the implantation of gold beads into dogs with hip dysplasia. Vet Rec 2006;158(21):722–6.
25. Hielm-Bjorkman A, Raekallio M, Kuusela E, et al. Double-blind evaluation of implants of gold wire at acupuncture points in the dog as a treatment for osteoarthritis induced by hip dysplasia. Vet Rec 2001;149:452–6.
26. Teixeira LR, Luna SP, Matsubara LM, al at. Owner assessment of chronic pain intensity and results of gait analysis of dogs with hip dysplasia treated with acupuncture. JAVMA 2016;249(9):1031–9.
27. Laim A, Jaggy A, Forterre F, et al. Effects of adjunct electroacupuncture on severity of postoperative pain in dogs undergoing hemilaminectomy because of acute thoracolumbar intervertebral disk disease. JAVMA 2009;234(9):1141–6.
28. Marques VI, Cassu RN, Nascimento FF, et al. Laser acupuncture for postoperative pain management in cats. Evid Based Complement Alternat Med 2015; 2015:653270.
29. Ribeiro MR, de Carvalho CB, Pereira RHZ, et al. Yamamoto new scalp acupuncture for postoperative pain management in cats undergoing ovariohysterectomy. Vet Anaesthes Analges 2017;44(5):1236–44.
30. Gakiya HH, Silva DA, Gomes J, et al. Electro-acupuncture versus morphine for the postoperative control pain in dogs. Acta Cir Bras 2011;26:346e351.
31. Xie H, Colahan P, Ott EA. Evaluation of electroacupuncture treatment of horses with signs of chronic thoracolumbar pain. JAVMA 2005;227(2):281–6.
32. Rungsri P, Trinarong C, Rojanasthien S, et al. Effectiveness of electroacupuncture on pain threshold in sport horses with back pain. Am J Trad Chin Vet Med 2009;4:22–6.
33. Faramarzi B, Lee D, May K, et al. Response to acupuncture treatment in horses with chronic laminitis. Can Vet J 2017;58(8):823–7.
34. Mathews K, Kronen PW, Lascelles D, et al. Guidelines for recognition, assessment and treatment of pain: WSAVA global pain council members and co-authors of this document. J Small Anim Pract 2014;55:E10–68.
35. Jung WM, Shim W, Lee T, et al. More than DeQi: spatial patterns of acupuncture-induced bodily sensations. Front Neurosci 2016;10:462.

36. Chen Z, Ma C, Xu L, et al. Laser acupuncture for patients with knee osteoarthritis: a systematic review and meta-analysis of randomized placebo-controlled trials. Evid Based Complement Alternat Med 2019;2019:6703828.

37. Cantwell SL. Traditional Chinese veterinary medicine: the mechanism and management of acupuncture for chronic pain. Top Companion Anim Med 2010; 25(1):53–8.

38. Yu JB, Dong SA, Luo XQ, et al. "Role of Ho-1 in protective effect of electro-acupuncture against endotoxin shock-induced acute lung injury in rabbits.". Exp Biol Med (Maywood) 2013;238(6):705–12.

39. Zhai L, Wen SE, Huang WM. "[Research on Energy Metabolism Enzyme in Liver of the Rabbit During Hemorrhagic Shock and Effect of Acupuncture at "Renzhong" Acupoint by Quantitative Histochemistry].". Zhen Ci Yan Jiu 1989;14(no. 4):431–4.

40. Zhang SH, Cheng ZD. Effects of Electroacupuncture on Cyp7a1 expression in liver of rabbits with atherosclerosis. Zhongguo Zhen Jiu 2019;39(no. 1):59–64.

41. Zhang W, Gao Y, Guo C, et al. Effect of acupotomy versus electroacupuncture on ethology and morphology in a rabbit model of knee osteoarthritis. J Tradit Chin Med 2019;39(no. 2):229–36.

42. Zhou ZF, Du MY, Wu WY, et al. Effect of intracerebral microinjection of naloxone on acupuncture- and morphine-analgesia in the rabbit. Sci Sin 1981;24(no. 8): 1166–78.

43. An P, Sun WS, Wu XL, et al. Effect of acupuncture on renal function and pathologic changes of kidney in rabbits with nephritis. Zhongguo Zhen Jiu 2012; 32(9):819–23.

44. Shi X, Yu W, Wang T, et al. Electroacupuncture alleviates cartilage degradation: improvement in cartilage biomechanics via pain relief and potentiation of muscle function in a rabbit model of knee osteoarthritis. Biomed Pharmacother 2020;123: 109724.

45. Yu C, Zhang K, Lu G, et al. Characteristics of acupuncture meridians and acupoints in animals. Rev Sci Tech 1994;13(no. 3):927–33.

46. Blair J Bumblefoot. A Comparison of clinical presentation and treatment of pododermatitis in rabbits, rodents, and birds. Vet Clin North Am Exot Anim Pract 2013; 16(no. 3):715–35.

47. Lao L, Wong RH, Berman B, et al. Electroacupuncture reduces morphine-induced emesis in ferrets: a pilot study. J Altern Complement Med 1995;1(no. 3):257–61.

48. Cerreta AJ, Walker ME, Harrison TM. Evaluation of acupuncture points governing vessels 1 and 26 on anesthetic recovery of eastern box turtles (Terrapene carolina carolina). J Zoo Wildl Med 2018;49(no. 4):870–4.

49. Goe A, Shmalberg J, Gatson B, et al. Epinephrine or Gv-26 electrical stimulation reduces inhalant anesthestic recovery time in common snapping turtles (Chelydra serpentina). J Zoo Wildl Med 2016;47(no. 2):501–7.

50. Fernandes TM, Lopes FC, Santana Gcom, et al. Identification and mapping of real acupoints in the anatomical topography of boa constrictor. Braz J Biol 2019;79(no. 2):243–7.

51. Coke R. Electro acupuncture in the management of osteoarthritis in a Komodo Dragon. ExoticsCon Proc 2015;53–5.

52. West C. TCVM for avian species: introduction, general overview, acupuncture point locations, indications and techniques. In: H., Trevisanewllo Xie L, editors. Application of traditional Chinese veterinary medicine in exotic animals. Reddick (FL): Jing Tang Publishing; 2011. p. 53–71.

53. Choi KH, Buhl G, Ponder J. Raptor acupuncture for treating chronic degenerative joint disease. J Acupunct Meridian Stud 2016;9(6):330–4.

Physical Rehabilitation in Zoological Companion Animals

Ronald B. Koh, DVM, MS, Dipl. ACVSMR[a],*,
Jessica Rychel, DVM, Dipl. ACVSMR[b], Lindsey Fry, DVM, cVMA, CVPP, CCRP[b]

KEYWORDS

- Zoological companion animals ● Physical rehabilitation ● Tissue healing stages
- Rehabilitation phases ● Multifactorial rehabilitation planning ● Manual therapy
- Therapeutic modality ● Therapeutic exercises

KEY POINTS

- Animal physical rehabilitation aims to decrease pain, reduce edema, promote tissue healing, restore gait and mobility, regain strength, prevent further injury, and promote quality of life.
- A thorough understanding of the biology and stages of tissue healing is imperative to develop and safely implement the phases of rehabilitation.
- Rehabilitation program should be a multifactorial planning with ergonomics, therapeutic modalities, manual therapy, and therapeutic exercise to achieve specific goals.
- Rehabilitation program should be individualized to address the following: pain, swelling, range of motion, flexibility, proprioception and balancing, muscle strength, endurance, and functional activities.
- A successful rehabilitation program requires the therapist to continually assess, identify problems to be addressed, screen treatment options, create goals, implement treatment plans, and reassess.

INTRODUCTION

Animal physical rehabilitation (APR) is one of the fast-growing fields in veterinary medicine in recent years. It has become increasingly common in small animal practice and will continue to emerge as an essential aspect of veterinary medicine that plays a vital role in the care of animals with physical impairments or disabilities from surgery, injuries, or diseases.[1] This is true now more than ever because of the increasing advances in lifesaving treatments, the increased lifespan of companion animals, and

[a] William R. Pritchard Veterinary Medical Teaching Hospital, University of California, Davis, School of Veterinary Medicine, 1 Garrod Road, Davis, CA 95616, USA; [b] Red Sage Integrative Veterinary Partners, 1027 West Horsetooth, Suite 101, Fort Collins, CO 80526, USA
* Corresponding author.
E-mail address: rbkoh@ucdavis.edu

Vet Clin Exot Anim 26 (2023) 281–308
https://doi.org/10.1016/j.cvex.2022.07.009
1094-9194/23/© 2022 Elsevier Inc. All rights reserved.

the growth of chronic conditions, of which many are associated with movement disorders.[2,3] The American Association of Rehabilitation Veterinarians (AARV) defines APR as "the diagnosis and management of patients with painful or functionally limiting conditions, particularly those with injury or illness related to the neurologic and musculoskeletal systems."[4] Rehabilitation not only focuses on recovery after surgical procedures, but also on improving the function and quality of life in animals suffering from debilitating diseases such as arthritis or neurologic disorders. The overall goal of APR is to decrease pain, reduce edema, promote tissue healing, restore gait and mobility to its prior activity level, regain strength, prevent further injury, and promote optimal quality of life (**Box 1**).[1,5] Typically, a multimodal approach with pharmaceutical and nonpharmaceutical interventions is used by APR therapists to manage patients during their recovery. Before incorporating APR into practice settings, veterinarians, veterinary technicians, physical therapists, and physical therapy assistants should receive formal training in APR. Veterinary or canine physical rehabilitation certification courses are offered at several institutions in the United States, Europe, and Asia (**Box 2**). Residency programs in veterinary sports medicine and rehabilitation are also offered for veterinarians who are interested in becoming diplomates in veterinary sports medicine and rehabilitation.

Many zoologic companion animals (ZCA) with functional impairments from diseases, injury, or surgery will greatly benefit from rehabilitation;[6] however, treatment guidelines and protocols for rehabilitation in ZCA are sparse. The purpose of this article aims to provide knowledge and guidance on physical rehabilitation to help veterinarians in the proper return of their patients with ZCA safely after injury and/or surgery.

Current Evidence in Zoological Companion Animals

Although there is evidence for canine physical rehabilitation being effective in the treatment of mobility impairments due to injuries, diseases, or surgeries,[7,8] the evidence of APR in ZCA is scarce. Several case reports and studies have demonstrated the benefits of APR related to postoperation, osteoarthritis, chronic torticollis, uncontrolled neuropathic pain, and muscles contractures in exotic animals.[9–13]

In a case report a Lotharinger rabbit underwent extracapsular techniques in both stifle joints after cranial cruciate ligament ruptures and showed no signs of discomfort and has normal use of both rear legs after a 3-month rehabilitation program intended

---

Box 1
Goals of animal physical rehabilitation in zoologic companion animals

1. Decrease pain

2. Reduce inflammation and edema

3. Promote tissue healing

4. Restore range of motion

5. Restore gait and mobility

6. Improve balance and proprioception

7. Regain strength

8. Minimize risk of reinjury

9. Maintain cardiovascular fitness

10. Promote optimal quality of life

Box 2
Resources on animal physical rehabilitation

a. Institutes that offer animal physical rehabilitation training and certification programs (listed alphabetically):
   1. Canine Rehabilitation Institute: caninerehabinstitute.com
   2. Chi University: chiu.edu
   3. Healing Oasis Wellness Center: healingoasis.edu
   4. University of Tennessee: utvetce.com

b. Nonprofit organizations that promote the art and science of veterinary rehabilitation:
   1. American Association of Rehabilitation Veterinarians (AARV): rehabvets.org
   2. American College of Veterinary Sports Medicine and Rehabilitation (ACVSMR): vsmr.org

c. Advanced certification in veterinary rehabilitation:
   1. American College of Veterinary Sports Medicine and Rehabilitation (ACVSMR): vsmr.org
   2. Academy of Physical Rehabilitation Veterinary Technicians (APRVT): aprvt.com

---

to increase muscle strength.[9] The rehabilitation exercises primarily involve walking on a leash and harness in a straight line on a hard surface for 5 minutes initially and then it was gradually increased to 15 minutes during the next 3 months. Another case report showed that physical therapy as an adjunctive therapy has effectively managed severe osteoarthritis in a 20-year-old Komodo dragon (*Varanus komodoensis*) that did not respond well to oral analgesics.[10] After 10 weekly rehab therapy sessions, the Komodo dragon showed marked improvement in pain level, gait, and function, and increased responsiveness to his environment, which continued to improve over the subsequent sessions. Rehabilitation has also been reported to be effective and beneficial in treating Aves with pain and physical impairments.[11–13] In a case-control study, physical therapy (especially passive range of motion and soft tissue therapy) resulted in better resolution of the trauma-induced chronic torticollis and increased likelihood of release back into the wild.[11] A multi multimodal approach including low-level laser therapy successfully controlled pain and healed wounds in a raptor suffering from uncontrolled neuropathic pain and self-inflicted wounds, secondary to right metacarpus fractures and surgical repair. The falcon was successfully released after treatments.[12] Additionally, therapeutic ultrasound, another common therapeutic modality used in APR, significantly prevented and reversed the loss of wing extension caused by bandaging-associated contractures in racing pigeons.[13]

Rehabilitation Assessment

The primary step toward developing rehabilitation protocols is to perform a thorough assessment of the patient at frequent intervals and before the progression of therapeutic interventions. A comprehensive assessment should include medical history, complete physical examination, orthopedic or musculoskeletal examination, neurologic examination, pain assessment, and functional examination. Functional evaluation can be divided into passive and active assessments which can be found in **Table 1**.[1,8] Regardless of the species presented, the ability to assess pain in an individual patient is essential before beginning any form of rehabilitation. A discussion of pain recognition and traditional pharmacologic analgesia in ZCA is beyond the scope of this article, but the reader is referred to previous work on this subject.

As with any species, an accurate history provides essential information in diagnosing and treating disease. Before the appointment, the rehabilitation therapist should review the medical record and diagnostic test results thoroughly and communicate with the referring veterinarian to discuss the reason and expectation for referral

Table 1
Passive and active functional assessments commonly performed in animal physical rehabilitation[1,8]

Exam	Type	Description
Passive Functional Assessments		
Passive Range of Motion	Subj. asst.	Assessment of pain and the amount of osteokinematic motion available when the patient's joint is moved through the ROM without the patient's assistance (eg, flexion, extension, abduction, and adduction).
End-feel	Subj. asst.	Characteristic sensation perceived by the examiner when the end of joint ROM is reached to determine the cause of articular, muscle, or connective tissue restrictions in motion.
Goniometry	Obj. asst.	Measurement of joint angles (eg, flexion, and extension) using a goniometer ruler.
Joint play	Subj. asst.	Assessment of accessory movement (arthrokinematic motion) available within a joint (ie, rolling, spinning, and gliding).
Flexibility	Subj. asst.	Assessment of the passive extensibility (the ability of the muscle to stretch) of the contractile and connective tissue components of the muscle.
Muscle girth	Obj. asst.	Measurement of muscle circumferential measurements with a tape measure.
Myofascial exam	Subj. asst	Assessment of myofascial dysfunction, pain, taut bands, or trigger points by applying gentle pressure on facia and muscles.
Active Functional Assessments		
Posture	Subj. asst.	Assess the ability of the animal to maintain a normal or symmetry posture and stability during standing, sitting, sternal recumbency, walking, and so forth.
Gait/Mobility	Subj. and obj. asst.	Assess subjective and objective gait. The subjective analysis involved the observation of gait, balance, and capability of mobility during walk, trot, or run. The objective gait analysis requires special equipment & software to quantitatively measure the kinetics (forces generated during movement) and kinematics (motion that occurs during ambulation) of the animal.
Transfer	Subj. asst.	Assess the ability of the body to move from one posture to another (eg, sit-to-stand, lie-to-stand, step-up & down).
Strength (Muscle) Test	Subj. asst.	Evaluate the strength capacity of the muscle by observing the ability of a limb to maintain a static standing position (ie, the ability to support against gravity), when the contralateral limb is lifted off the ground.

Abbreviations: Asst, assessment; Obj, objective; ROM, range of motion; Subj, subjective.

and the owner's goals. After taking the history from the owner, the rehabilitation assessment may be started. Performing and interpreting rehabilitation assessment in ZCA can present a particular clinical challenge due to the significant variation in species, temperament, and cooperation levels in this group of patients. To get the most information possible from the rehabilitation assessment, it is important that the therapist is familiar with all aspects of the normal patient physical examination alongside the basic anatomy of the species.

As with any patient, it is important to assess the patient before handling. Generally, posture, gait, transfer, and balance assessments can be performed by observing the patients move around in the examination room or cage without any handling or restraint. It is important to provide a nonslip surface with yoga or rubber mats for the patient. An animal that feels unsteady is more likely to panic, become uncooperative, and may even injure itself or staff during restraint. After that, passive ROM, flexibility and myofascial assessments can be performed with minimal handling or restraint. If the therapist is unfamiliar with the best approach to restrain any ZCA, seeking advice from an experienced handler or having a skillful handler restrain the patients for assessment will allow for the most thorough examination. If needed, use an appropriately sized towel for each animal. A calming cap or hood may decrease the visual stimulation and stress of certain animals during handling.

The therapist should approach the patients calmly, and then gently palpate the musculoskeletal system to detect heat, pain, swelling, wound, joint stiffness, soft tissue tightness, and myofascial trigger points if adequate musculature is readily available. With most ZCA, handling time should be kept to a minimum to avoid stress on the animal and potential injury. Assessment must be discontinued immediately when the patients show increased signs of stress or distress. After the assessment, any abnormal findings should be recorded to aid in formulating an individualized rehabilitation plan for the patient based on the phases of tissue healing which will be discussed later in discussion. Lastly, the discussion of examination findings and treatment plan should be made with the owner and referring veterinarian to ensure that everyone fully understands the strategy and plans, and the owner is committed to pursue the rehabilitation program.

Stages of Tissue Healing

First and foremost, rehabilitation programs, whether from a conservative or surgical management, must be based on the basic science and stages of tissue healing. The phases of rehabilitation closely match the stages of healing.[8,14] These principles are applicable or generalizable across species. The therapist must have a thorough understanding of the sequence of the various stages of the healing process to develop and implement an effective and safe rehabilitation program.

The healing process consists of the inflammatory stage, reparative (fibroblastic) stage, and remodeling (maturation) stage.[8,14] These processes are a continuum and overlap one another with no definitive beginning or end points. Each tissue type (skin, muscle, tendon, ligament, bone, and so forth) will follow a predictable sequence and time frame of healing, regardless of species; however, the amount of time spent in each stage may vary depending on the type of tissue injury.[8] Therefore, a rehabilitation program should be individualized and primarily based on recognizing the stages of tissue healing, the type of injured tissue, and the clinical signs of an individual patient. It must also be stressed that inappropriate therapy selected at any stage could possibly inhibit its healing progress or inflict further injury which may further jeopardize the patient's recovery. **Table 2** shows the healing stages of tissue corresponding to the phases of rehabilitation.

Phases of Rehabilitation

The patient-specific rehabilitation program is a multifactorial strategy that combines 4 main interventions: ergonomics, manual therapy, therapeutic exercise, and electrophysical (therapeutic) modalities.[5] The use of these interventions during rehabilitation varies over time and is primarily based on the three phases of tissue healing within the rehabilitation program. Each rehabilitation phase has specific goals to accomplish before

Table 2
The 3 stages of tissue healing correspond to the 3 phases of rehabilitation and its proposed rehabilitation intervention

Healing Stage	Rehabilitation Phase	Rehabilitation Goals	Rehabilitation Intervention
Inflammatory stage	Acute or Inflammatory phase	• Protect healing tissues • Relieve pain • Reduce inflammation and edema • Maintain joint ROM	• Confinement/immobilization • Pain medication • Manual therapy • Cryotherapy, PBM[a], PEMF, acupuncture • PROM, assisted standing and walking, weight shifting
Reparative (Proliferative) stage	Subacute or Transition phase	• Promote weight bearing and joint function • Reeducation of muscle • Regain ROM • Regain flexibility and strength	• Promote tissue strength • Manual therapy • Heat therapy, PBM[a], PEMF, TUS[a], acupuncture • Muscle reeducation, gait patterning, and exercises to improve weight bearing, balancing, and active ROM
Remodeling (Maturation) stage	Chronic or Strength/Function phase	• Restore full ROM and flexibility • Improve muscle mass and strength • Improve proprioception • Regain endurance • Return functional activities	• Protect healing tissues • Manual therapy • Exercises to improve muscle and core strength, proprioception, endurance, and functional activities • PBM[a], PEMF, TUS[a], ESW[a], acupuncture as needed

Abbreviations: ESW, extracorporeal shockwave therapy; PBM, photobiomodulation; PEMF, pulsed electromagnetic field therapy; ROM, range of motion; TUS, therapeutic ultrasound.
[a] Settings are varied depending on injury type, tissue type, and injured tissue region.
Adapted from Kirkby Shaw K et al. 2020 with modifications.[8]

progressing to the next phase, rather than being based on a time frame of the injury. In general, the initial focus in the inflammatory phase would be on ergonomics (eg, nursing care, ambulation assistance), therapeutic modalities (cryotherapy, electrostimulation, photobiomodulation, therapeutic ultrasound), and manual therapy to control pain and edema, rather than therapeutic exercise due to the delicacy and fragility of healing tissues in the early phase.[5] As pain and edema have improved in the subacute phase, the focus on ergonomics and therapeutic modalities would remain, with an increase of emphasis toward manual therapy and therapeutic exercises to promote weight bearing and active range of motion (ROM). In the chronic phase, therapeutic exercises should be the focus of rehabilitation to improve strength, proprioception, and endurance to return to normal function and activity.[5] **Table 2** shows the characteristics of each rehabilitation phase and its proposed rehabilitation intervention.

Acute or inflammatory phase
Goals in this phase include:

- Protect healing tissues
- Relieve pain
- Reduce inflammation and edema

- Maintain joint ROM

This phase starts from the moment of the injury or surgery up to 7 days post-injury or surgery.[8] Clinical signs include edema, inflammation, pain, hemorrhage, ecchymosis, loss of joint ROM, acute paresis or plegia, and lameness when a weight-bearing limb is affected.[8,14] Rehabilitation starts immediately after injury or surgery with the focus on protecting the healing tissues and controlling pain and inflammation. Multifaceted use of pain medication remains the cornerstone of pain control in this phase, although many rehabilitation modalities can contribute to a well-managed, comfortable patient. These rehabilitation modalities shine in ZCA who may not tolerate analgesic medications well or who need to maintain normal appetite and gastrointestinal function throughout their recovery. Short-term mandatory crate rest and immobilization can be a critical component of recovery for patients with injury or surgery in this initial phase of rehabilitation.[14] Although this phase typically last 3 days, clinical signs of inflammation (heat, pain, redness, edema) should be used to gauge the end of this phase, as inflammation can be ongoing or intermittent throughout future phases.

In the inflammatory phase, manual therapy with gentle effleurage, stretching, passive range of motion (PROM), and low-grade joint mobilization (gliding, traction, and compression) can be performed 2 to 3 times daily to reduce edema, relax muscles, relieve pain, promote joint motion, prevent stiffness, and reduce the anxiety of the patient. Because the tensile strength of the injured tissues remains poor in this phase, therapeutic exercises should be minimized to avoid further tissue damage. Instead, gentle pain-free assisted standing of weight-bearing limbs may be initiated 2 to 3 times per day to prevent stiffness and promote edema reduction (through muscle contraction and enhanced lymphatic drainage) (**Fig. 1**). In patients with neck or back pain, a gentle active range of motion of the neck and back can be performed by using a treat or a toy to lure the patient to bend its neck and back to the side to improve flexibility. Therapeutic modalities that should be considered in this phase to control pain, reduce edema, and promote healing include cryotherapy, photobiomodulation therapy, nonthermal therapeutic ultrasound, pulsed electromagnetic field therapy, and acupuncture.[7] Detailed information on the use of manual therapy, therapeutic modalities, and therapeutic exercises commonly used in animal rehabilitation could be found in later in discussion paragraphs.

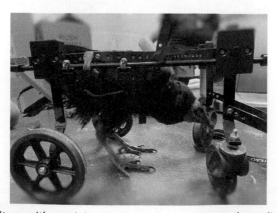

Fig. 1. A black vulture with postinjury paraparesis was supported standing in a cart.

Subacute or motion phase

The goals of this phase include:

- Promote weight bearing and joint function
- Reeducation of muscle
- Regain range of motion
- Regain flexibility and strength

This phase starts once the pain and edema are under control. At this time, the connective tissue is still immature, but it begins to gain tensile strength and can sustain a certain amount of stress or load, which is necessary to regain strength.[14] Weight bearing or joint motion should be encouraged when applicable as soon as possible to attain an optimal outcome. It has been shown that joint immobilization or failure to bear weight on a limb can lead to deleterious changes in cartilage, bone, and muscle.[8,14]

Over the next 2 weeks, the patient receiving proper rehabilitation should gradually progress from nonweight bearing to full weight bearing or from impaired joint to regained joint movement by approximately 4 weeks. Before exercises, manual therapy with soft tissue and joint mobilizations should be performed to improve flexibility and stimulate proprioceptors within the joint. When choosing therapeutic exercises, the therapist should be creative and choose appropriate exercises based on the form of the locomotion of the ZCA that is quadruped, biped, or serpentine. When applicable, weight bearing and balancing exercises such as weight shifting on a flat ground or an uneven surface (such as pillows, mattress, or balancing disc) can be initiated 2 to 3 times per day. All joints in the affected limb should be placed through a pain-free range of motion exercises. An introduction to more normal movement patterns (eg, getting up from lying down) can be gently introduced in this phase. In birds, perch exercises can be performed either on a perch stand or on the handler's hand. If needed, the handler could gently but firmly hold the toes of the bird to provide more stability to the bird (**Fig. 2**). To promote the joint motion of the affected wing, the handler's hand can gently drop to force the bird to flap the wings to promote wing ROM. Additionally, therapeutic modalities can be progressed from cryotherapy to thermotherapy to promote circulation to the injured tissue. Photobiomodulation, acupuncture, and

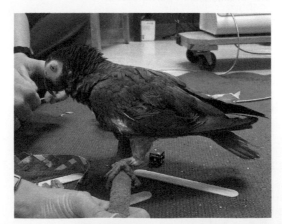

Fig. 2. A parrot with suspect multifocal vascular events receiving perch exercises on a stand for his paraparesis, followed by wing flapping exercises by slightly dropping the stand to stimulate his right-wing function with neurologic deficit.

pulsed electromagnetic field therapy can be continued to relieve pain and enhance healing. To advance to the next phase, the patient should have consistent full weight bearing during a normal gait pattern or pain-free range of motion.

Chronic or strength and function phase

The goals of this phase include:

- Restore full ROM and flexibility
- Improve muscle mass and strength
- Improve proprioception
- Regain endurance
- Return to functional activities

The final phase of the rehabilitation process is the strength/function phase. This phase is the longest spanning from months to years depending on the type of injured tissue. For example, bone is normally expected to regain full strength in approximately 12 weeks, but tendon and ligament are generally less vascular and may take up to 1 year or longer to resume full strength.[8]

Depending on the severity of the injury and the activity level of the ZCA, this phase may be approached by subdividing into an early phase that focuses on strength and stability, a midphase that emphasizes endurance, and a late phase that targets functional skills and activities. The transition from the early to late chronic phase to the next phase should be gradual to prevent reinjury. To a great extent, pain and swelling will dictate the rate of progression. Any exacerbation of pain or swelling during or after a specific exercise or activity indicates that the load is too great for the level of tissue strength. The therapist must assess the patient frequently during the early period of this phase and make proper adjustments to the rehabilitation program accordingly based on the patient's pain and functional status. It is also important to know that some patients may never achieve a preinjury level of function and activity. Therefore, every rehabilitation protocol or program should be individualized to the specific needs of the patient and owner, and it should also follow the general tissue healing principles outlined above.

In this phase, reduced strength, muscle atrophy, and poor proprioception that results from a period of immobility are generally a concern. Controlled strengthening exercises and proprioceptive training are the keys to increase muscle mass, strength, and balance, as outlined later in the therapeutic exercise section of this article. If soft tissue flexibility is reduced or joint motion remains restricted, soft tissue and joint mobilization techniques should be considered, respectively. Therapeutic modalities such as photobiomodulation, acupuncture, and pulsed electromagnetic field therapy can be used as needed for chronic pain in this phase.[15] Thermotherapy and therapeutic ultrasound before exercises help increase circulation and improving the extensibility of soft tissues, thus reducing joint stiffness, and leading to increased ROM.[16] Extraxcorporeal shockwave therapy is beneficial for managing chronic tendinopathies, nonunion fractures, open wounds, and chronic pain associated with degenerative joint disease.[7]

As the patient becomes stronger, the frequency, duration, and intensity of strengthening exercises should be gradually increased, with an increase of emphasis on endurance and controlled functional training. The degree of endurance training will differ based on the expected activity level of the patient following therapy. The last step of this phase is to gradually return to normal function and activity, and the patient can safely perform routine activities, such as playing, chasing, running, hopping, or jumping.

Multimodal Rehabilitation Interventions

Manual therapy

Manual therapy (MT) is a skilled, specific hands-on approach used by clinicians or therapists to treat soft tissues, joints, and nerves of various etiologies. The goals of treatment are to produce relaxation, improve circulation, relieve muscle tension, reduce pain, increase flexibility of soft tissues, and restore joint mobility.[17,18] The exact therapeutic mechanism by which MT works is not fully understood and probably represents a combination of physiologic, bio-mechanical or physical, and psychological effects.[18,19] (**Table 3**) The physiologic effects of MT include the reduction of pain via the pain gate theory and stimulation of the descending inhibitory tracts leading to pain inhibition and tissue relaxation.[20,21] MT may also directly affect inflammatory mediators (ie, TNF-α, IL-1β) and peripheral nociceptors (ie, β-endorphin, anandamide, N-palmitoylethanolamide, serotonin, endogenous cannabinoids) that interact in the healing process and pain perception.[22–24] The biomechanical effects of MT include altering tissue extensibility and fluid dynamics when soft tissue and joint capsule are mechanically pressured and mobilized, thus facilitating tissue repair and remodeling and improving tissue functions.[19] Lastly, the psychological effects of MT which has direct physical contact, such as massage, decreases stress and anxiety, produces relaxation, and improves emotional well-being in some ZCA.[18,25] ZCA that are unsocialized to human or easily distressed on physical contact might not be candidates for any form of MT.

Recent meta-analysis and systemic reviews have shown that MT is an effective treatment of human patients with pain and dysfunction due to knee osteoarthritis,[26] cervical radiculopathy,[27] and upper quarter musculoskeletal disorders.[28] While MT is an important component of the rehabilitation for many patients, there is a paucity of studies substantiating its clinical benefits in animals. Two recent studies suggest that MT alone or with acupuncture might be effective and safe for improving pain, physical function, and quality of life in dogs suffering from degenerative diseases, chronic pain, or musculoskeletal pain.[29,30] The authors' collective experiences suggest that this form of treatment either as a sole or combined other form of treatment (eg, therapeutic modalities or exercises) can be highly effective in managing musculoskeletal pain and mobility impairments, including in ZCA who may tolerate a shorter duration of MT, but can benefit from the biomodulatory benefits just as other species.

Manual treatments generally include soft tissue mobilization and joint mobilization. Soft tissue mobilization uses many different hand techniques, such as effleurage, petrissage, tapotement, stretching, friction, and myofascial release, to induce relaxation, lessen pain, reduce swollen, improve extensibility, prevent or break up scar tissue, and prevent muscle shortening or contracture of the affected soft tissues, that is, fascia, muscle, tendons, and ligaments.[17–19] Joint mobilization, such as joint gliding,

Table 3	
Clinical benefits of soft tissue mobilization and joint mobilization	
Soft Tissue Mobilization	**Joint Mobilization**
• Induce soft tissue relaxation • Lessen soft tissue pain • Provide sensory stimulation • Improve circulation • Improve soft tissue extensibility • Prevent or break up scars • Prevent muscle shortening or contracture	• Maintain joint mobility and nourishment • Reduce joint pain • Address joint restriction • Restore joint optimal motion and function • Provide sensory stimulation • Prevent connective tissue adhesions

traction and compression, on the other hand, focuses on continuum of passive move-ments to the joint complex with the intent to promote joint nourishment, reduce pain, provide sensory stimulation, and restore optimal motion and function of the affected joints.[31] Joint mobilization requires extra-coursework and hands-on training before application on animals, thus it is beyond the scope of this article, but the reader is referred to previous work on this subject.[31] Contraindications and precautions of MT include direct mechanical pressure over an open wound, infected tissue, sites of recent trauma, fractures, malignancy, and acute nerve or neuralgia. Clinical benefits of both soft tissue and joint mobilizations are listed in **Table 3**. Common techniques of soft tissue mobilization and their goals are listed in **Table 4**.

Given these positive effects and the safety of conscientiously performed soft tissue manual therapy, certain gentle techniques such as effleurage, rolling and lifting of the skin, and myofascial release play a prominent role in caring for many ZCA, such as small mammals, birds, reptiles, and so forth, experiencing myofascial pain and me-chanical dysfunctions associated with musculoskeletal or neurologic disorders. When performing soft tissue mobilization, the therapist often starts with gentle effleur-age for relaxation and to assess soft tissue for stiffness, inflammation, swelling, trigger point, or masses (**Fig. 3**). It is then followed by other techniques for the treatment of the soft tissues which are listed in **Table 4** and **Figs. 4–6** along with special considerations when applying these techniques on ZCA. Generally, effleurage is also conducted at the end of each session. All manual therapies must be administered with caution in pa-tients that are easily stressed to avoid further injury to the patients. Manual therapy in amphibians should be extremely cautious or be avoided altogether due to their deli-cate and highly glandular nature of skin that is very sensitive to handling.

Cryotherapy

Cryotherapy, the application of cold therapy to an injured region, is commonly used to reduce pain and inflammation during the acute phase of injury.[8] Animal models have demonstrated that tissue cooling can have significant beneficial effects on postoper-ative or postinjury pain, inflammation and swelling by reducing or delaying the infiltra-tion of white blood cells and subsequent inflammatory cytokines within injured tissue.[32–34] Rabbits, ferrets, and other small mammals tend to tolerate postoperative or postinjury cryotherapy well, and improvement in incisional outcomes have been subjectively noted.[6] Trends toward the use of cryotherapy after intraoral procedures is becoming more widely used in human dentistry,[35,36] and because dental interven-tions are common in some ZCA, this is another place to consider the use of cryo-therapy in these animals after the procedure.

Several important considerations must be made when applying cryotherapy to ZCA. The first is their size and the propensity for large changes in tissue and body temper-ature. Large changes can contribute to postprocedure hypothermia and create changes in the muscle than are intended or achieved in other species. For this reason, cryotherapy should be avoided in reptiles, amphibians, and fishes because of their ectothermic physiology.[6] Secondly, Takagi and colleagues showed some evidence that even a single cryotherapy event after a muscular crush injury in a rat can delay and even inhibit muscular regeneration with the application of a crushed ice pack directly to the skin postmuscular injury.[34] Ultimately, clinical recommendations should include a brief period of cryotherapy immediately following an injury, taking into ac-count body size and temperature as to avoid hypothermia or over-cooling of the soft tissues. Based on the periods of healing, this therapy should only be instituted in the first several hours to days after injury or surgery to avoid delaying tissue healing. Our current recommendation is to consider 3 to 4 sessions of cryotherapy with a

Table 4
Treatment techniques, goals, and applications of soft tissue mobilization in ZCA

STM Technique	Description and Effect	Applications in ZCA
Effleurage	Gliding or sliding the palms, fingertips, and/or thumbs over the skin in a rhythmic circular pattern with varying degrees of pressure depends on the size and clinical conditions of the patients. Goals: relaxation, reduce pain and swelling, stimulate lymphatic drainage.	MT starts with effleurage for relaxation and assessment. It is also conducted at the end of each session (see **Fig. 3**).
Petrissage	Kneading or wringing of soft tissues in a circular motion with hands, or pressing, rolling, or lifting of the tissues with fingers and thumbs. Goals: relaxation, stimulate circulation and tissue pliability, decrease adhesions.	Pressing, skin rolling, or skin lifting along the neck, back, thigh, quadriceps, and triceps in any size of ZCA (see **Fig. 4**). Kneading or wringing on a large muscle group, such as the neck, shoulder, and hip in large mammals (see **Fig. 5**).
Stretching	Passive stretching techniques applied by the therapist to muscle groups for a period of 10–30 s. Goals: promote muscle elongation and flexibility, improve ROM.	Stretching is well tolerated by most ZCA, but it should be performed slowly (see **Fig. 6**).
Myofascial release	Slow, gentle press and stretch to the fascia to elongate and release the restricted fascial tissue. Goals: relax tissue tension, reduce pain, restore tissue extensibility.	Myofascial release is well tolerated by most ZCA and can be performed in between other techniques.
Friction Massage	A circular, longitudinal, or transverse pressure applied by the finger or thumb to small area tissues or tendons. Goals: breakdown scar tissue, loosen ligaments, relieve trigger points.	Friction massage is often uncomfortable and therefore light pressure initially is recommended. Despite this, it is an effective treatment of tendonitis or tendinopathy, and trigger points in ZCA (see **Fig. 10**).
Tapotement or Percussion	Various parts of the hand including fingers striking the tissues (hacking, clapping, beating, tapping, vibration) at varying pressure and rate on stiff or weak muscles. Goals: stimulate circulation, muscle reflexes, and muscle tone.	Tapping and vibration techniques with fingers are generally safe and easy to perform in any size of ZCA with care. Hacking or clapping can be performed with cautions on a large muscle group in large mammals.

Abbreviations: MT, manual therapy; ROM, range of motion; STM, soft tissue mobilization; ZCA, zoologic companion animals.

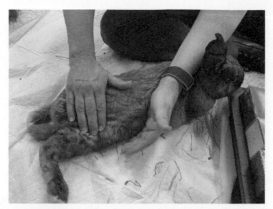

Fig. 3. An ambulatory paraparetic rabbit due to myelopathy receiving gentle effleurage for calming and muscle relaxation.

duration of 3 to 7 minutes in the first 24 hours up to 72 hours, dependent on the body size of the ZCA. The application of cryotherapy should only be applied to a patient once its body temperature is normal and stable postprocedure or injury.

Photobiomodulation therapy

Photobiomodulation (PBM) or therapeutic laser is the application of irradiation with certain wavelengths of red or near-infrared light over lesions or injured tissues to produce a range of physiologic effects in cells and tissues.[37,38] In veterinary practice, it is commonly used for analgesia, tissue healing, and enhancing neurologic function.[37] PBM therapy is also frequently used in the treatment of swelling, edema and local inflammation, as it can attenuate inflammatory cytokine production and influx of inflammatory cells into an injured region.[38–40] In addition, it improves tissue healing process by upregulating fibroblast populations and enhancing collagen production and organization for soft tissue and bone regeneration,[41,42] likely due to the result of PBM-induced osteogenesis and angiogenesis.[43] Overall, photobiomodulation therapy is a safe and effective treatment to be used throughout the healing stages of injured tissue aimed at controlling pain, reducing inflammation and edema, and enhancing

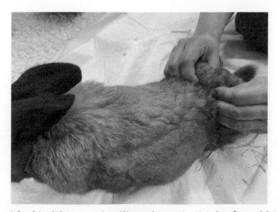

Fig. 4. Petrissage with skin lifting and rolling along the back of a rabbit with paraparesis with back pain to relieve pain and muscle tension.

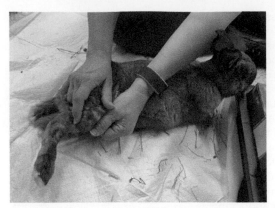

Fig. 5. Petrissage with kneading on the thigh muscle of a rabbit with paraparesis to increase circulation and tissue flexibility.

tissue healing in ZCA. Besides, PBM reduces both inflammatory and neuropathic pain, making it an excellent tool for use in the acute and chronic settings.[44] The benefits of PBM therapy can significantly impact outside need for drugs, and sometimes prevent more invasive procedures in the case of orthopedic and soft tissue injuries in these species.

In recent years, PBM with light-emitting diodes (LED) is gaining both scientific evidence and popularity among the medical community.[38,40] Because ZCA are generally small, LED therapy may represent a noninvasive, inexpensive, and safe approach to laser devices, for clinical and home use, in these species. Clinical recommendations for PBM in ZCA aim for judicious use of laser or LED therapy, either in the clinic or for home use.

At this time, optimal treatment doses have yet to be identified. The World Association of Laser Therapy (WALT) recommends a dose of 4 to 6 J/cm^2.[45] Because of the small body and limb size of these species, it is important to remember that a dose ranging from 1 to 5 J/cm^2 is probably optimal for wound healing or superficial lesions, whereas a higher dose ranging from 1 to 20 J/cm^2 may be an appropriate range for osteoarthritis, deep lesions, pain conditions, and other chronic ailments.[46] It is worth

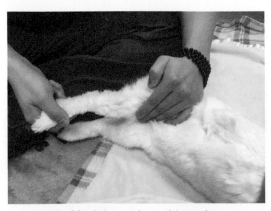

Fig. 6. Stretching of the right hip joint and quadriceps in a paraparetic rabbit due to myelopathy.

noting that excessive PBM dosing has been shown to delay wound healing and reduce fibroblast metabolism in certain injury types, indicating that a lower-level energy or power densities may be more appropriate in some cases.[47] Additionally, Alves *and colleagues* showed a superior reduction in inflammation in rats with joint injuries with use of 50 milli-Watt therapy compared with 100 mW therapy.[39] For best results, treatment is applied not only directly over the existing injury, but also to address compensatory muscle soreness and surrounding myofascial trigger points, nerves innervating the painful region and lymph nodes receiving the inflammatory waste from the affected tissue.[48] The frequency of treatment can vary greatly, from every 1 to 2 days to once a week, depending on the severity of the lesion. Several PBM therapy sessions (up to 10 sessions) may be necessary over a few weeks to elicit a successful outcome. Consideration of pet owners using lower-level laser therapy or LED therapy in the home setting may be a way for these species to receive more regular care than frequent appointments with a rehabilitation therapist. The only absolute clinical contraindication for PBM therapy is direct or reflected exposure through the pupil onto the retina.[46] The animal's eyes can be protected by covering them with a dark cloth or towel. Another well-known contraindication for PBM therapy is in the presence of known or suspected neoplasia, due to the ability of PBM to enhance cell proliferation which can contribute to aggression in certain cancer types.[41] Because PBM increases microcirculation in tissue, treatment of actively hemorrhaging lesion should be avoided. **Fig. 7** showed a Sulcata tortoise receiving photobiomodulation (laser) therapy for an injured foot from the dog bite.

Acupuncture
Acupuncture is the most frequently used rehabilitation modality in veterinary patients including ZCA, and also has the largest accompanying body of efficacy literature in

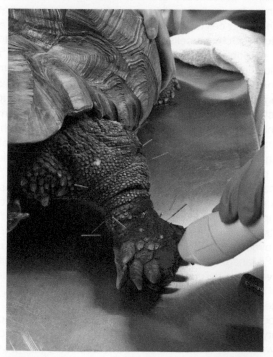

Fig. 7. A Sulcata tortoise receiving photobiomodulation (laser) therapy for its injured foot.

these species.[49–51] Its safety has also been well established when used by a trained practitioner, and treatments are generally well tolerated by patients.[50,52] Acupuncture is an essential component of rehabilitation treatment plans in ZCA, and provides significant benefit for patients pursuing rehabilitation for a wide variety of conditions, such as pain, osteoarthritis, orthopedic diseases, neurologic disorders, and gastrointestinal disorders.[50,52] In particular, enhanced analgesia or management of complex pain is frequently a goal of a rehabilitation plan. A more detailed discussion of acupuncture in ZCA is beyond the scope of this article, but the reader is referred to the article "Acupuncture in Zoologic Companion Animals" in the same issue.

Pulsed electromagnetic field therapy

Pulsed electromagnetic field (PEMF) therapy has grown in popularity and accessibility in veterinary rehabilitation medicine over the past decade and offers a compelling noninvasive therapy for the management of wound healing, bone healing, neurologic recovery, swelling and edema reduction, and pain management.[53] PEMF involves the flow of electricity through a coil or antenna which in turn generates a magnetic field that can then be directed at tissues for therapeutic effects.[53] The parameters of the electromagnetic field (frequency, duration, and amplitude) will determine the magnitude and likely correlate with various biologic functions and ultimately the efficacy and safety of treatment.[53] The ideal parameters for therapeutic effect remain nebulous and inconsistent among research studies. While PEMF affects numerous cellular functions and the exploration into these effects continues, there are a few well-recognized mechanisms of action that apply directly to its use in the rehabilitation setting.[7] PEMF exposure alters calcium release and binding with calmodulin which can impact metabolism, inflammation, cell death, blood pressure/vascular tone, gene activation, immune function, cAMP production, and nervous signal transduction.[54] There are shifts in the inflammatory cell signaling mediators, such as IL-6, TNF-alpha, heat phase proteins, and other cell mediators. There are also significant effects on certain cell types, specifically, Schwan cells and other neurologic support cells, fibrocytes, endothelial cells, osteoblasts, and chondroblasts which can all impact recovery from musculoskeletal or neurologic injury and disease.[54,55]

PEMF therapy has shown significant promise in the management of wounds which can pose challenges in rehabilitation patients and limit progress if not addressed. Through its impact on angiogenesis, fibroblast migration, and inflammatory modulation, and pain management, PEMF therapy enhances wound healing on many levels.[55,56] Additionally, PEMF therapy has a role to play in bone healing and osteoarthritis management. Bone turnover, osteoblast, and chondroblast activity, as well as inflammation and pain can all be augmented with the use of PEMF.[57] PEMF therapy has also proven especially useful in nonunion fractures in numerous species. In rabbits, turkeys, and rats, PEMF therapy has sped recovery and improved bone health after disuse osteopenia, acute fractures, and nonhealing fractures.[58] In osteoarthritis management, pets' owners have reported better quality of life scores, lowered pain scores, and improved gait analysis with PEMF treatment when compared with the control group.[59,60] Managing these painful conditions with the addition of PEMF will likely speed recovery and reduce pain, therefore, reducing dependence on medications and length of time needed to stay confined, immobilized, or hospitalized-frequent challenges for ZCA.

Much of the recent data exploring PEMF use in veterinary medicine have been related to recovery from neurologic injury and surgery.[61,62] The groundwork for this clinical research was laid by numerous studies in laboratory animals with both peripheral and spinal cord injuries (including crush, transection, and contusion induced injuries), which have revealed that PEMF treatment results in less neuronal apoptosis and cytotoxicity, reduced neurogenic inflammation, and improved axonal recovery and resilience.[63–65] Therefore, it stimulates the rapid recovery of sensory and motor function and enhances pain control,[66] so that animals can potentially return to a more normal function and mobility earlier. As previously mentioned, it is critical to speed the functional recovery of ZCA with neurologic injury as it would help minimize their stress or distress level due to prolonged immobilization and confinement.

A variety of veterinary-specific PEMF devices are available including wearable loops and beds or mats. PEMF can be included for ZCA when additional analgesia is needed, there is a need for faster healing, or there are neurologic deficits secondary to injury in the central or peripheral nervous system. PEMF devices (loops or mats) can be incorporated into a bandage, recovery enclosure, or habitat, or placed in direct contact with the patient for a treatment session (**Fig. 8**). Duration, parameters, and frequency of treatment are flexible, but titrating to effect and tolerance can lead to good clinical outcomes. Depending on delivery protocols for commercially available products, PEMF can be applied continuously in a bandage, or intermittently in treatment sessions, with as little as 15 to 30 minutes daily providing benefit.

Extracorporeal shockwave therapy

Extracorporeal shockwave (ESW) therapy has expanded from its original indication for the treatment of kidney stones into the realm of physical rehabilitation and the management of myofascial, tendon, ligament, and boney disorders.[67] The application of unique high-pressure acoustic waves to tissues results in a cascade of physiologic changes with significant potential therapeutic effects. When the wave passes through

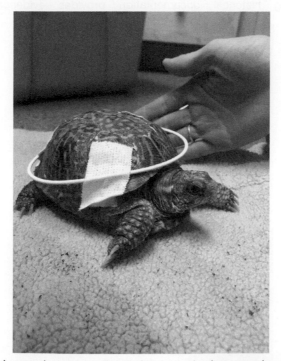

Fig. 8. A Western box turtle receiving PEMF Therapy with a loop taped to his carapace after a dog bite injury left the carapace damaged and his left hindlimb injured.

tissues of different densities, energy dissipates and is greater when there is a larger difference in density (like between bone and cartilage) inducing some of the clinical effects of shockwave. There is also mechanical compression and cavitation that can exert biological effects.[67] Generating this energy can be conducted through a variety of types of shockwave units including electrohydraulic, electromagnetic, and piezoelectric and these vary in how the energy wave is generated and also the amount of energy delivered.[67] Although ESW treatments are generally very sage, there is some risk of cell damage with over exuberant dosing, frequency, and intensity.

As with above-mentioned modalities, ESW therapy also offers a convincing noninvasive method for a variety of musculoskeletal problems such as wound healing, osteoarthritis, tendinopathy, and bone healing, based on experimental and clinical research.[68–72] One of the primary effects of ESW treatment is analgesia and, in both humans and horses has been documented to have a biphasic pattern. There is initial pain relief that will last days and then pain can return to then again be relieved after 3 to 4 weeks. The initial pain relief is hypothesized to be more related to effects on local nociceptors and altering in cell signaling/growth factors, whereas the later pain relief effect is associated with the modification of inflammation and changes in tissue matrix and structure.[73,74] During the application of ESW therapy, it is important to recognize signs of discomfort that are species specific. Treatment sites and parameters (dosing, frequency, and intensity) should be appropriately adjusted if needed. Sedation may be needed in some cases. **Fig. 9** showed a rabbit receiving ESW therapy for chronic spinal cord injury.

Therapeutic exercise

Animal physical rehabilitation uses a combination of the discussed modalities, as well as addresses the importance of movement and strengthening to treat injury and illness.[1,4] Strong historical documentation provides evidence that tissue

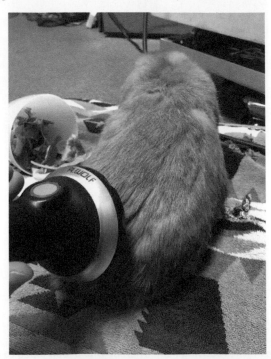

Fig. 9. A rabbit receiving ESW therapy to treat a chronic spinal cord injury.

immobilization leads to atrophy of bone, ligament, tendon, cartilage, and muscle, significantly impacting injury outcomes and the long-term health of the tissue.[7,75] This can be the result of bulky external coaptation for the treatment of wounds and fractures, particularly challenging in zoologic companion species, or the result of overly enthusiastic confinement in an attempt to encourage healing.

Therapeutic exercise can be used for nearly every type of musculoskeletal and neurologic injury, and even during recovery from illnesses such as pneumonia or dysbiosis.[76,77] Much of the evidence for the types and applications for therapeutic exercise is adapted from human medicine. Therapeutic exercise is challenging to study in the veterinary realm due to the lack of funding for this topic, individualized patient challenges/motivations and a great variety of underlying injury types. When recovering from musculoskeletal injury, considering the phase of tissue healing discussed above a patient is likely experiencing and then building a therapeutic exercise program based on that phase is the primary goal. Protecting the injury early in therapy, during the acute phase of healing, while ensuring that muscle and joint contracture are prevented, and generalized bone and soft tissue atrophy are avoided is the way to start. By introducing voluntary, active weight-bearing and movement, therapeutic exercise will help maximize positive outcomes. Incentivizing voluntary participation in therapeutic exercise with rewards will improve the outcome for the participating patient,[78] and is helpful in ensuring the patient has a good experience and will enjoy continuing with the activity throughout their recovery. Once the patient has passed the acute phase of tissue healing, a broader approach to rehabilitation can be taken. Several categories of therapeutic exercise help to customize therapeutic exercise programs for ZCA and help the rehabilitation practitioner in clinical planning for these patients.

Balance and proprioceptive exercise. The first category is aimed at improving balance, stability, and proprioception. Balance and proprioceptive exercises can be initiated in the reparative stage or subacute phase, and continue throughout the remodeling stage or chronic phase. Working on unstable and uneven surfaces and requiring the engagement of core musculature, as well as muscular proprioception, will help a patient reestablish enhanced conscious proprioception in the central nervous system and proprioceptive function in the peripheral tissues.[76] Muscle spindles and Golgi tendon organs play an important role and can be positively impacted by therapeutic exercise that encompasses an element of balance with the challenge of instability of weight bearing.[79] The active function of these muscular proprioceptors is also important in achieving the best possible morphology in healing bone after a fracture.[80] Balance work and even posture coordinating with visual function, can help in the common situation of head tilt or head trauma in a variety of ZCA. Clinical examples of balance-oriented exercises (**Figs. 10** and **11**) include navigating an uneven surface during gait (mattress, pillow, sand, stones, grass, or balance equipment), weight-bearing strength exercise performed on an unstable or vibrating surface, and navigating a variety of surfaces, gait patterns, and postures while the visual system on moving (treats, toys, cotton ball) or fixed objects (horizon, pet owner, exit door).

Strength exercise. Once the patient can bear weight consistently without overtly painful or discomfort, the strength and function phase (remodeling stage) begins, and strengthening exercises should be slowly introduced to the patient. Muscular strength can be difficult to achieve with ZCA, as it requires a creative approach and the voluntary and repetitive participation of the patient. Strength exercises should always be designed with the stage of tissue healing in mind, patient goals, and baseline abilities for a given species or individual. Strength training usually does not include external

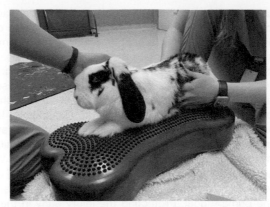

Fig. 10. Weight bearing and balancing exercises on a nonambulatory paraparetic rabbit due to myelopathy using a balancing disc.

weight, but rather strengthening using eccentric, concentric, or isometric contraction against the patient's own body weight. Using the previously discussed rewards systems as an incentive is essential to get these animals to participate in strength training exercises.

Strength training in elderly humans is known to improve outcomes after traumatic or pathologic fracture and can help ameliorate the sarcopenia and loss of muscle

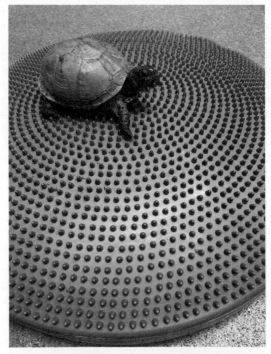

Fig. 11. A three-toed box turtle working on balancing exercise during convalescence from a head and ocular injury.

strength and function that are seen with aging and the degenerative processes that accompany aging.[81] Strength training, and beginning with gentle isometric or "static" strengthening, has also been shown across multiple trials to relieve pain and improve outcomes for osteoarthritis in humans.[82] Animal models also show good evidence that strength training can help mitigate profound muscle atrophy after injury, surgical intervention and significant lameness or disuse.[83–85]

For clinical considerations in this grouping of exercises, patient comfort and motivation are the key, as well as injury type. For example, avian patients with a leg or foot injury who will eventually need to feel comfortable on a perch should incorporate digital flexion and extension into their exercise program. Weight-bearing static work usually progresses into more challenging and intensive "hill work," single-limb weight bearing accomplished by stepping over an obstacle (Cavaletti rails) or holding up 1 to 2 limbs, and eventually even considering more explosive work like hopping up onto an elevated surface (**Figs. 12** and **13**).

Endurance and repetitive locomotor exercise. Being able to comfortably move in an environment independently for a reasonable amount of time is a tenant of quality of life for most ZCA. Additionally, neuroplasticity and the ability to regeneration function in brain, spinal cord, and peripheral nerves after trauma, is achieved through locomotor therapeutic exercise.[78,86,87] Medium intensity, low to moderate impact repetitive locomotor exercise is also great for maintaining mobility in degenerative joint and other musculoskeletal injuries.[9] Locomotor therapeutic exercise includes wheel exercise for interested small mammals, leash walking on stable surfaces, or any other repetitive weight-bearing activity that helps reestablish normal movement patterns. Providing surfaces that are safe and easy for the patient to navigate early in recovery is essential for safety as well as voluntary participation. Again, food motivation or other positive training rewards are very helpful for enticing a patient to participate, and will yield improved clinical outcomes.[86] It should also be noted that an uncomfortable patient will be less likely to participate, so adequate pain management is important.

Determining a patient's rehabilitation plan should always be based on the phases of healing, but for aerobic or endurance exercise, it is especially important to note that for approximately 3 days after a traumatic injury, during the peak of the acute inflammatory phase, aerobic activity should be avoided. The focus during this time should instead be limited to modalities that reduce inflammation and pain. During the remodeling stage or strength and function phase, frequent locomotor activity is the best tool

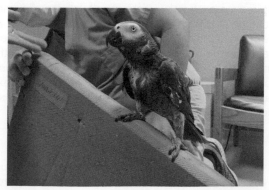

Fig. 12. The same parrot in **Fig. 2** was receiving incline exercises in the chronic phase to improve strength and proprioception.

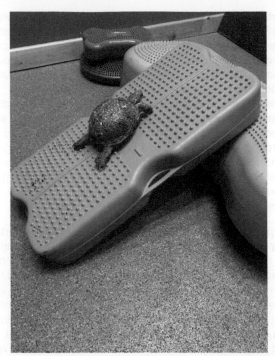

Fig. 13. A Western box turtle participating in a progression of therapeutic exercise to a steeper incline with the introduction of instability in the equipment, allowing progressive strength and proprioceptive function for a return to an outdoor habitat.

to maintain neuroplasticity and encourages full recovery to normal patterns of gait and movement. Conversely, patients who are restrained and kept "quiet" or immobilized after injury do not recover the motor function of their limbs and even when allowed to return to more normal activity late, never achieve complete recovery.[78] Even dragging paretic limbs in a safe habitat after spinal cord injury provides enough locomotor retraining that much more complete recovery can happen in comparison to small mammals kept on strict activity or movement restriction.[88]

Stretching exercise. Stretching has been shown to maintain the length of muscle fibers as well as help reduce back pain, improve gait, improve inflammation in laboratory animals, and can be active with participation from the ZCA.[89] Active stretching (patient initiated, as part of a therapeutic exercise) is often superior to passive stretching (a passive stretch performed by therapist or pet owner), both from a patient handling standpoint, as well as the patient's ability to lengthen muscle and improve flexibility.[90,91] Passive stretching can also be helpful in enhancing flexibility in patients better suited to that intervention, as long as it is not a source of stress or creating too much force on a contracted or fibrotic muscle.[92]

SUMMARY

It is vital to assess the underlying cause for injury or illness in ZCA, just as it is in other species. Once the underlying condition has been identified and appropriate treatment is instituted, the recovery process begins. Animal physical rehabilitation plays an essential role in the recovery process for many ZCA that are affected by injury or trauma. Rehabilitation can also be used to improve pain, mobility, and quality of life in geriatric patients or patients with ongoing or progressive medical conditions. Rehabilitation should begin as soon as the patient stabilizes to minimize the deleterious impacts of rest and immobilization. The optimal rehabilitation plan involves a thorough patient assessment to identify musculoskeletal or neurologic impairment, then uses the combination of the 4 main rehabilitation therapies (ergonomics, manual therapy, therapeutic exercise, and therapeutic modalities), and lastly reassessment at regular time intervals to monitor patient progress. With proper training, rehabilitation can be easily implemented in a clinical setting to improve health and outcomes for ZCA with functional impairments. Nonetheless, research involving well-designed clinical studies is needed to expand the knowledge and efficacy of rehabilitation in these unique patients.

CLINICS CARE POINTS

- Animal physical rehabilitation plays an essential role in the recovery process for many ZCA that are affected by injury, trauma, aging, or ongoing and progressive medical conditions.
- The ideal rehabilitation plan should be based on the three phases of rehabilitation (Inflammatory, Transition, and Strength/Function phases), which are corresponding to the 3 stages of tissue healing (Inflammatory, Reparative, and Remodeling stages, respectively.)
- A multimodal approach to rehabilitation is strongly recommended—emphasizing a combination of ergonomics, manual therapy, acupuncture, therapeutic exercise, and therapeutic modalities when developing a rehabilitation program.
- Given the significant variation in species and cooperation levels in ZCA, the therapist should always think "out of the box" and be creative when designing and implementing a treatment plan in zoologic companion patients, when developing a therapeutic exercise program.
- Mindfulness should be granted toward low-stress and fear-free handling and techniques when performing any form of rehabilitation therapy on ZCA.

DISCLOSURE

The authors of this article have no commercial or financial conflicts of interest.

REFERENCES

1. Kramer A, Hesbach AL, Sprague S. Introduction to Canine Rehabilitation. In: Zink C, Van Dyke JB, editors. Canine sports medicine and rehabilitation. 2nd edition. Wiley Blackwell; 2018. p. 96–119.
2. Bays TB. Geriatric Care of Rabbits, Guinea Pigs, and Chinchillas. Vet Clin North Am Exot Anim Pract 2020;23(3):567–93.
3. Frye C, Carr BJ, Lenfest M, et al. Canine Geriatric Rehabilitation: Considerations and Strategies for Assessment, Functional Scoring, and Follow Up. Front Vet Sci 2022;9:842458.
4. AARV (American Association of Rehabilitation Veterinarians). What is Rehabilitation?. Available at: http://rehabvets.org/what-is-rehab.lasso. Accessed April 25, 2022.
5. Marcellin-Little DJ, Levine D, Millis DL. Multifactorial Rehabilitation Planning in Companion Animals. Adv Small Anim Care 2021;(2):1–10.
6. Rychel JK, Johnston MS, Robinson NG. Zoologic companion animal rehabilitation and physical medicine. Vet Clin North Am Exot Anim Pract 2011;14(1):131–40.

7. Millis DL, Ciuperca IA. Evidence for canine rehabilitation and physical therapy. Vet Clin North Am Small Anim Pract 2015;45(1):1–27.

8. Kirkby Shaw K, Alvarez L, Foster SA, et al. Fundamental principles of rehabilitation and musculoskeletal tissue healing. Vet Surg 2020;49(1):22–32.

9. van Zuijlen M, Vrolijk P, van der Heyden M. Bilateral successive cranial cruciate ligament rupture treated by extracapsular stabilization surgery in a pet rabbit (Oryctolagus cuniculus). J Exot Pet Med 2012;(19):245–8.

10. Wolfe TC, Stringer E, Krauss S, et al. Physical therapy as an adjunctive treatment for severe osteoarthritis in a Komodo dragon (Varanus komodoensis). J Zoo Wildl Med 2015;46(1):164–6.

11. Nevitt BN, Robinson N, Kratz G, et al. Effectiveness of Physical Therapy as an Adjunctive Treatment for Trauma-induced Chronic Torticollis in Raptors. J Avian Med Surg 2015;29(1):30–9.

12. Shaver SL, Robinson NG, Wright BD, et al. A multimodal approach to management of suspected neuropathic pain in a prairie falcon (Falco mexicanus). J Avian Med Surg 2009;23(3):209–13.

13. Wimsatt J, Dressen P, Dennison C, et al. Ultrasound therapy for the prevention and correction of contractures and bone mineral loss associated with wing bandaging in the domestic pigeon (Columba livia). J Zoo Wildl Med 2000; 31(2):190–5.

14. Henderson A, Millis D. In: Millis DL, Levine D, editors. Canine rehabilitation and physical therapy. 2nd edition. Elsevier; 2014. p. 79–91.

15. Canapp DA. Select modalities. Clin Tech Small Anim Pract 2007;22(4):160–5.

16. Hanks J, Levine D, Bockstahler B. Physical agent modalities in physical therapy and rehabilitation of small animals. Vet Clin North Am Small Anim Pract 2015; 45(1):29–44.

17. Hesbach AL. Manual therapy in veterinary rehabilitation. Top Companion Anim Med 2014;29(1):20–3.

18. Corti L. Massage therapy for dogs and cats. Top Companion Anim Med 2014; 29(2):54–7.

19. Sutton A, Whitlock D. Massage. In: Millis DL, Levine D, editors. Canine rehabilitation and physical therapy. 2nd edition. Elsevier; 2014. p. 464–83.

20. Abraira VE, Ginty DD. The sensory neurons of touch. Neuron 2013;79(4):618–39.

21. Bialosky JE, Beneciuk JM, Bishop MD, et al. Unraveling the Mechanisms of Manual Therapy: Modeling an Approach. J Orthop Sports Phys Ther 2018; 48(1):8–18.

22. Teodorczyk-Injeyan JA, Injeyan HS, Ruegg R. Spinal manipulative therapy reduces inflammatory cytokines but not substance P production in normal subjects. J Manipulative Physiol Ther 2006;29:14–21.

23. Degenhardt BF, Darmani NA, Johnson JC, et al. Role of osteopathic manipulative treatment in altering pain biomarkers: a pilot study. J Am Osteopath Assoc 2007; 107:387–400.

24. McPartland JM, Giuffrida A, King J, et al. Cannabimimetic effects of osteopathic manipulative treatment. J Am Osteopath Assoc 2005;105(6):283–91.

25. Downing R. The role of physical medicine and rehabilitation for patients in palliative and hospice care. Vet Clin North Am Small Anim Pract 2011;41(3):591–608.

26. Anwer S, Alghadir A, Zafar H, et al. Effects of orthopaedic manual therapy in knee osteoarthritis: a systematic review and meta-analysis. Physiotherapy 2018; 104(3):264–76.

27. Borrella-Andrés S, Marqués-García I, Lucha-López MO, et al. Manual Therapy as a Management of Cervical Radiculopathy: A Systematic Review. Biomed Res Int 2021;2021:9936981.

28. Schenk R, Donaldson M, Parent-Nichols J, et al. Effectiveness of cervicothoracic and thoracic manual physical therapy in managing upper quarter disorders - a systematic review. J Man Manip Ther 2022;30(1):46–55.

29. Riley LM, Satchell L, Stilwell LM, et al. Effect of massage therapy on pain and quality of life in dogs: A cross sectional study. Vet Rec 2021;189(11):e586.

30. Lane DM, Hill SA. Effectiveness of combined acupuncture and manual therapy relative to no treatment for canine musculoskeletal pain. Can Vet J 2016;57(4): 407–14.

31. Saunders DG, Walker JR, Levine D. Joint Mobilization. In: Millis DL, Levine D, editors. Canine rehabilitation and physical therapy. 2nd edition. St. Louis, MO: Elsevier; 2014. p. 447–63.

32. Kwiecien SY, McHugh MP. The cold truth: the role of cryotherapy in the treatment of injury and recovery from exercise. Eur J Appl Physiol 2021;121(8):2125–42.

33. Vieira Ramos G, Pinheiro CM, Messa SP, et al. Cryotherapy Reduces Inflammatory Response Without Altering Muscle Regeneration Process and Extracellular Matrix Remodeling of Rat Muscle. Sci Rep 2016;6:18525.

34. Takagi R, Fujita N, Arakawa T, et al. Influence of icing on muscle regeneration after crush injury to skeletal muscles in rats. J Appl Physiol (1985) 2011;110(2): 382–8.

35. Fayyad DM, Abdelsalam N, Hashem N. Cryotherapy: A New Paradigm of Treatment in Endodontics. J Endod 2020;46(7):936–42.

36. Gundogdu EC, Arslan H. Effects of Various Cryotherapy Applications on Postoperative Pain in Molar Teeth with Symptomatic Apical Periodontitis: A Preliminary Randomized Prospective Clinical Trial. J Endod 2018;44(3):349–54.

37. Hochman L. Photobiomodulation Therapy in Veterinary Medicine: A Review. Top Companion Anim Med 2018;33(3):83–8.

38. Heiskanen V, Hamblin MR. Photobiomodulation: lasers vs. light emitting diodes? Photochemical Photobiological Sci 2018;17(8):1003–17.

39. Alves AC, de Paula Vieira R, Leal-Junior EC, et al. Effect of low-level laser therapy on the expression of inflammatory mediators and on neutrophils and macrophages in acute joint inflammation. Arthritis Res Ther 2013;15(5):1.

40. Pigatto GR, Silva CS, Parizotto NA. Photobiomodulation therapy reduces acute pain and inflammation in mice. J Photochem Photobiol B: Biol 2019;196:111513.

41. Tam SY, Tam VC, Ramkumar S, et al. Review on the cellular mechanisms of low-level laser therapy use in oncology. Front Oncol 2020;10:1255.

42. Khadra M, Rønold HJ, Lyngstadaas SP, et al. Low-level laser therapy stimulates bone–implant interaction: an experimental study in rabbits. Clin Oral Implants Res 2004;15(3):325–32.

43. Bai J, Li L, Kou N, et al. Low level laser therapy promotes bone regeneration by coupling angiogenesis and osteogenesis. Stem Cel Res Ther 2021;12(1):1–8.

44. de Andrade AL, Bossini PS, Parizotto NA. Use of low level laser therapy to control neuropathic pain: a systematic review. J Photochem Photobiol B: Biol 2016;164: 36–42.

45. Bjordal JM. Low level laser therapy (LLLT) and World Association for Laser Therapy (WALT) dosage recommendations. Photomed Laser Surg 2012;30(2):61–2.

46. Riegel RJ. Laser therapy in veterinary medicine: photobiomodulation. Chichester, West Sussex: John Wiley & Sons Inc; 2018. p. 285–312.

47. Bjordal JM, Couppé C, Chow RT, et al. A systematic review of low level laser therapy with location-specific doses for pain from chronic joint disorders. Aust J Physiother 2003;49(2):107–16.
48. Cotler HB, Chow RT, Hamblin MR, et al. The Use of Low Level Laser Therapy (LLLT) For Musculoskeletal Pain. MOJ Orthop Rheumatol 2015;2(5):00068.
49. Magden ER. Spotlight on Acupuncture in Laboratory Animal Medicine. Vet Med Res Rep 2017;8:53–8.
50. Harrison TM, Churgin SM. Acupuncture and Traditional Chinese Veterinary Medicine in Zoological and Exotic Animal Medicine: A Review and Introduction of Methods. Vet Sci 2022;9(2):74.
51. Shmalberg J, Memon MA. A retrospective analysis of 5,195 patient treatment sessions in an integrative veterinary medicine service: patient characteristics, presenting complaints, and therapeutic interventions. Veter Med Int 2015;2015:983621.
52. Robinson NG. Veterinary acupuncture, an ancient tradition for modern times. Altern Comp Therap 2007;13(5):259–65.
53. Gaynor JS, Hagberg S, Gurfein BT. Veterinary applications of pulsed electromagnetic field therapy. Res Vet Sci 2018;119:1–8.
54. Wade B. A review of pulsed electromagnetic field (PEMF) mechanisms at a cellular level: a rationale for clinical use. Am J Health Res 2013;1(3):51–5.
55. Yadollahpour A, Jalilifar M. Electromagnetic fields in the treatment of wound: a review of current techniques and future perspective. J Pure Appl Microbio 2014;8(4):2863–77.
56. Scardino MS, Swaim SF, Sartin EA, et al. Evaluation of treatment with a pulsed electromagnetic field on wound healing, clinicopathologic variables, and central nervous system activity of dogs. Am J Vet Res 1998;59(9):1177–81.
57. Cai J, Shao X, Yang Q, et al. Pulsed electromagnetic fields modify the adverse effects of glucocorticoids on bone architecture, bone strength and porous implant osseointegration by rescuing bone-anabolic actions. Bone 2020;133:115266.
58. McLeod KJ, Rubin CT. The effect of low-frequency electrical fields on osteogenesis. J Bone Joint Surg Am 1992;74(6):920–9 [Erratum in: J Bone Joint Surg Am 1992;74(8):1274].
59. Pinna S, Landucci F, Tribuiani AM, et al. The effects of pulsed electromagnetic field in the treatment of osteoarthritis in dogs: clinical study. Pak Vet J 2013;33(1):96–100.
60. Sullivan MO, Gordon-Evans WJ, Knap KE, et al. Randomized, controlled clinical trial evaluating the efficacy of pulsed signal therapy in dogs with osteoarthritis. Vet Surg 2013;42(3):250–4.
61. Alvarez LX, McCue J, Lam NK, et al. Effect of targeted pulsed electromagnetic field therapy on canine postoperative hemilaminectomy: a double-blind, randomized, placebo-controlled clinical trial. J Am Anim Hosp Assoc 2019;55(2):83–91.
62. Zidan N, Fenn J, Griffith E, et al. The effect of electromagnetic fields on postoperative pain and locomotor recovery in dogs with acute, severe thoracolumbar intervertebral disc extrusion: a randomized placebo-controlled, prospective clinical trial. J Neurotrauma 2018;35(15):1726–36.
63. Hei WH, Byun SH, Kim JS, et al. Effects of electromagnetic field (PEMF) exposure at different frequency and duration on the peripheral nerve regeneration: in vitro and in vivo study. Int J Neurosci 2016;126(8):739–48.
64. Crowe MJ, Sun ZP, Battocletti JH, et al. Exposure to pulsed magnetic fields enhances motor recovery in cats after spinal cord injury. Spine 2003;28(24):2660–6.

65. Ross CL, Syed I, Smith TL, et al. The regenerative effects of electromagnetic field on spinal cord injury. Electromagn Biol Med 2017;36(1):74–87.

66. Das S, Kumar S, Jain S, et al. Exposure to ELF-magnetic field promotes restoration of sensori-motor functions in adult rats with hemisection of thoracic spinal cord. Electromagn Biol Med 2012;31(3):180–94.

67. Durant A, Millis DL. Applications of Extracorporeal Shockwave in Small Animal Rehabilitation. In: Millis DL, Levine D, editors. Canine rehabilitation and physical therapy. 2nd edition. St. Louis, MO: Elsevier; 2014. p. 381–92.

68. Wang CJ, Huang KE, Sun YC, et al. VEGF modulates angiogenesis and osteogenesis in shockwave-promoted fracture healing in rabbits. J Surg Res 2011; 171(1):114–9.

69. Chow DH, Suen PK, Huang L, et al. Extracorporeal shockwave enhanced regeneration of fibrocartilage in a delayed tendon-bone insertion repair model. J Orthop Res 2014;32(4):507–14.

70. Wang CJ, Sun YC, Wong T, et al. Extracorporeal shockwave therapy shows time-dependent chondroprotective effects in osteoarthritis of the knee in rats. J Surg Res 2012;178(1):196–205.

71. Becker W, Kowaleski MP, McCarthy RJ, et al. Extracorporeal shockwave therapy for shoulder lameness in dogs. J Am Anim Hosp Assoc 2015;51(1):15–9.

72. Mueller M, Bockstahler B, Skalicky M, et al. Effects of radial shockwave therapy on the limb function of dogs with hip osteoarthritis. Vet Rec 2007;160(22):762–5.

73. Klonschinski T, Ament SJ, Schlereth T, et al. Application of local anesthesia inhibits effects of low-energy extracorporeal shock wave treatment (ESWT) on nociceptors. Pain Med 2011;12(10):1532–7.

74. Wilner JM, Strash WW. Extracorporeal shockwave therapy for plantar fasciitis and other musculoskeletal conditions utilizing the Ossatron–an update. Clin Podiatr Med Surg 2004;21(3):441–viii.

75. Millis DL. Responses of Musculoskeletal Tissues to Disuse and Remobilization. In: Canine rehabilitation and physical therapy. 2nd edition. St. Louis, MO: Elsevier; 2014. p. 92–153.

76. Drum MG, Marcellin-Little DJ, Davis MS. Principles and applications of therapeutic exercises for small animals. Vet Clin North Am Small Anim Pract 2015;45(1): 73–90.

77. Manning AM, Vrbanac Z. Physical Rehabilitation for the Critically Injured Veterinary Patient. In: Canine rehabilitation and physical therapy. 2nd edition. St. Louis, MO: Elsevier; 2014. p. 652–8.

78. Loy K, Bareyre FM. Rehabilitation following spinal cord injury: how animal models can help our understanding of exercise-induced neuroplasticity. Neural Regen Res 2019;14(3):405–12.

79. Kröger S. Proprioception 2.0: novel functions for muscle spindles. Curr Opin Neurol 2018;31(5):592–8.

80. Blecher R, Krief S, Galili T, et al. The Proprioceptive System Regulates Morphologic Restoration of Fractured Bones. Cell Rep 2017;20(8):1775–83.

81. Mayer F, Scharhag-Rosenberger F, Carlsohn A, et al. The intensity and effects of strength training in the elderly. Dtsch Arztebl Int 2011;108(21):359–64.

82. Anwer S, Alghadir A. Effect of isometric quadriceps exercise on muscle strength, pain, and function in patients with knee osteoarthritis: a randomized controlled study. J Phys Ther Sci 2014;26(5):745–8.

83. Drum M, McKay E, Levine D, et al. The Role of Strengthening in the Management of Canine Osteoarthritis. Adv Small Anim Care 2021;(2):1–10.

84. Hurst JE, Fitts RH. Hindlimb unloading-induced muscle atrophy and loss of function: protective effect of isometric exercise. J Appl Physiol (1985) 2003;95(4): 1405–17.
85. Canapp S, Acciani D, Hulse D, et al. Rehabilitation therapy for elbow disorders in dogs. Vet Surg 2009;38(2):301–7.
86. Greenwood BN, Foley TE, Le TV, et al. Long-term voluntary wheel running is rewarding and produces plasticity in the mesolimbic reward pathway. Behav Brain Res 2011;217(2):354–62.
87. van den Brand R, Heutschi J, Barraud Q, et al. Restoring voluntary control of locomotion after paralyzing spinal cord injury. Science 2012;336(6085):1182–5.
88. Caudle KL, Brown EH, Shum-Siu A, et al. Hindlimb immobilization in a wheelchair alters functional recovery following contusive spinal cord injury in the adult rat. Neurorehabil Neural Repair 2011;25(8):729–39.
89. Corey SM, Vizzard MA, Bouffard NA, et al. Stretching of the back improves gait, mechanical sensitivity and connective tissue inflammation in a rodent model. PloS one 2012;7(1):e29831.
90. Park DJ, Park SY. Long-term effects of diagonal active stretching versus static stretching for cervical neuromuscular dysfunction, disability and pain: An 8 weeks follow-up study. J back Musculoskelet Rehabil 2019;32(3):403–10.
91. Meroni R, Cerri CG, Lanzarini C, et al. Comparison of active stretching technique and static stretching technique on hamstring flexibility. Clin J Sport Med 2010; 20(1):8–14.
92. Winters MV, Blake CG, Trost JS, et al. Passive versus active stretching of hip flexor muscles in subjects with limited hip extension: a randomized clinical trial. Phys Ther 2004;84(9):800–7.

Moving?

Make sure your subscription moves with you!

To notify us of your new address, find your **Clinics Account Number** (located on your mailing label above your name), and contact customer service at:

Email: journalscustomerservice-usa@elsevier.com

800-654-2452 (subscribers in the U.S. & Canada)
314-447-8871 (subscribers outside of the U.S. & Canada)

Fax number: 314-447-8029

Elsevier Health Sciences Division
Subscription Customer Service
3251 Riverport Lane
Maryland Heights, MO 63043

*To ensure uninterrupted delivery of your subscription, please notify us at least 4 weeks in advance of move.

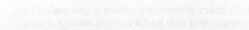

Printed and bound by CPI Group (UK) Ltd, Croydon, CR0 4YY

03/10/2024

01040470-0010